Empathy in Patient Care

Mohammadreza Hojat, Ph.D.

Empathy in Patient Care

Antecedents, Development, Measurement, and Outcomes

Mohammadreza Hojat
Center for Research in Medical Education and Health Care
Jefferson Medical College
1025 Walnut Street
Philadelphia, Pennsylvania 19107
mohammadreza.hojat@jefferson.edu

Library of Congress Control Number: 2006924590

ISBN-13: 978-0-387-33607-7 e-ISBN-13: 978-0-387-33608-4
ISBN-10: 0-387-33607-9 e-ISBN-10: 0-387-33608-7

Printed on acid-free paper.

9 8 7 6 5 4 3 2 1

springer.com

In dedication to those who devote their professional lives to
understanding human suffering,
eliminating pain,
eradicating disease and infirmity,
curing human illnesses, and
improving the physical, mental, and social well-being
of their fellow human beings.

Foreword

Empathy for me has always been a feeling "almost magical" in medical practice, one that brings passion with it, more than vaunted equanimity. Empathy is the projection of feelings that turn *I **and** you* into *I **am** you,* or at least *I **might be** you.* Empathy grows with living and experience. More than a neurobiological response, it brings feelings with it. Empathy helps us to know who we are and keeps us physicians from sterile learned responses. Originally the emotion generated by an image, empathy began as an aesthetic concept, one that should have meaning for medical practices now become so visual.

Empathy comes in many different guises. Empathy can be looking out on the world from the same perspective as that of the patient: to understand your patients better, sit down beside them, to look out at the world from their perspective. But empathy can be far more, therapeutic even, when physicians try to help their sick patients.

As a gastroenterologist, I have always been interested in what people feel, more than in what their gut looks like. When the flexible endoscopes began to change our vision in the 1960s, I gave up doing "procedures." Taking care of patients with dyspepsia or diarrhea up to that time had been a cognitive task: We deduced what might be seen from what our patients told us. Fortunately for our confidence, few instruments tested the truth of what we thought. The endoscopes I disdained proved forerunners of more discerning apparatus that now makes it easy for physicians to "see" an abnormality they can equate with the diagnosis. Gastroenterologists no longer trust what they hear—but only what they can see.

"Imaging," as X-ray studies have been renamed, has vastly improved medical practice. In the twenty-first century, surgeons are more likely to take out an inflamed appendix than they were in the twentieth century, thanks to the ubiquitous CAT scans that depict the offending organs. Cancer of the pancreas once was allowed to grow unchallenged in the belly when physicians had only a "barium meal" to hint at a malign process, but now they can see it at a much earlier stage. Paradoxically, such prowess makes the patients' story more important than ever: CAT scans uncover so many harmless anatomical abnormalities that, more than ever, the physician must be sure that what is to be removed from the patient will prove to be the origin of his or her complaints.

"Imaging," so seductive to the physician, sometimes stands in the way of the empathy that this book is all about. One of my favorite aphorisms, of untraceable provenance, holds that ***"The eye is for accuracy, but the ear is for truth."*** It is easy to see a cancer of the pancreas in a CAT scan as you jog by the view-box, but it takes far longer to listen to the anguish of the patients at the diagnosis which encapsulates their abdominal pain. And modern physicians have so little time.

Moreover, this enhanced ability to see what is amiss has turned many minor symptoms into diseases, in a frenzy of reification. "Heartburn," which patients once talked about, has now been renamed "GERD," gastro-esophageal reflux *disease,* which doctors must see to recognize. That once innocuous complaint, which boasted the badge of duty but could be banished by a little baking soda, has become a disease requiring treatment, not just a change of heart or mind. And it has become almost universal, thanks to the media hype magnifying attention to every little qualm of digestion.

The triumphs of medical instrumentation have led some medical students to worry that the physicians they will become may have little to do for patients as the twenty-first century moves on. They point to the "Turing experiment": Talking to someone behind a curtain, can you detect whether the answers come from a living person or a computer? Sooner or later, they fear, patients will talk to a computer with about as much idea of what or who is responding as Dorothy before the Wizard of Oz. How will tomorrow's physicians compete with the all-knowing and all-seeing "Doc in the Box!"

I hope they will learn that the sick need the right hand of friendship, for neither robots nor computers can compete with humans when it comes to empathy, sympathy, or even love for those in trouble or despair. Empathy is a crucial component of being truly human and an essential characteristic of the good physician. Yet critics assert that modern physicians lack empathy. If that is true, the selection process may be at fault: Physicians are winnowed by victories, from the competition to get into college and then the struggle to get into medical school. Having clambered up the greasy pole, students may have little feeling left for the defeated, the humble, those who have not made it to the top. Once in medical school, they don white coats—unwisely I think—helped to see themselves separate from their patients and the world. As they learn to be experts fixing what is damaged, they learn the primacy of the eye over the ear.

Sadly, current medical school education squeezes empathy out of the students who learn the body and forget the spirit/mind, while their teachers inculcate more detachment from the "still sad music of humanity." Later, the experience of postgraduate hospital training quenches the embers of empathy, as they see young lives cut too short by disease and old lives suffering too long. They learn to talk about the case rather than the person, medical writing is objective and impersonal, and imperturbability becomes their watchword. Medical students, so many studies have shown repeatedly, lose their empathy as they go through medical school training that "clinical medicine" has been relabeled "cynical medicine."

That is what this book is intended to counter, just as the program it depicts has changed medical education at Jefferson.

In *Empathy in Patient Care*, Dr. Mohammedreza Hojat expands on what we physicians do not see, but can only imagine. **The Jefferson Longitudinal Study of Medical Education,** which he has headed for so long, provides the bedrock for this volume. He and his colleagues have studied how empathy begins—how medical students develop—and how empathy affects "outcomes"—how patients fare. We humans are social beings who need to live with others and who depend on interpersonal relationships for support. That need for human relationship, Hojat finds essential to the patient–physician dyad, as much as to the work of the ministry. Basing his conclusions on data obtained by the research instruments he has utilized and perfected, Dr. Hojat does not just talk about empathy, he measures it.

A Ph.D. psychologist of estimable attainment, Dr. Hojat has been drawn to viewing empathy as integral to the practice of medicine. The whole aim of this longitudinal study is to select medical students who will be empathic practitioners and to keep them empathic throughout life. "Attainment" and "success" provide the benchmarks of this long-term comprehensive psychosocial study of what makes for successful medical students and turns them into good physicians.

Teachers must find paths to refresh students' feeling for the human condition early; for that, the humanities loom so important. Beginning in college, premedical students—at least those who are not committed to a career in research—should focus less on the hard sciences and far more on the social sciences and literary fields. Liberal studies should make it easier for them to fold real human emotions into the care they give and—just as important—into their character. The humanities are not forgotten in this book, which recommends more experience with poetry and literature to nurture an empathic attitude in medical students.

It may be easier to recognize the absence of empathy than its presence. Knowing that it had its first openings in the Nazi concentration camp at Theresienstadt (Terezin), I cannot watch the play *Brundibar* without anguish. Its children/actors sing a song of defiance and survival on stage, but they know, Maurice Sendak its illustrator avers, that at its end they will be shipped to Auschwitz, to burn in the ovens of the death camps. Where was the empathy that makes us human in the German guards and officials of that place? In other concentration camps, it is said, prisoners who were musicians were ordered to play chamber music for the guards and officials who, afterwards, would send them off to be gassed. Not much empathy there. Pleasure in music, but no humanity.

Empathy is both rational *and* emotional, for many physicians. Dr. Hojat devotes attention to how much empathy comes from thinking—what the trade calls cognition—and how much from emotion. When we reason, he asks, do we also have emotions appropriate to our thoughts? Surely the answer must depend on what we are thinking about, but here I yield to his appraisal of the data.

His distinction between empathy as a cognitive act and sympathy as an emotional attribute physicians may find more daring, since for us sympathy involves compassion. We physicians, licensed by the state and more knowledgeable than our patients because of experience, try to feel what they experience. Can we feel too much? Get too involved? Can doctors take care of friends? Is it possible for a physician to manage the medical problems of spouse or children? Are people better off being taken care of by a friend who treats them as patient than by a stranger? Such questions arise from reflecting on his studies.

Dr. Hojat's strong views on human connections are echoed by the phrase, "A *friend* a day keeps the doctor away!" Friends, marriage, all social arrangements help; falling sick, illness, and disease test those relationships. Aging tests them too, especially in the loss of friends, so few left for the funeral. Dr. Hojat attends to some optimistic psychological studies from California claiming that emotional support for women with breast cancer improves their longevity—but, I must caution, most of the time, prognosis depends more on the presence of metastases in lymph nodes than on the circuits of the brain, or even on the spirit.

Hojat finds the roots of empathy nourished by the mother–child relationship, even as he elucidates the nature–nurture conflict. Emotional support in childhood must be enormously fruitful, and the nurturing of infants crucial in establishing a model. Culture must have equal influence, along with the central role of genetic endowment.

Hospital chaplains understand the importance of connections when they talk about "being there" with the patient; no need for talk, just being there, actively present. Dr. Hojat traces the physiological path of that clinical mystery, as he puts it, a gift to the patient. Or is it our duty?

His words on brain imaging bring everything into balance, as up-to-date as possible. Nevertheless, I wonder whether psychiatry as talk-therapy will survive the burgeoning skills of computers. Neurobiology seems to suggest that the mind is like a secretion from the brain, like insulin from the pancreas, that the tide of neurotropic drugs can sweep clean. I prefer to dream that the mind arises from the brain more like smoke from a burning log, to obey quite different physical laws. Just as smoke flies free from its earth-bound roots, so from our protoplasm springs poetry, from the circuits of the brain our hope for a Creator. Yet Leibnitz wisely asked, if we could stroll through a brain as through a room, where would we find charity, love, or ambition? A Creator may have fashioned the channels, but will we ever locate them in that gray matter of the brain? Much depends on culture and environment, as the author so wisely points out.

Empathy is crucial to clinical practice, to treatment especially, though not all physicians agree. Some time ago, an essay "*What is empathy and can it be taught?*" was quickly rejected by a well-known journal of opinion, its editor observing that "Empathy has no place in medical practice." After the essay appeared in a less austere journal, however, many supportive letters and comments encouraged a book on that topic, one that welcomed the return of emotion to medicine.

Hojat sees empathy as largely cognitive, but some will think of empathy as present at birth, innate, waiting to be developed but unlikely to be created by any act of will. That could be too much like play-acting, for if the physician–patient relationship is as central to practice as I believe, there are mystical relationships not yet pictured by our models.

Psychologists will find much of interest in the chapters on techniques and testing. A remarkable collection of abstracts from the Jefferson Longitudinal Study, published in 2005, supports the conclusions in this book. One hundred fifty-five of those abstracts eventuated in papers published elsewhere provide the outcome data that has changed much at Jefferson. Some, unfamiliar with such studies, will wonder about psychometrics, and how often answers can be "socially desirable," as Dr. Hojat puts it. They remember that to test how well a subject bears pain in a laboratory setting cannot replicate the state of mind of a patient lying in a bed despairing of unfamiliar abdominal pain and wondering what will happen next. Knowing that an experimenter is causing your pain makes it a lot easier to bear than when you are in the dark. Psychometrics is a complicated science.

The "wounded healer" represents a model. Something good has to be said for the narcissistic satisfactions that comes from patient–physician relationships: working with patients, caring for them and sharing their emotional life but respecting boundaries. That can be therapeutic for physicians. The physician who has been sick is more likely to be empathic in future practice. Physicians who have had their own troubles have confessed that they have found surcease in talking with patients. Physicians who "burn out" or are bored are often, I imagine, those who regard their tasks as purely medical and technical. Countertransference can play a dynamic therapeutic role for physicians, at times.

The social revolutions of the late twentieth century brought the physician–patient relationship from the distant "professional" ideal of William Osler to one that encourages an intimacy that must vary with the cultural norms. Physicians of the twenty-first century in America ask about sexual habits and proclivities, questions which once were taboo. With the fading of parentalism, we are far more frank about the uncertainties of our practices. Prudently, Dr. Hojat has studied the influence of culture and environment, the expectations that mold our behavior. As educators, we might wish to have had empathy poured into our students before they come to medical school, but, as the Jesuits knew, for that we would have to train them from early childhood. The habits and norms of physicians vary with the passage of time; the ideal of what is proper for a physician to do or say also has varied remarkably: Sometimes touching the patient is appropriate and comforting, and sometimes it is misunderstood and inappropriate.

Empathy varies with age and experience. Am I more empathic now than 40 years ago because I have experienced so much more? Does empathy develop? Or does it atrophy or weaken? In recognizing the differences between men and women, Hojat comes down firmly on the side of women as more empathic than men, at least in Western culture. Women are new in medicine, at least in America still finding their way; and the data may change with the "maturation" of their medical practices.

Not all physicians need empathy, for patient–physician encounters comprise many different relationships. Chameleon-like, physicians have to vary with circumstances. Treating a patient with pneumonia is quite different from evaluating someone with abdominal pain of uncertain origin. Their faith in the efficiency of computers has convinced some physicians that empathy is an unnecessary addition to their character. Time is at such a premium; family care doctors complain that they do not get paid for being nice to patients. They have to see more patients ever more briefly just to pay expenses. That must be why fewer graduates are choosing primary-care or even internal medicine.

Analysis of videotaped interviews must be a good way to refresh and recover the empathy that students bring to medical school. They can relearn empathy in discussing why patients have asked certain questions, and what answers are most fitting, and what comfortable phrases may make patients feel better. Rita Charon and others have gotten medical students to write about diseases from their patient's perspective; a very appropriate stimulus to empathy and understanding, the "narrative competence" that Hojat praises.

That also requires the reading of stories and novels, the discussion of narratives, and it certainly requires more collegiality than trainees tell about in the beginning of the twenty-first century. Empathy can be strengthened through stories. I have no wish to add to what others have written about the medical school curriculum, but I am convinced that rhetoric—the equivalent of persuasion—needs a rebirth in medical practice. We physicians are more than conduits of pills and procedures, we need to build bridges between our medical practice and the world of suffering around us. Conversation is essential, continuing discussions about patient–doctor relationships, about human relationships in general. We can fan the passion of empathy in medicine by both science and poetry, reason and intuition; we can provide more than the robots and computers, for only men and women are capable of empathy.

Team medicine, now looming so large, may supply that remedy in some other member of the group. A nurse or medical student, someone other than a doctor, can readily ask questions and provide the comfort that the physicians on the team do not always find the time to give. Now that hospitalists go from one desperately sick patient to the next, medical practice in the hospital has become too complex for any one person, and the emotional burdens of hospital care cannot be any less trying.

As technology takes over the physicians' task of making diagnoses, empathy will need more attention than equanimity. What physicians can do in the twenty-first century is vastly more effective than before. But physicians no longer find the time to talk to each other, let alone their patients. Conversation helps to develop empathy, empathy overcomes our isolation and in empathy we rediscover ourselves.

Dr. Hojat wisely provides an agenda for future research ranging from selecting prospective medical students for their empathy to evaluating the neurobiological components of empathy and compassion. He and his coworkers are keen to provide measurements that will predict clinical competence and clinical empathy to help in the selection of medical students. But it may be a long time before the personal qualities of prospective medical students will trump their scientific know-how or their desirably high scores in the MCAT. Gentleness does not loom as captivating as high science grades to most deans of admission. Hojat's utopia wisely provides goals which medical practitioners and teachers can ponder and try to reach for in their daily activities. We are in his debt.

Howard Spiro, M.D.
Emeritus Professor of Medicine
Yale University School of Medicine

Preface

All human beings are in truth akin,
all in creation share one origin.
When fate allots a member pangs and pain,
no ease for other members then remains.
If, unperturbed, another's grief canst scan,
thou are not worthy of the name of human.

—Saadi (classic Persian poet, 1210–1290 AD)

Although the primary intention of this book is to describe the antecedents, development, measurement, and consequences of empathy in the context of patient care, some of the material presented goes beyond that purpose. For the sake of a more comprehensive analysis, one cannot isolate such a complex and dynamic entity as empathy in patient care from a string of determining factors (e.g., its evolutionary, genetic, developmental, and psychodynamic aspects) and multiple consequences (e.g., physical, mental, and social well-being). Thus, to achieve a broader understanding of empathy in patient care, I discuss the issue in the wider context of a dynamic system, the function of which rests on the following six premises:

- Human beings are social creatures.
- The human need for affiliation and social support has survival value.
- Interpersonal relationships can fulfill the human need for affiliation and social support.
- The interpersonal relationship between clinician and patient is a special case of a "mini" social system that can fulfill the need for affiliation and support.
- Empathy in patient care contributes to the fulfillment of the need for affiliation and support.
- An empathic clinician–patient relationship can improve the physical, mental, and social well-being of the clinician as well as the patient.

Human beings are designed by evolution to form meaningful interpersonal relationships through verbal and nonverbal communication. There is a system of needs in human beings for social affiliation—for bonding and attachment, for forming a social network, for feeling felt, for understanding and being understood. The grand principle is the same whether the individual is an infant, a child, an adolescent, or an adult or whether the individual is male or female or is healthy or ill: *Being connected is beneficial to the human body and mind.*

The aforementioned principle is indeed the theme underlying all 12 chapters of this book. In some chapters, it may seem that I take my eyes off the intended target of patient care, but I always return to the underlying theme to link the discussion to the clinician–patient relationship. When appropriate, I frequently use the terms "clinician" and "client," rather than "doctor," "physician," and "patient," to make the discussion more general and thus applicable to all health care professions, not to medicine alone.

Empathy is viewed in this book from a multidisciplinary perspective that includes evolution; neurology; clinical, social, developmental, and educational psychology; sociology; medicine; and medical education. Some theoretical aspects of antecedents, development, and outcomes of empathy are discussed, and relevant experimental studies and empirical findings are presented in support of the theoretical discussion. The book is based on my years of research on empathy in medical education and practice at Jefferson Medical College that resulted in the development and validation of the Jefferson Scale of Physician Empathy, a psychometrically sound instrument that is being used by many researchers in the United States and in other countries (see Chapter 7).

The book is written for a broad audience that includes physicians, residents, medical students, and students and practitioners of other health professions including the disciplines of nursing, psychology, and clinical social work. In particular, faculty involved in the education and training of health professionals can use the book as a reference in their courses. The book is divided into two parts. The first part consists of Chapters 1 through 5, in which empathy is discussed from a broader perspective in the general context of human relationships. This part lays the foundation for the second one, without which the discussion of empathy in the second part would look like a structure without supporting pillars.

In the second part, consisting of Chapters 6 through 12, the focus shifts more specifically to empathy in the context of patient care. The two parts are closely interrelated, evident by frequently referring readers to different chapters in the other part to avoid redundancies. Each chapter begins with a preamble presenting the highlights of the text and ends with a recapitulatory paragraph that provides a global view of the chapter.

Because the book is intended to serve as a reference source on the topic of empathy in patient care, on many occasions I have cited multiple references for critical issues for those who need to further review the issues beyond what I have presented in this book. Although a critical review of the literature was not among the intended purposes of the book, occasionally when appropriate I reported additional information such as the measuring instruments, and described the sample used in the cited research to help readers judge the validity of the findings.

Chapter 1 presents a historical background about the concept of empathy and discusses the ambiguity associated with the definitions and descriptions of empathy. The longstanding confusion between empathy and sympathy is described and specific features of each construct are listed to distinguish between the two. In addition, distinctions are made between cognition and emotion and between understanding and feeling. Finally, the implications of such distinctions are outlined to avoid confusion about the conceptualization and measurement of empathy in the context of patient care.

Chapter 2 is based on the assumption that human beings are evolved to connect together for survival. Thus, the importance of making and breaking human connections in health and illness is emphasized. The beneficial effects of a social support system on health and the detrimental effects of loneliness are presented to underscore the nature, mechanisms, and consequences of interpersonal relationships. The chapter concludes with a notion that the relationship between clinician and patient is formed by the drive for human connectedness and serves as a special kind of social support system, with all its beneficial healing power.

In Chapter 3, empathy is viewed from an evolutionary perspective, and the psycho-socio-physiological function of empathic engagement is described. Also discussed in this chapter are recent findings from neuroimaging studies on the brain and a new line of research on the mirror neurons in the brain that hold promise of increasing our understanding of the neuroanatomy of empathy and how we perceive other people's experiences, feelings, and emotions. In addition, the chapter discusses the genetic studies of empathy and the link between neurological impairment and deficiencies in empathy. The chapter ends with the notion that the foundation of the capacity for empathy developed during the evolution of the human race and that the neurological basis of empathy is hard-wired.

Chapter 4 discusses the psychodynamics of empathy by emphasizing the importance of prenatal, perinatal, and postnatal factors in the development of prosocial and altruistic behaviors. In particular, the effects of the early rearing environment, especially the mother's availability and responsiveness, in the development of internal working models that operate in a person's later interpersonal relationships are described. Experimental studies are presented to show that early relationships with a primary caregiver influence the regulation of emotions that becomes an important factor in interpersonal relationships in general and in empathic engagements in particular.

Chapter 5 briefly describes several instruments that researchers have used most often to measure empathy in children and adults. The contents of the items in these instruments indicate that most of these instruments are useful for measuring empathy in the general population, but their relevance in the context of patient care is limited. Thus, a psychometrically sound instrument, developed specifically to measure empathy in the context of patient care was needed to satisfy an urgent need to measure empathy among students and practitioners of the health care professions.

In Chapter 6, empathy in patient care is discussed in relation to the World Health Organization's definition of health and the triangular biopsychosocial paradigm of illness. In that context, empathy in patient care is defined, and three key features in the definition are emphasized: cognition, understanding, and communication. The chapter concludes with the point that the patient's recognition of the clinician's empathy through verbal and nonverbal communication plays an important role in the outcome of empathic engagement.

Chapter 7 describes in detail the developmental phases and psychometric properties of the Jefferson Scale of Physician Empathy (JSPE), which was developed specifically to measure empathy among students and practitioners in the medical and other health-related professions. Empirical evidence is presented to support the validity (face, content, construct, and criterion-related) and reliability (internal consistency and score stability) of both the student version (S-Version) and the health professional version (HP-Version) of the JSPE. The chapter ends with the thought that the evidence supporting the scale's validity and reliability should instill confidence in those who are searching for a psychometrically sound instrument that can be used in empirical research on empathy among students being educated for the health professions or among individuals already practicing in those professions.

Chapter 8 discusses the interpersonal dynamics involved in an empathic relationship between clinician and patient, and proposes that both can benefit from empathic engagement. The chapter presents several experimental studies that describe how role expectations, the tendency to bind with others for survival, uncritical acceptance of and compliance with authority figures, and the effects of the clinical environment can influence clinicians' and patients' behavior in clinical encounters. In addition, the chapter argues that such psychological mechanisms as identification, transference, and countertransference, plus placebo effects, and cultural factors, personal space, and boundaries make clinician–patient encounters unique. The chapter ends with a notion that for achieving a better empathic engagement, the clinician should learn to listen with the "third ear" and to see with the "mind's eye."

Chapter 9 describes the link between empathy, sex, psychosocial variables, clinical performance, career interest, and choice of specialty. It is argued that women may be endowed at an early age with a greater sensitivity to social stimuli and a better understanding of emotional signals that can result in a greater capacity for empathic engagement. This argument is reflected in studies reporting sex differences in the practice styles of male and female physicians. The chapter also reports a number of desirable personality attributes that are positively correlated with empathy and a number of undesirable personal qualities that are negatively correlated with empathy. Data reported in this chapter suggest that high scores on measures of empathy are associated with greater clinical competence and interest in people-oriented specialties as opposed to technology- or procedure-oriented specialties.

Chapter 10 reports the theoretical link between empathy and positive patient outcomes and provides evidence concerning the quality of clinician–patient relationships that lead to more accurate diagnoses, and to patients' greater satisfaction with their health care providers, better compliance with clinicians' advice, firmer commitment to treatment plans, and a reduced tendency to file malpractice suits. The reported studies in this chapter confirm the link between clinician–patient empathic engagement and positive patient outcomes.

Chapter 11 describes obstacles to the development of empathy in medical education and practice—the cynicism that students develop during their professional education, the changes evolving in the health care system, and the current overreliance on technology. The chapter also presents some evidence suggesting that empathy is amenable to change by targeted educational programs and describes a variety of approaches used in psychological and health education research to enhance empathy: interpersonal skills training, perspective taking, role playing, exposure to role models, imagining, exposure of students to activities resembling patients' experiences while hospitalized or during encounters with health care providers, the study of literature and the arts, development of narrative skills, and the Balint approach to training physicians.

In Chapter 12, the final chapter, empathy in the context of patient care is viewed from the broad perspective of systems theory. I suggested that a systemic paradigm of empathy in patient care includes the following subsets that interactively operate in the system: the clinician-related, nonclinician-related, social learning and educational subsets. The elements within each subset and the interactions of the elements within and between subsets during clinical encounters that lead to functional (positive) or dysfunctional (negative) patient outcomes are discussed. Finally, an outline of an agenda for future research on seven topics involving empathy in patient care is presented. The chapter concludes that the implementation of remedies for enhancement of empathy is a mandate that must be acted upon and that any attempt to enhance empathic understanding among people is a step toward building a better civilization.

It is my hope that this book can help to improve our understanding of empathy in the context of patient care. A problem that is well understood is a problem that is half solved. The more that health professionals understand the importance of empathy in patient care, the better the public is served.

Acknowledgments

I am indebted to many for their influence on my thoughts, for inspiring me to pursue this line of research, and for their encouraging and supporting my research ideas and activities. Because of space constraints, I cannot name them all.

There is a popular saying in the Persian language: "Forever remain my masters those from whom I have learned." Following this piece of advice, I must begin with my mother—that angel from whom I heard before taking my first breath, who taught me to say my first word, who is engraved vividly in my mind as the foremost symbol of love, care, and empathic understanding.

Then there are others: among them, those who are the most valuable of all human resources, the teachers. There are many of them, but I would like to mention two of my undergraduate psychology teachers, Professors Reza Shapurian and Amir Hooshang Mehryar, who not only opened up a window for me to the study of human behavior but also instilled self-confidence in me by asking me, when I was a novice undergraduate student, to write a critical review of their book for publication.

There are others who trained me on the job and encouraged me in my professional development, particularly in medical education research. Among them are Joseph S. Gonnella, M.D., and Carter Zeleznik, Ph.D. Joe Gonnella is one of the best and brightest role models of an exemplary clinician-academician, teacher, leader, scholar, and researcher in medical education, who is my mentor in medical education research. His great advice to me that "perfectionism is an obstacle to progress" has made my research career productive. Carter Zeleznik often says, humorously I hope, that his worst mistake was to hire me at Jefferson! His ideas, kind heart, and sense of humor made medical education research fun for me. He is now enjoying the golden years of retirement.

Enormous appreciation is due to colleagues at Jefferson Medical College who have contributed intellectually and instrumentally to the inception and development of the Jefferson physician empathy project. This book is an offshoot of that project. Those colleagues are (in alphabetical order) Clara A. Callahan, M.D., Associate Dean for Admissions, Jefferson Medical College; James B. Erdmann, Ph.D., Dean of Jefferson College of Health Professions; Joseph S. Gonnella, M.D., Emeritus Dean of Jefferson Medical College, Distinguished Professor of Medicine, and Founder and Director of the Center for Research in Medical Education and Health, Jefferson Medical College;

Daniel Louis, M.S., Managing Director, Center for Research in Medical Education and Health Care; Thomas J. Nasca, M.D., Dean of Jefferson Medical College and Senior Vice President of Thomas Jefferson University; Salvatore Mangione, M.D., Associate Professor of Medicine, Course Director for Physical Diagnosis, Jefferson Medical College; and Jon Veloski, M.S., Chief of the Medical Education Research Division, Center for Research in Medical Education and Health Care, Jefferson Medical College. Throughout the book, I have frequently used the plural pronoun "we," rather than the singular "I." Such phrases as "our research findings," rather than "my research findings," reflect my acknowledgment of the contributions of these colleagues.

The Jefferson physician empathy project has been supported over the past four years by a grant from the Pfizer Medical Humanities Initiative, Pfizer Inc., New York. Mike Magee, M.D., who was Director of the Pfizer Medical Humanities Initiative and a member of the Jefferson physician empathy project, provided me with continued support, intellectual input, and encouragement in my pursuit of this line of research. At the beginning, I could not imagine that a modest financial support could lead to such an important project. I also received an unrestricted grant from the Pfizer Medical Humanities Initiative for complementary copies of this book to send to the deans of all allopathic and osteopathic medical schools in the United States and to the directors of some residency programs in psychiatry.

Several colleagues reviewed different chapters of this book and made valuable suggestions for improvement. Dr. Gonnella was kind enough to review all the chapters; Herbert Adler, M.D., Ph.D., reviewed Chapters l and 6; James Erdmann, Ph.D., reviewed Chapters 5 and 7; A. M. Rostami, M.D., Ph.D., reviewed Chapter 3; and Jon Veloski, M.S., reviewed Chapters 1, 5, 6, and 7. All of these colleagues made valuable comments to improve the chapters, but I take full responsibility for any possible shortcomings in the text.

Kaye Maxwell has played a major role in the development of computer scanning forms, compiling the User's Guide for the Jefferson Scale of Physician Empathy (see Chapter 7), and preparing computerized reports for the scale. Elizabeth Bowman kindly assisted me with editorial polishing of the text, and Bethany Brooks helped me in copy editing the manuscript. I chose Springer Science + Business Media over other book publishers, not only because of its reputation as a publisher of scholarly books, but also because of the professional manner in which Janice Stern, the acquisitions editor, responded to my book proposal. I was pleased and impressed by her initial and encouraging feedback—she would seek an expert to endorse the value of the book, rather than offering the standard response that the book's merit must first be judged by the publisher's reviewers. Scholarly publishers need more editors like her who empathically understand the strong bond that exists between authors and their intellectual property.

Felix Portnoy, the production editor, had a leading role in the book's design aspects and cosmetic improvements. He also made useful suggestions about improving the organization of the chapters. Arvind Sohal, the typesetting project manager kindly worked with me to incorporate last minute changes I made in the text, and also helped me in compiling the Author and Subject indices. Jason Robeson assisted me in preparing the initial indices.

I would like to express my sincere gratitude to everyone I have acknowledged so far and to those colleagues at the Jefferson Medical College who offered me a sabbatical leave to pursue the self-rewarding endeavor of writing this book.

My children, Arian, Anahita, and Roxana, filled me with additional joy and energy by repeatedly asking: "Dad! How is your book going?" Last, but certainly not the least, I would like to thank my wife, Mimi, who provided me with all I needed to work in an atmosphere full of peace and love at home during my sabbatical to write this book.

A Personal Odyssey

Life is full of surprises!

—(A popular cliché)

A mother and her young daughter sat in the examination room, waiting for the doctor to show up. They looked anxiously at the closed door, expecting a stranger in a white coat to open it at any moment. Time seems to stand still when a patient is waiting for a doctor to come. It is interesting that patients always view a doctor as the most trusted of all strangers unless a strange thing happens, usually during their first encounter.

At the recommendation of the pediatrician, the mother brought her 13-year-old daughter to this pediatric cardiologist to be examined for heart palpitations. The pediatrician had indicated that, at age 13, occasional palpitations were not necessarily a serious cause for concern: They could be a result of too much caffeine for a coffee-lover like that young girl, a sign of test-taking anxiety at school, or a sign of a transitory emotional state. However, to eliminate the possibility of a serious heart condition, the pediatrician referred the girl to an expert in cardiology.

Here they were waiting for the expert to deliver the final verdict—either a clean bill of health or a long-term treatment that eventually could involve surgical procedures. The fear of the unknown that always haunts human beings was escalating with the passage of time. Finally, the doctor entered the room shadowed by a young woman also wearing a white coat. He pointed to her and said, "This is my resident." No greetings were exchanged, and the doctor seemed indifferent and in a rush. The encounter was cold. Without looking at the mother or the girl, he opened the medical chart the pediatrician had sent him and announced that additional tests were needed. The test he suggested was a heart monitor the girl would wear 24 hours a day, 7 days a week, for at least a month. After each abnormal heartbeat, the device would transmit the recorded signals to a monitoring center via a telephone line connected to the monitor.

When the anxious mother asked the doctor how her daughter could be hooked up to a heart monitor for a month without missing her classes, the cardiologist said the monitor was light and could be attached to a belt around her waist and connected to a watch-like device on her wrist. The only additional information he offered was that the monitor could be rented for a month and that the expense might not be covered by insurance. He seemed to be more concerned about how the monitor would be paid for than about the mother's and daughter's need for comforting comments.

The doctor informed the mother that the next appointment would be in a month or so, after the heart monitor test was completed. The anxious mother expected, to no avail, more information about her young daughter's condition, some sign from the doctor that would make her daughter, who was looking hopelessly into the doctor's emotionless eyes, feel a little hopeful at least. As the doctor and his resident were leaving the examination room (where no examination had been performed), the mother, with a despairing look, asked the doctor: "Is my daughter's heart condition really serious enough to need constant monitoring for a month? Couldn't her condition be transitory?" The doctor looked at his resident and mumbled, "We've got another doctor in here," and the two left the room, leaving mother and daughter feeling desperate and confused.

The mother did not trust the expert, never rented the monitor, and the heart palpitation stopped abruptly when the daughter stopped drinking coffee. However, memories of cold encounters can last forever.

It is interesting that an adverse event occurring when a person is in a heightened state of emotional arousal tends to leave a deeper scar in the sufferer's mind than it would otherwise. Or it may be that a lack of empathic understanding has a more lasting effect than the presence of a "detached concern." Is it any wonder that many patients hate to go to a doctor's office? (By the way, that mother happened to be my wife and the 13-year-old happened to be my daughter.)

***

This event, plus my long-standing curiosity about and fascination with the two opposing poles of human connectedness versus lack of connectedness—namely, interpersonal relationship versus loneliness—compelled me to embark on a journey that would lead to a better understanding of why empathy is so important in patient care.

Since my college years, I have been curious about why people behave as they do in making or breaking human connections. What are the foundations on which human beings build, or fail to build, the capacity to form meaningful interpersonal relationships? Has human evolution included development of the ability to form interpersonal connections? What roles do genetic predisposition, rearing environment, personal qualities, and educational experiences play in achieving personal and professional success, in clinician–patient encounters, or in student–teacher relationships, or even in achieving likeability or attaining the qualities of professional, educational, or political leadership?

While earning my master's degree at the University of Tehran, I attempted to satisfy my curiosity about the personal attributes leading to success by examining the qualities of popular students using a sociometric methodology.

I found that the human attribute of likeability, or popularity, was rooted in the early rearing environment and was also linked to positive personality traits, such as self-esteem. Furthermore, academic and professional success is the end result of these social skills. This research culminated in my master's thesis, *An Empirical Study of Popularity.*

While earning my doctoral degree at the University of Pennsylvania several years later, I continued to pursue my research interests, which eventually resulted in my doctoral dissertation, *Loneliness as a Function of Selected Personality, Psychosocial and Demographic Variables.* During this period, I studied factors contributing to loneliness, an indication of an inability to form meaningful interpersonal relationships. The findings showed that a set of personality factors, early experiences in the family environment, perceptions of the early relationship with a primary caregiver, early relationships with peers, and later living environment could predict experiences of loneliness in adulthood.

From the results of both studies, I learned that a common set of psychosocial attributes contributes to the development of a capacity (or incapacity) to make (or break) human connections. These psychosocial attributes are similar to the elements of "emotional intelligence," such as social competency and the ability to understand the views, feelings, and emotions of others: that is, the capacity for empathic understanding.

***

As a psychologist by academic training, I entered a new territory of medical education research more than two decades ago. At the beginning, I was not sure whether my interests, knowledge, skills, and academic background in psychology could serve the purpose of medical education research. However, I soon discovered that the field of medical education research was a rich and challenging territory at the crossroad of several disciplines, including psychology, education, and sociology as well as medicine. As a result of learning more about the field, I became convinced that both the art of medicine and the alleviation of human suffering would flourish by incorporating ideas from the behavioral and social sciences into the education of physicians.

I started my career in medical education research at a great academic medical center, Jefferson Medical College of Thomas Jefferson University, where I was charged with administrative and research responsibilities for the Jefferson Longitudinal Study of Medical Education. This now well-known longitudinal study retrieves data about Jefferson's medical students and graduates from the most comprehensive, extensive, and uninterrupted longitudinal database of medical education maintained in a single medical school. The Jefferson Longitudinal Study was initiated under the supervision of Joseph S. Gonnella, M.D., a decade before I joined the faculty. Joe was then the Director of the Office of Medical Education and later the Dean of Jefferson Medical College and Senior Vice President of Thomas Jefferson University.

Currently, he is Emeritus Dean, Distinguished Professor of Medicine, and Director of The Center for Research in Medical Education and Health Care. Joe initiated the study because he had a vision (he jokingly says that schizophrenic patients have visions!) concerning the need to assess the outcomes of medical education at a time when most medical faculty members did not believe in the value of such an expensive and extensive study and thus were unwilling to devote resources to it.

My involvement with the Jefferson Longitudinal Study not only opened up a new research opportunity for me but also proved to be an extremely interesting beginning to my professional life. I enjoyed the freedom bestowed on me to add new dimensions (e.g., personality and psychosocial measures) to the longitudinal database to address psychosocial aspects of academic success in medical school. To me, that green light, which allowed me to include personality and psychosocial measures in the longitudinal study, was analogous to offering a cool glass of water to a thirsty man in the heat of a desert! The job provided me with a golden opportunity to incorporate my ideas about personality attributes into research on the contribution of those attributes to the academic attainment of medical students and to the professional success of physicians. So far, this highly productive research enterprise has resulted in more than 150 publications in peer-reviewed journals. Meanwhile, my long-term interest in why people behave as they do in making or breaking human connections shifted to a more specific interest in empathy in patient care. Then the question became: Why are some physicians more capable than others of forming empathic relationships with their patients? More important, how can empathy be conceptualized and quantified in the context of patient care? How does the capacity for empathy develop? How can it be measured? And what are the antecedents and consequences of empathy in the context of patient care?

A few years ago, in pursuit of answers to these questions, I began to develop an instrument for physicians that measures empathy in patient care (see Chapter 7). During that time, I was fortunate to benefit from the intellectual input and instrumental support of the group of medical education scholars and practicing physicians making up the team of the Jefferson Medical College physician empathy project (see Acknowledgments).

All the elements in this interrelated chain of events brought me to the uncharted terrain of empathy in patient care. Interestingly, empathy has proved to be an extremely rich area of research requiring a multidisciplinary approach that links views, concepts, theories, and data from diverse disciplines, such as evolutionary psychiatry; ethology; developmental, clinical, and social psychology; psychoanalysis; sociology; neuroanatomy; philosophy; art; and literature. What prompted me to embark on a search for the answers to my questions about how empathy develops and what its antecedents and outcomes are in the health professions was fascination with the richness of this uncharted territory, in combination with my long-time interest in the mysteries of interpersonal relationships, my academic background in the behavioral and social sciences, and my professional experience in medical education research.

If a fortune-teller had told me at the beginning of my college years that I would end up with a career as a researcher in medical education, I would have laughed uproariously in disbelief! And that wise fortune-teller probably would have responded by saying, "Well, young man! Life is full of surprises." It is indeed!

Contents

Part I

Empathy in Human Relationships

Definitions and Conceptualization

1

To be one in heart is enchanting,
more than to be one in tongue.

—Rumi (Persian mystical poet and philosopher, 1207–1273 AD)

Preamble

Empathy, a translation of the German word *Einfühlung*, has been described as an elusive and slippery concept with a long history marked by ambiguity and controversy. There is no consensus on the definition of empathy. However, there has been an ongoing debate about the construct of empathy, described sometimes as a cognitive attribute featuring understanding of experiences of others; at other times, as an emotional state of the mind featuring sharing of feelings; and at still other times as a concept involving both cognition and emotion. Distinctions are made in this chapter between cognition and emotion and also between understanding and feeling. Subsequently, the unsettled issue of the differences between empathy and sympathy is addressed by viewing empathy as a predominantly cognitive attribute featuring understanding of others' concerns that has a positive and linear relationship with patient outcomes and by viewing sympathy as a primarily emotional concept featured by sharing emotions and feelings that has a curvilinear relationship (an inverted U shape) with patient outcomes. Distinctions between cognition and emotion, understanding and feeling, and empathy and sympathy have important implications not only for the conceptualization and measurement of empathy in patient care but for the study of patient outcomes as well.

Introduction

The notion of "empathy" has a long history marked by ambiguity, discrepancy, and controversy among philosophers and behavioral, social, and medical scholars (Aring, 1958; Basch, 1983; Preston & deWaal, 2002; Wispe, 1978, 1986). Because of conceptual ambiguity, empathy has been described as an "elusive" concept (Basch, 1983)—one that is difficult to define and hard to measure (Kestenbaum, Farber, & Sroufe, 1989). Eisenberg and Strayer

(1987a, p. 3) described empathy as a "slippery concept . . . that has provoked considerable speculation, excitement, and confusion." Also, because of the ambiguity associated with the concept of empathy, Pigman (1995) suggested that empathy has come to mean so much that it means nothing! More than half a century ago, Theodore Reik (1948, p. 357), the prominent psychoanalyst, made a similar comment: "The word empathy sometimes means one thing, sometimes another, until now it does not mean anything at all."

Because of the conceptual ambiguity, Wispe (1986) suggested that the outcomes of empathy research may not be valid because empathy means different things to different investigators, who may believe they are studying the same thing but actually are referring to different things! As a result, Lane (1986) suggested that empathy may not even exist in reality after all. Later, Levy (1997) proposed that the term should be eliminated and replaced by a less ambiguous one.

Despite the conceptual ambiguity, it is interesting to note that empathy is among the most frequently mentioned humanistic dimensions of patient care (Linn, DiMatteo, Cope, & Robbins, 1987). Many successful clinicians know intuitively what empathy is without being able to define it. In that respect, empathy may be analogous to love, which many of us have experienced without being able to define it! Thus, while we all have a positive image of the concept of empathy and a preconceived idea about its positive outcomes in interpersonal relationships, we wonder how to define it operationally. Needless to say, no concept can be subject to scientific scrutiny without an operational definition.

The Origin and History of the Term *Empathy*

The concept of empathy (not the English term) was first discussed in 1873 by Robert Vischer, a German art historian and philosopher who used the word *Einfühlung* to address an observer's feelings elicited by works of art (Hunsdahl, 1967; Jackson, 1992). According to Pigman (1995), the word was used to describe the projection of human feelings onto the natural world and inanimate objects. However, the German term was originally used not to describe an interpersonal attribute but to portray the individual's feelings when appreciating a work of art, specifically when those feelings blurred the distinction between the observer's self and the art object (Wispe, 1986).

In 1897, the German psychologist-philosopher Theodore Lipps brought the word *Einfühlung* from aesthetics to psychology. In describing personal experiences associated with the concept of *Einfühlung*, Lipps indicated that "when I observe a circus performer on a hanging wire, I feel I am inside him" (cited in Carr, Iacoboni, Dubeau, Mazziotta, & Lenzi, 2003, p. 5502). In 1903, Wilhelm Wundt, the father of experimental psychology, who established the first laboratory of experimental psychology in 1879 at the University of Leipzig in Germany, used *Einfühlung* for the first time in the context of human relationships (Hunsdahl, 1967). In 1905, Sigmund Freud (1960) used *Einfühlung* to describe the psychodynamics of putting oneself in another person's position (cited in Pigman, 1995).

The English term "empathy" is a neologism coined by psychologist Edward Bradner Titchener (1909) as an English equivalent or the translation of the meaning of *Einfühlung*. The term empathy derives from the Greek word *empatheia*, which means appreciation of another person's feelings (Astin, 1967; Wispe, 1986).

Although Titchener (1915) used the term empathy to convey "understanding" of other human beings, Southard (1918) was the first to describe the significance of empathy in the relationship between a clinician and a patient for facilitating diagnostic outcomes. Thereafter, American social and behavioral scientists have often used the concept of empathy in relation to the psychotherapeutic or counseling relationship and in the discussion of prosocial behavior and altruism (Batson & Coke, 1981; Carkhuff, 1969; Davis, 1994; Eisenberg & Strayer, 1987b; Feshbach, 1989; Feudtner, Christakis, & Christakis, 1994; Hoffman, 1981; Ickes, 1997; Stotland, Mathews, Sherman, Hansson, & Richardson, 1978). Empathy also has been discussed frequently in the psychoanalytic literature (Jackson, 1992) and in social psychology, counseling, and clinical psychiatry and psychology (Berger, 1987; Davis, 1994; Eisenberg & Strayer, 1987c; Ickes, 1997).

Definitions, Descriptions, and Features

A review of the literature indicates that there is more disagreement than agreement among researchers about the definition of empathy. Presenting a long list of definitions and descriptions of empathy would take us far beyond the intended scope and space constraints of this book. I have deliberately chosen a few definitions and descriptions that seem to be most relevant to the theme of the book and also can provide a framework for the conceptualization and definition of empathy in the context of patient care that will be presented in Chapter 6.

Carl Rogers (1959, p. 210), the founder of client-centered therapy, suggested the following often-cited definition of empathy as an ability "to perceive the internal frame of reference of another with accuracy as if one were the other person but without ever losing the '*as if*' condition" (emphasis added). In addition, Rogers (1975) described the experience of empathy as entering into the private perceptual world of another person and becoming thoroughly at home in it. Similarly, in one of the first psychoanalytic studies of empathy, Theodore Schroeder (1925, p. 159) suggested that "empathic insight implies seeing *as if* from within the person who is being observed" (emphasis added).

George Herbert Mead (1934, p. 27) suggested the following definition of empathy more than seven decades ago: "The capacity to take the role of another person and adopt alternative perspectives." About half a century ago, Charles Aring (1958) described empathy as the *act* or *capacity* of appreciating another person's feelings *without* joining those feelings. Robert Hogan (1969, p. 308) defined empathy as "the intellectual or imaginative apprehension of another's condition or state of mind *without* actually experiencing that person's feelings" (emphasis added). Clark (1980, p. 187) defined empathy as "the unique capacity of the human being to feel the experience, needs, aspirations, frustrations, sorrows, joys, anxieties, hurt, or hunger of others *as if* they were his or her own" (emphasis added). These definitions by Hogan and Clark are in line with Rogers's (1959) "as if" condition in describing empathy and with Aring's (1958) "without joining" feature of empathy described earlier. I will assert later in this chapter that the "as if" condition is a key feature that distinguishes empathy from sympathy.

Wispe (1986, p. 318) described empathy as "the attempt by one self-aware self to comprehend nonjudgmentally the positive and negative experiences of another self." Baron-Cohen and Wheelwright (2004) described empathy as the "glue" of the social world that draws people to help one another and stops them from hurting others. Levasseur and Vance (1993, p. 83) described empathy as follows: "Empathy is not a psychological or emotional experience, nor a psychic leap into the mind of another person, but an openness to, and respect for, the personhood of another." Similarly, Shamasundar (1999) described empathy as related to open-mindedness and tolerance for ambiguity and complexity.

Mead (1934) described empathy as an element of social intelligence. This description resembles the notion of emotional intelligence introduced originally by Salovey and Mayer (1990) and later by Goleman (1995) who proposed that empathy, as an ability to recognize emotions in others, is one domain of emotional intelligence. The proposition that empathy has a significant overlap with measures of emotional intelligence and social skills has been supported (Schutte et al., 2001).

Greif and Hogan (1973) described empathic development as a parallel function of moral maturity. Schafer (1959, p. 343) defined empathy as "the inner experience of sharing and comprehending the momentary psychological state of another person." Stefano Bolognini (1997, p. 279) described empathy as "a state of complementary conscious-preconscious contact based on separateness and sharing." William Ickes (1997, p. 183) defined empathy as "a state of our mind upon which we reflect." Bellet and Maloney (1991, p. 183) defined empathy as "the capacity to understand what the other person is experiencing from within the other person's frame of reference, i.e., the capacity to place oneself in another's shoes." Hamilton (1984, p. 217) defined empathy as a "vehicle for understanding one another in a meaningful way."

Levasseur and Vance (1993, p. 82) described empathy as "a mode of caring," adding that "Empathy is not for those who are flourishing or happy.... Empathy is for those who need help or are suffering or struggling in some way." Similarly, Shamasundar (1999) suggested that the intensity of empathic resonance is deeper for negative states, such as sadness, anger, and hostility. These descriptions portray the importance of empathy in situations where others are suffering or are sad. Thus, the importance of empathic relationships in patient encounters is apparent.

Recently, empathy has been described as the neural matching mechanism constituted of a mirror neuron system in the brain that enables us to place ourselves in the "mental shoes" of others (Gallese, 2001, 2003). Briefly, mirror neurons are brain cells (not visual cells) that are activated when we observe another person who is performing a goal-directed action as if we are performing that act (Carr et al., 2003; Gallese, 2001; Iacoboni et al., 1999). Imaging studies have shown that watching on a television screen a needle prick a specific hand muscle influences the same hand muscle in the observer (Singer & Frith, 2005). These new studies suggest the possibility that, in the future, empathy may be defined in neuroanatomical terms and be measured by physiological indicators (see Chapter 3 for a more detailed discussion).

Empathy Viewed from the Cognitive and Emotional Perspectives

In general, empathy has been described as a cognitive or an emotional (or affective) attribute or a combination of both. Cognition is mental activities involved in acquiring and processing information for better understanding, and emotion is sharing of the affect manifested in subjectively experienced feelings (Colman, 2001). Two types of empathy, cognitive empathy and emotional empathy, fit these descriptions.

Cognitive Perspective

Rosalind Dymond (1949) viewed empathy as a cognitive ability to assume the role of another person. Heins Kohut (1971, p. 300) described empathy as "a mode of *cognition* that is specifically attuned to the perception of a complex psychological configuration" (emphasis added). Basch (1983) also described empathy as a complex cognitive process involving cognitive functions, such as judgment and reality testing. MacKay, Hughes, and Carver (1990, p. 155) described empathy as "the ability to understand someone's situation without making it one's own."

Cognitive activities, such as perspective taking and role taking, are among the features some authors have presented in their definition of empathy. For example, Dymond (1949, p. 127) defined empathy as "the imaginative transposing of oneself into the thinking, feeling, and acting of another, and so structuring the world as he does." Blackman, Smith, Brokman, and Stern (1958) defined empathy as an ability to step into another person's shoes and to step back as easily into one's own shoes again when needed. Those who advocate the cognitive view of empathy, place more emphasis on understanding and social insight than on emotional involvement (Rogers, 1975).

Emotional Perspective

Some authors have defined empathy as an emotional response by generating identical feelings and sharing emotions between people. For example, Batson and Coke (1981, p. 169) defined empathy as "an emotional response elicited by and congruent with the perceived welfare of someone else." Rushton (1981, p. 260) defined empathy as "experiencing the emotional state of another." Eisenberg (1989) described it as "an emotional response that stems from the apprehension of another's emotional state or condition and is congruent with the other's emotional state or condition" (p. 108). Halpern (2001, p. xv) described empathy as "a form of emotional reasoning with risks of error that such reasoning involves." Katz (1963, p. 26) defined it as "the inner experience of feeling oneself to be similar to, or nearly identical with the other person." Kalisch (1973, p. 1548) defined it as "the ability to enter into the life of another person, to accurately perceive his current feelings and their meaning"; and Hoffman (1981, p. 41) defined it as "a vicarious affective response to someone else's situation rather than one's own." However, Underwood and Moore (1982) suggested that an emotional perspective is not a sufficient condition to define empathy. I will describe later that emotional empathy is analogous to sympathy.

A number of researchers, however, believe that empathy involves both cognition and emotion (Baron-Cohen & Wheelwright, 2004; Davis, 1994). For example, Bennett (2001, p. 7) defined empathy as "a mode of relating in which one person comes to know the mental content of another, both *affectively* and *cognitively*, at a particular moment in time and as a product of the relationship that exists between them." Mark Davis (1994) believes that cognitive and affective facets of empathy interact in his organizational model of empathy. He defined empathy as "a set of constructs having to do with the responses of one individual to the experiences of another. These constructs specifically include the process taking place within the observer and the affective and non-affective outcomes which results from those processes" (Davis, 1994, p. 12). Hodges and Wegner (1997, p. 313) suggested that "empathy can have either an emotional component . . . or a cognitive component, or both."

Cognition and Emotion

Silvan Tomkins (1962, 1963) viewed cognition and emotion as two separate systems working side by side to process incoming data. The processing of cognitive information often involves specific mental activities, such as reasoning and appraisal (Tausch, 1988). In contrast, emotional mental processing often entails an affective response experienced spontaneously without involvement of the higher mental processes that are activated in reasoning (Basch, 1996). Therefore, *reasoning* and *appraisal* are the features of cognitive responses, and *spontaneity* and *arousal* are the hallmarks of emotional responses. Solomon's (1976) description of the wisdom of "reason" against the treachery of the "passions" is somewhat analogous to the nature of a cognitive response as opposed to an emotional one.

Emotions and their expressions, as Charles Darwin (1965) was first to note, are universally similar regardless of cultural factors, personal background, and educational experiences. On the contrary, the processing of cognitive information is not culture free and is heavily dependent on personal background, learning, and educational experiences. Thus, the contribution of learning is more significant in a cognitive response (e.g., empathy) than it is in an emotional reaction (e.g., sympathy). Manifestation of cognitive behaviors is more *effortful*, and its behavioral roots are more *advanced*. The same is true of empathy. Expression of emotion is *effortless*, and its behavioral roots are more *primitive*. The same is true of sympathy. An emotional response is colored more by subjective judgments, leading to a less accurate interpretation than would result from a cognitive response.

At the neuroanatomical level, different brain mechanisms appear to be involved in the processing of cognitive and emotional input (Nathanson, 1996). Cognitive mental processing is primarily an *advanced intellectual process* that often involves social perception, analysis of information, and generation of appropriate responses based on one's understanding of another person and the situation. Emotional responses consist primarily of more *primitive* mental processes, wherein the person responds, through a process of contagion, with emotions similar to the emotions of others who are present (Mehrabian, Young, & Sato, 1988). Thus, emotion often is contagious in interpersonal exchanges, but cognition is not.

Despite these differences between cognition and emotion, some authors do not make such distinctions and assign equal weight to both cognition and emotion in the construct of empathy (Bennett, 2001). Freud (1958a, 1958b), for example, emphasized the intellectual or cognitive component while recognizing emotion as another important aspect of empathy in forming empathic relationships between clinician and patient.

It is indeed virtually impossible to treat emotion and cognition as two completely independent entities because one cannot fully exist without the other. For practical reasons, however, the distinction between the two is important to avoid confusion between the concepts of understanding and feeling (and thus between empathy and sympathy) that I will discuss in the following sections.

Understanding and Feeling

The distinction between cognition and emotion provides a context for distinguishing between the two other interrelated concepts of understanding and feeling, which are often used interchangeably. In the context of interpersonal relationships, however, it is useful to define understanding as the awareness of meaning (Sims, 1988) and to define feeling as the perception of emotions. All meaningful social relationships are based on both mutual understanding of one another and feeling of emotions.

Understanding is often based on *tangibility* and *objectivity*, whereas feeling is more a product of *subjectivity* and thus can be subject to *prejudice*. *Accuracy in judgment* is more likely to emerge from effortful mental activities associated with understanding than from spontaneous and effortless emotional arousal. Understanding is more likely to be based on learning and requires active efforts, whereas feeling is more likely to be *innate* and *effortless* (Wispe, 1986). A higher mental processing is involved when attempting to understand another person's concerns, whereas a primitive mental processing is involved in feeling another person's emotions. Empathy is associated more with cognitive response and understanding, whereas sympathy is associated more with emotions. To be empathic, according to Bellet and Maloney (1991, p. 1831) "the physician does not have to experience the intense feelings or emotions that grip the patient . . . but only to understand these feelings and relate to them while maintaining a sense of self." According to Shamasundar (1999), the less empathy between individuals, the more difficult it is to reach a mutual understanding of each other regardless of the use of a larger and more precise vocabulary.

Empathy and Sympathy

Both empathy and sympathy are important components of interpersonal relationships. Sympathy derives from the Greek *sym* (being with) and *pathos* (suffering, pain) (Black, 2004). The two distinct concepts of empathy and sympathy are often mistakenly tossed into the same terminological basket in empathy research—a mistake that has created conceptual confusion and debates for years but has never been settled (Black, 2004; Chismar, 1988; Gruen & Mendelsohn, 1986; Wispe, 1986; Zhou, Valiente, & Eisenberg, 2003). It has even been suggested that sympathy is an empathy-related response (Zhou et al., 2003). However, evidence suggests that the two constructs of empathy and sympathy reflect different human qualities that have different measurable influences on clinicians' professional behavior, utilization of resources, and clinical outcomes (Nightingale, Yarnold, & Greenberg, 1991; Yarnold, Greenberg, & Nightingale, 1991).

According to Decety and Jackson (2004, p. 85) "an essential aspect of empathy is to recognize the other person as like self while maintaining a

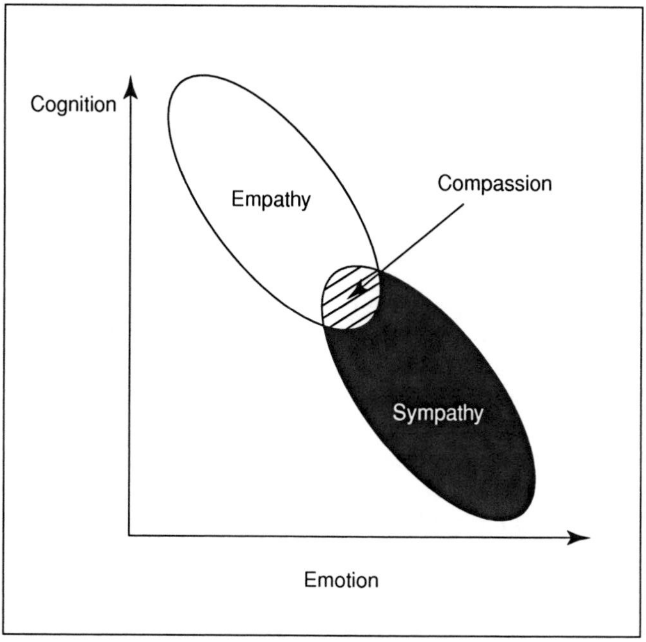

Figure 1.1 Empathy and sympathy as related to cognition and emotion.

clear separation between self and other." The key feature of empathy is the preponderance of *cognitive* information processing that distinguishes it from the predominantly *emotional* mental processing involved in sympathy (Brock & Salinsky, 1993; Streit-Forest, 1982; Wolf, 1980). One cannot claim that empathy and sympathy are fully independent from cognition and emotion, but one can argue that the degree of cognitive and emotional involvement is different in the two concepts of empathy and sympathy. Figure 1.1 is a graphic presentation showing the relative contribution of cognition and emotion in empathy and sympathy and the overlap between them. (My colleague Jon Veloski came up with the idea for this graphic presentation.) As it is shown in the figure, empathy is in the area of higher cognition than emotion. Conversely, sympathy is in the area of higher emotion than cognition. Compassion, I propose, resides in the area of the overlap between empathy and sympathy, where both of these attributes are expressed in a moderate amount.

Empathy is an *intellectual* attribute, whereas sympathy is an *emotional* state of mind (Gruen & Mendelsohn, 1986). Empathy refers to one person's attempt to comprehend nonjudgmentally another person's experiences (Wispe, 1986). Self-awareness is augmented in empathy, but it is reduced in sympathy. Whereas the aim of empathy is to *know* another person's concerns better, the aim of sympathy is to *feel* another person's emotions better. The empathic relationship implies a *convergence* of understanding between two people, and the sympathetic relationship implies a *parallelism* in the feelings between the two (Buchheimer, 1963). According to Kohut (1984), empathy is a "value-neutral" mode of observation. Similarly, Olinick (1984) believed that empathy is an affect-free phenomenon, whereas sympathy involves an affect-laden perception.

The underlying behavioral motivation in empathy is likely to be altruistic, but is more likely to be egoistic in sympathy. The ultimate goal of altruistically motivated helping behavior is to reduce another person's distress without any expectation of reward, whereas the primary goal in egoistically motivated helping behavior is to reduce one's own level of stress, to avoid adverse feelings, or to receive rewards (Coke, Batson, & McDavis, 1978). A genuine attempt to understand the experiences of another person—or *empathic understanding*—increases the likelihood of altruistic helping behavior. However, feeling the emotions of others, or sympathetic sharing of emotions, leads to physiological arousal, thus increasing the likelihood of egoistic behavior to reduce emotional arousal and avoid aversive experiences.

In clinical encounters, empathy involves an effort to *understand* the patient's experiences without joining them, whereas sympathy involves an effortless feeling of *sharing* or joining the patient's pain and suffering (Aring, 1958). Olinick (1984) suggested that empathy entails separateness and sympathy entails closeness; empathy "feels into" and sympathy "feels with." Titchener (1915), who first coined the term empathy, distinguished empathy from sympathy by describing empathy as a tendency to perceive another person's experiences and by describing sympathy as "feeling together" with another person. McKellar (1957, pp. 220–221) suggested that "One can, however, empathize without necessarily experiencing sympathy for the other person; empathy involves understanding rather than 'siding with.'" Wilmer (1968) described empathy as entering into the sufferer's mind and understanding his pain from within as if the pain were ours but remains his own. In contrast, sympathy, according to Wilmer, is sharing feelings together with the patient as if the pain were ours and remains so.

Hinshelwood (1989) wrote that empathy, in contrast to sympathy, involves a sophisticated mental operation in which two interacting people are clearly separated, but one conceives of the other person's mental landscape without losing sight of reality and his or her own identity. Similarly, Black (2004) believes that empathy is a sophisticated and conscious act and that sympathy is an involuntary propensity that makes affective attunement possible.

Understanding the *kind* and *quality* of the patient's experiences is the territory of empathy, whereas feeling the *degree* and *quantity* of the patient's concerns falls within the terrain of sympathy. A patient will feel felt if the clinician understands the kind and quality, not the degree and quantity, of the patient's experiences (Greenson, 1960). Whereas empathy is an internal cognitive process that should be communicated, sympathy seems to be more transparent. Benjamin Disraeli described the transparency of feelings in the following statement: "Never apologize for showing feelings. When you do so, you apologize for the truth" (retrieved February 2005 from http://www.wisdomquotes.com).

Empathy has been described as the art of understanding (Agosta, 1984; Starcevic & Piontek, 1997). This notion of empathic understanding is reflected in different features attributed to empathy, such as perspective taking, role playing, standing in another person's shoes, tolerance, openness, uncritical judgment, and unconditional acceptance.

The difference between empathy and sympathy is more than a semantic one because each involves different mental activities during information processing (Gruen & Mendelsohn, 1986). The predominantly cognitive nature of empathy and the primarily emotional nature of sympathy imply additional differences between the two terms that go beyond semantics. A cognitive response (in empathy) is more likely to be nonspontaneous because it is influenced by the regulatory process of *appraisal*. An affective reaction (in sympathy) is more likely to be spontaneous because it is influenced by the psychological regulatory process of *arousal* (Siegel, 1999).

Also, empathy as a cognitive response is characterized by an *inhibitory* energy-conserving state in the *parasympathetic* branch of the neurological regulatory process. However, sympathy as an emotional reaction is characterized by an *excitatory* energy-consuming state related to the *sympathetic* neurological regulatory process (Siegel, 1999).

Despite the differences between empathy and sympathy, they cannot be completely independent from one another. For example, in one of our studies (Hojat et al., 2001b), we found a moderate correlation between measures of the two constructs ($r = 0.45$, $p < 0.01$). A correlation of this magnitude indicates that the overlap between the two concepts is approximately 20% (coefficient of determination: $r^2 = 0.45^2 = 20\%$). More empirical research is needed to examine the degree of overlap between measures of empathy and sympathy.

Empathy and Sympathy in the Context of Patient Care

The distinction between sympathy and empathy has important implications for the clinician–patient relationship because joining the patient's emotions, a key feature of sympathy, can impede clinical outcomes. A clinician should feel the patient's feelings only to a limited extent to improve his or her understanding of the patient without impeding professional judgment (Starcevic & Piontek, 1997). When experiencing empathy, individuals are able to disentangle themselves from others, whereas individuals experiencing sympathy have difficulty maintaining a sense of whose feelings belong to whom (Decety & Jackson, 2006).

Ehrlich and Jaffe (2002) indicated that empathy must be distinguished from sympathy and sentimentalism because neither of the latter two concepts is desirable in the context of patient care. Starcevic and Piontek (1997) argued that because a clinician, as a separate human being, can never fully share the patient's feelings, perfect sympathy can never be achieved. Furthermore, as Truax and Carkhuff (1967) suggested, it would be undesirable for the clinician to feel the patient's emotions too strongly. Black (2004) points out that sympathy is a concept that psychoanalysts avoid, in contrast to empathy, which they use with pride. Wilmer (1968, p. 246) compared the outcomes of pity, sympathy, and empathy in the patient-care context and concluded that "pity rarely helps, sympathy commonly helps, empathy always helps."

Because of the emotional nature of sympathy, its overabundance can be overwhelming and therefore can impede the clinician's performance. This notion about the restraints in sympathetic clinician–patient relationships and clinical outcomes implies that the relationship between sympathy and a clinician's performance is likely to be *curvilinear*—an inverted U function

Table 1.1 Features of empathy and sympathy

Feature	Empathy	Sympathy
Contribution of learning	More significant	Less significant
Contribution of cognition	More significant	Less significant
Contribution of affects	Less significant	More significant
Contribution of innate or genetic factors	Less innate	More innate
Objectivity vs. subjectivity	More objective	More subjective
Likelihood of accuracy	More accurate	Less accurate
Behavioral roots	Advanced	Primitive
Required efforts	More effortful	More effortless
Relation to clinician's performance	Linear	Inverted U shape
Reaction time	Nonspontaneous	Spontaneous
Patient's emotions	Appreciated without joining	Perceived by joining
Feeling felt	The kind and quality of the patient's feelings	The degree and quantity of the feelings
Brain processing area	Predominantly neocortex	Predominantly limbic system
Psychological regulatory process	Appraisal	Arousal
Neurological regulatory process	Parasympathetic (inhibitory)	Sympathetic (excitatory)
Psycho-physiological state	Energy conserving	Energy consuming
Behavioral motivation	Altruistic	Egoistic
State of mind	Intellectual	Emotional
Typical expression to patient	I understand your suffering	I feel your pain
Key mental-processing mechanism	Cognitive/intellectual/ understanding	Affective/emotional/ feeling

similar to that between anxiety and performance on achievement tests. Although a certain amount of anxiety can improve performance, too much anxiety can hinder it by disrupting cognitive functioning. Thus, to a certain degree, sympathy can be beneficial in clinician–patient encounters—beyond that however, it can interfere with clinical objectivity and professional effectiveness. The relationship between empathy and a clinician's performance however, is considered to be *linear*. That is, the more empathic the relationship, the better the clinical outcomes. Therefore, the general conclusion is that sympathy must be restrained in clinical situations, whereas empathy needs no restraining boundary (Hojat, Gonnella, Mangione, Nasca, & Magee, 2003b).

The differences in features between empathy and sympathy are summarized in Table 1.1. I described some of these differences when discussing the notions of cognition and emotions and of understanding and feelings that correspond to empathy and sympathy, respectively.

In the context of patient care, when expressed in abundance, empathy would be an "enabling" factor, whereas sympathy in excess would be a "disabling" factor. As I indicated previously, the two concepts of empathy and sympathy have been used interchangeably as if one can replace the other without any serious consequences. However, in the context of patient care, the two terms must be used in their proper context because of their different patient outcomes. It is my hope that the differences described in Table 1.1 can help to settle the longstanding debate about empathy and sympathy. I will return again to the issues of empathy's definition and differences between empathy and sympathy in the context of patient care in Chapter 6.

Recapitulation

Empathy is a vague concept that has been described sometimes as a cognitive attribute, sometimes as an emotional state of mind, and sometimes as a combination of both. The ambiguity associated with the definition of empathy obstructs our view to clearly see what we intend to study, and hinders our ability of how to measure it in the context of patient care. Also, we should realize that the fundamental differences that exist between cognition and emotion, between understanding and feeling, and between empathy and sympathy have important implications not only for the conceptualization and measurement of empathy in patient care but also for the assessment of patient outcomes. Research findings on empathy can be subject to serious challenges if the conceptualization, definition, and measurement issues remain unsettled.

2

Human Connection in Health and Illness

Hear the reed's complaining wail!
Hear it tell its mourning tale!
Torn from spot it loved so well,
Its grief, its sighs our tears compel.

—Rumi (Persian mystical poet and philosopher, 1207–1273 A.D.)

It is not good for man to be alone.

—(Genesis 2:18)

Preamble

Human beings are evolved to connect together for survival. Among the factors that fulfill the human need for affiliation and connectedness are social institutions, such as marriage, family, and the social support network, including clinician–patient empathic relationships. Human connection serves to promote health and prevent disease. Conversely, an absence of satisfactory human connection, experienced as loneliness, is detrimental to physical, mental, and social well-being. The mechanisms involved in linking the quality of human connection to health or illness are not well understood. However, opportunities for empathic engagement and involvement of a multisystem of psychoneuroimmunology may provide some explanations for the beneficial effects of human connections. The clinician–patient relationship is formed by the drive for connectedness that increases with illness. The empathic connection between clinician and patient can serve as a special kind of social support system with beneficial healing power.

Introduction

Human beings are evolved to be social. We are, according to Larson (1993) "pre-wired" to be connected by evolutionary design for the sake of survival. Our survival depends on our ability to understand others and skills to communicate our understanding. Social relationships provide opportunities for empathic engagement, which in turn reinforces human connections, a cycle that has always been in motion in the evolution of humankind. In the often-cited list of basic needs proposed by psychologist Henry Murray (1938), the need for "affiliation" as well as the needs for "understanding" and "succorance" (to be gratified by being understood) are listed among the human being's basic psychosocial needs. Without fulfillment of those needs, Murray said, self-actualization cannot be fully achieved.

In this chapter, I describe the importance of human ties in health and illness and describe the consequences of making and breaking human connections on one's physical, mental, and social well-being. Also, I will attest that clinician–patient empathic engagement is the epitome of human connection.

The Need for Connectedness

Human connection is the bedrock of empathic growth. The urge for connectedness arises from the human need for affiliation. That basic need prompts us to fall in love, marry and establish a family, raise children, associate with other people, enjoy the company of others, and develop interpersonal relationships with help seekers and help providers. The need for affiliation has survival advantages and is deeply rooted in the evolutionary history of humankind.

Feeling connected leads not only to psychological pleasure but also to biophysiological changes and activities in the endocrine system. For example, female students living together in university dormitories noticed that their menstrual cycles had become synchronized, and this hormonal synchronization occurred not only among roommates but among networks of close friends as well (McClintock, 1971).

People interacting with one another often show behavioral synchronization, usually unconsciously, that is reflected in such nonverbal clues as "facial mimicry" and the "motor mirroring" reaction (see Chapter 4). These signals are not necessarily learned; they seem to be the outcomes of a built-in behavioral repertoire that facilitates interpersonal exchanges (see Chapter 8).

The Making of Connections

It is now widely recognized that making connections has a powerful effect on the maintenance of health and that breaking connections can lead to the development of illness (Cohen, 1988). This recognition is not new, however. Early research by the French sociologist Emile Durkheim on factors contributing to suicide found that erosion of the capacity for social integration and human connection was the triggering factor for social miseries, including people's attempt to end their lives (Durkheim, 1951).

In their widely cited epidemiological research conducted more than a quarter century ago, Berkman and Syme (1979) showed that the absence of human connections was significantly linked to an increase in disease and mortality. So much evidence has been accumulating that it is now beyond doubt that being connected and feeling felt are beneficial to physical, mental, and social well-being, the three pillars of health defined by the constitution of the World Health Organization (WHO, 1948) (see Chapter 6). Social connections in epidemiological research are typically defined in terms of marital status, family, friends and peer relationships and membership in social or religious groups (Cacioppo et al., 2002). In this context, marriage, family, and social network as well as clinician–patient empathic engagement have a common denominator: They connect people together and serve as social support systems.

Marriage and the Family

Traditionally, the family is built on the covenant of marriage for the purpose of bringing couples together, to make a commitment to share their concerns, feelings, and experiences in health and illness and in happiness and sadness 'til death they do part. Thus, marriage and the family are important social support systems that can fulfill the human needs for affiliation, intimacy, and connectedness.

The social support system originates in the family, which is regarded as a secure base for the development of the capacity for human connection from cradle to grave. The relationships inside the family between spouses, between parents and children, and among other family members become prototypical or representational models of human connections outside the family, extending to friends, peers, and colleagues (see Chapter 4).

Consistent with the notion that fulfillment of the need for affiliation promotes health, research has shown that the mortality rate for medical causes of death is significantly lower for married couples than it is for single, separated, divorced, and widowed individuals (Goodwin, Hunt, Key, & Samet, 1987; Ortmeyer, 1974; Wiklund, Oden, & Sanne, 1988). In addition, married people are the healthiest group, with the lowest rates of chronic disease and disabilities, followed by single, widowed, divorced, and separated people in that order (Verbrugge, 1979).

The proportion of elderly people living in an assisted living or nursing home facility was highest among those who were single or divorced and lowest among married elderly people (Verbrugge, 1979). Research also indicates that married patients with cancer live longer than their single counterparts do (Goodwin et al., 1987).

Numerous studies indicate that spouses, children, other family members, and a network of friends play important roles in prevention of disease and maintenance of health. Among patients who underwent coronary angiography and had at least one blocked coronary artery, those who were not married or lacked a companion to talk to regularly were significantly more likely to die within 5 years after the procedure (Williams et al., 1992).

It has been suggested that a stable marriage and close family relationships can free a person from becoming entrapped in serious psychopathology (Valliant, 1977). Consistent with this suggestion, empirical data from a longitudinal study conducted in Sweden found that single people and those living alone had an elevated risk of dementia compared with married people living with their spouses (Fratiglioni, Wang, Ericsson, Maytan, & Winblad, 2000). In summarizing his family studies, Lewis (1998) pointed out that marriage and family have beneficial effects because couples often express their affects openly to one another and family members frequently communicate empathy, in particular, to one another.

It is interesting to note that although making a connection through marriage is beneficial for both men and women, men benefit more from marriage than women do. In addition, although breaking the marital connection is harmful for both men and women, men seem to suffer more than women do from separation, divorce, and spousal death (Glynn, Christenfeld, & Gerin, 1999). Sex differences in sociability, interpersonal skills, social behavior, and empathic capacity (see Chapter 9) can explain the differential effects of making and breaking human connections in men and women.

It also should be noted that because breakdown of human connections resulting from disruption of marriage, separation, and divorce is detrimental to physical, mental, and social well-being (Bloom, Asher, & White, 1978; Verbrugge, 1979), fragmentation of this important social institution raises a red flag for public health in society at large. Such a trend toward the breakdown of the family places additional responsibility on health care providers to fill the gap and serve as a social support. Having a supportive clinician who listens empathically to the patient's personal experiences with a "third ear" and sees patient's concerns with the "mind's eye" helps the patient sort out those experiences and is, in itself, therapeutic.

Social Support

Social support is defined as a multidimensional construct of social relationships that enhances well-being (Rodriguez & Cohen, 1998). It also has been described as the interpersonal resource people use to share understanding and emotions and to develop a sense of belonging (Wellman, 1998). A social support system provides psychological and material resources that benefit an individual's ability to cope with stress (Blumenthal et al., 1987; Cohen, 2004). A social support network of peers and friends is important for the well-being of both children and adults (Cohen, 2004; Hartup & Stevens, 1999). A substantial volume of accumulated evidence indicates the extent to which supportive social relationships are related to individuals' physical, mental, and social well-being (Berkman, 1995). Because of the benefits of a social support system in promoting health, Berkman (1995) suggested that social support networks, such as family, friends, and community, should be incorporated into treatment interventions. According to Morgan (2002), a functional social support network requires empathy.

Beneficial Outcomes of Making Connections

The association between social connection and health outcomes is fairly well established in epidemiological research (Glynn et al., 1999). Dean Ornish (1998) described the healing power of intimacy and social relationships in coronary artery disease, beyond drugs and surgery, as follows: "Our heart *is* a pump that needs to be addressed on a physical level, but our hearts are more than just pumps. A true physician is more than just a plumber, technician, or mechanic. We also have an emotional heart, a psychological heart, and a spiritual heart. Our language reflects that understanding." (p. 11)

Cohen (1988) reported that when research participants were exposed to the common cold virus, the perceived social connections served as a protective factor against the virus. Sociability and social activity were found to predict longer survival among women with breast cancer (Hislop, Waxler, Coldman, Elwood, & Kan, 1987), and it is widely recognized that one factor that contributes to improving the health of patients with cancer is social connection (Holland, 2001). The aforementioned studies support the notion that meaningful social relationships, manifested in empathic engagement, can enhance human immunocompetence to a miraculous degree.

Although the well-known Framingham Heart Study has concentrated primarily on physiological and life-style factors in heart disease (Levy, 1999), this and several other large-scale epidemiological studies provide strong support for the proposition that human connection is beneficial to health and a lack of it is an independent risk factor for illness. For example, in a study of the mortality rate caused by heart disease among Italian American residents in two adjacent towns in eastern Pennsylvania, the researchers found that the death rate among the residents of Roseto was higher than it was among the residents of Bangor (Egolf, Lasker, Wolf, & Potvin, 1992; Wolf, 1992). The researchers attributed this difference in mortality rates to changes in the social support system and to lower family and community cohesiveness among Italian-Americans in Roseto as a result of becoming a more "Americanized" community.

Remarkable recoveries from life-threatening diseases have been linked to the power of social connections, such as an enduring marriage, family relationships, and friendships (Hirshberg & Barasch, 1995). In a study of Japanese people who emigrated to the United States, Marmot and Syme (1976) found that the immigrants who maintained their traditional family ties had a low prevalence of heart disease similar to their counterparts living in Japan, but the immigrants who became acculturated by adopting the Western life-style were three to five times more likely to suffer from heart problems.

Another epidemiological study, conducted in Alameda County near San Francisco, found that perception of a lack of social network (family, friends, religious and other group affiliations) significantly increased the mortality rate from 1.9 to 3.1 during the 9-year follow-up period (Berkman, 1995; Berkman, Glass, Brissette, & Seeman, 2000; Berkman, Leo-Summers, & Horwitz, 1992; Berkman & Syme, 1979). Using residents of the same county, researchers found that during their 5-year study, the mortality rate for breast cancer was twice as high among the women who lacked a strong social connection (Raynolds, Boyd, & Blacklow, 1994).

Investigators in the Tecumseh Community Health Study conducted in Michigan found that during a period of 10–12 years, the morbidity rates for stroke, other cardiac problems, cancer, arthritis, and lung disease increased two to three times during the study period as a result of participants' weakening of social support systems (House, Robbins, & Metzner, 1982). Blazer (1982) found that people who expressed dissatisfaction with their social support system were more than three times as likely as their satisfied counterparts to die sooner of disease.

These and other epidemiological studies indicate that the risk of a physical illness doubles, at least, when a person's social connections become weak or fragmented (Kaplan, Salonem, & Cohen, 1988; Orth-Gomer & Johnson, 1987; Schoenbach, Kaplan, Fredman, & Kleinbaum, 1986; Seeman, Berkman, & Kohout, 1993). On the basis of the findings just described, it appears that vigilance, inquiries, and advice about patients' social connections not only can help clinicians find remedies that will improve their patients' health status but also can confirm the importance of empathic connection between clinician and patient as a prototype of a support system that in itself is therapeutic.

Pennebaker (1990) suggested that a social support system has a potent benefit because it serves as an outlet for people to talk about their concerns and feelings. Similarly, the healing power of "opening up" during consultations with a health care provider is facilitated by the provider's active listening and empathic interpersonal connection with the patient (see Chapter 8). Pennebaker, Kiecolt-Glaser, and Glaser (1988) reported that self-disclosure of past traumatic events during a clinician–patient encounter can have beneficial effects on the patient's immune system. The clinician's empathic understanding can strengthen the clinician–patient connection that leads the patient to self-disclose at deeper levels, which in turn results in a more positive health outcome. In support of this notion, Greenberg, Watson, Elliot, and Bohart (2001) suggested that an empathic relationship can help strengthen the self and free a person from isolation and loneliness.

The precise mechanisms that promote health as an outcome of human connection are not well understood. However, research suggests that some neurobiological as well as psychological mechanisms are involved. Berkman (1995) suggested that the immune and neuroendocrine systems are involved in the linkage of social connection and health outcomes. In a review article, Cohen (1988) concluded that health-promoting effects of social ties reflected in social integration (e.g., marriage, network of family and friends, group activities, and religious affiliation) are the combined outcomes of psychosocial factors (e.g., regulation of emotions, cognitive processes, life-style, and health behaviors) as well as biophysiological functions (e.g., neuroendocrine, immune, and cardiovascular systems).

Social connections are protective because of the satisfaction that results from human relationships—an important health-promoting factor. For example, Berkman (2000) emphasized that satisfaction with one's spouse, children, relatives, and friends is more important than is the frequency of contact with them. In other words, the perceived *quality* of one's social connections is more important than the *quantity* of such connections in maintaining health. Similarly, Seeman and Syme (1987) showed that the size of one's social network is less important than the quality of the interpersonal relationships within that network in lowering the risk of coronary artery disease. Evidence has been accumulating that social support serves as a protective "buffer" against fear and anxiety associated with stress (Cohen, 1988; LaRocco, House, & French, 1980), which in turn can prolong the lives of patients with breast cancer (Spiegel, Bloom, Kraemer, & Gottheil, 1989).

The health-promoting aspects of human connection could be a consequence of certain patterns of psychophysiological response involving the relaxing effect of affiliation, decreased sympathoadrenal activity, and hormonal and metabolic activities associated with human contact (Uvnas-Moberg, 1997). It appears that perceptions of interpersonal connection affect the nervous, endocrine, and immune systems (collectively called psychoneuroimmunology) and that the combined effects of the interactions of the three systems contribute to either health (when connections are satisfactory) or illness (when connections, such as negative or stressful relationships, are dissatisfactory).

According to the aforementioned studies, the risk of illness should be lower among people who have strong social connections in several domains, including the perception of support from their health providers. This is important for health care providers to know, because Berkman (2000) suggested that one type of social relationship can fill the gap for another. Thus, empathic engagement in clinician–patient encounters can serve as a substitute for, or an additional source of, human connection, with all its beneficial outcomes.

Detrimental Outcomes of Breaking Connections

Making and breaking human connections obviously will have opposite consequences for health. An inadequate social network is associated with a high degree of loneliness experiences (Seeman & Syme, 1987). Lonely people obviously are deprived of the beneficial effects of human connections. According to House and colleagues (House, Landis, & Umberson, 1988), social isolation is a significant risk factor for morbidity and mortality comparable to obesity, sedentary life-style, and even smoking. A detailed discussion of loneliness and its corrosive effects on human well-being is beyond the intended scope of this book. However, because loneliness reduces the likelihood of empathic engagement, I will briefly discuss its detrimental outcomes as well as its link to empathy.

Loneliness, defined as the perception that one lacks meaningful connections with others, is a complex phenomenon that is an outcome of many factors, including the early rearing environment, insecure attachment relationships in childhood, a dysfunctional social network, a nonfacilitative living environment, social forces, and the lack of interpersonal skills (Hojat & Crandall, 1989). These same factors also contribute to a deficient capacity for empathy (see Chapter 4).

Loneliness not only impedes psychosocial well-being but also has a negative effect on physical health through the pathway of the immune system (Kennedy, Kiecolt-Glaser, & Glaser, 1988). It has been shown that human disconnectedness, experienced as loneliness, leads to a compromised immune system and thus increases a person's vulnerability to infection and disease. For example, medical students who were lonely had poor immune function, as measured by decreases in the proportions of T-helper lymphocytes and in the number and function of natural killer cells (Kiecolt-Glaser et al., 1984).

Disconnected people lack social skills and are similar to people with deficient empathic capacity. For example, in one of our recent studies with medical students (Hojat et al., 2005b), we found that scores on the Jefferson Scale of Physician Empathy (see Chapter 7) were negatively correlated with scores on the UCLA Loneliness Scale (Russell, Peplau, & Cutrona, 2004) but were positively correlated with sociability scores on the Extraversion subscale of the Zuckerman–Kuhlman Personality Questionnaire (Zuckerman, 2002).

Research shows that lonely people are likely to score low on measures of positive aspects of personality that contribute to better interpersonal relationships (e.g., self-esteem, extraversion) (Hojat, 1982a, 1982b, 1983; Shapurian & Hojat, 1985). Conversely, lonely people are likely to score high on negative aspects of personality that are detrimental to interpersonal relationships (e.g., depression, anxiety, neuroticism, tough-mindedness) (Hojat, 1982a, 1982b, 1983; Hojat & Shapurian, 1986; Hojat, Shapurian, & Mehryar, 1986; Shapurian & Hojat, 1985). Disconnected people are less likely to trust others, as is indicated by a significant correlation between scores on the UCLA Loneliness Scale and scores on a scale measuring misanthropy or faith-in-people (Hojat, 1982a). The findings that lonely people lack the skills required to achieve interpersonal connections and tend not to trust others suggest that loneliness is not conducive to forming empathic relationships. In a recent study (Papadakis et al., 2005), it was found that impaired peer relationships during medical school could predict later disciplinary action by medical boards against physicians. Thus, capacity to connect can have a lasting effect on physicians' professional behavior.

In his intriguing book with the telling title *The Broken Hearts: The Medical Consequences of Loneliness*, James Lynch (1977, p. 181) proposed that "the lack of human companionship, the sudden loss of love, and chronic human loneliness are significant contributors to serious disease (including cardiovascular disease) and premature death." For example, being surrounded by family or friends reduced the likelihood of premature death by half among the elderly patients compared to the rate of death among those who were lonely (Penninx, van Tilburg, & Kriegsman, 1997).

Another study found that living alone was an independent risk factor in recurrent major cardiac events (Case, Moss, Case, McDermott, & Eberly, 1992). However, it is reported that feeling alone is more detrimental to health than living alone (Berkman, 2000; Hojat, 1992). A growing body of evidence in epidemiologic and psychosomatic medicine suggests that disconnectedness is a significant stressor that can be a causative element in the onset or exacerbation of a large and diverse number of medical illnesses, including asthma, cancer, congestive heart failure, diabetes mellitus, infectious hepatitis, leukemia, peptic ulcer, hypertension, hyperthyroidism, and rheumatoid arthritis and in the onset of medical catastrophes, such as sudden death after bereavement (for a review, see Hojat & Vogel, 1989). The perceived distress emerging from dissatisfaction with the social network adversely affects the psychoneuroimmune system, which leads to the progression of illness and deterioration of health (Keller, Shiflett, Schleifer, & Bartlett, 1994).

A number of studies have documented that patients who are lonely, single, or lack a confidant have a higher mortality rate after a myocardial infarction (Berkman et al., 1992; Case et al., 1992). Low levels of social resources were identified as important risk factors, independent of important medical prognostic factors, in patients medically treated for coronary artery disease, (Williams et al., 1992). The harmful outcomes associated with the lack of interpersonal connections result in a reduced ability to adapt to environmental changes, which can inflict damage on the cardiovascular, metabolic, and immune systems (McEwen, 1998).

A recent report indicates that myocardial stunning was an outcome of emotional stress resulting from the death of a family member or close friend in 47% of the patients with stress-related cardiomyopathy (Wittstein et al., 2005). The authors suggest that exaggerated sympathetic stimulation (or "broken heart" syndrome) as a result of overwhelming emotional stress after loss of a loved one might be central to the myocardial stunning.

Windholz, Marmar, and Horowitz (1985) reported that bereaved spouses were at greater risk for deteriorating health and had a higher mortality rate. In a longitudinal study of volunteers of mammography, Fox, Harper, Hyner, and Lyle (1994) found that experiencing the death of a spouse or another close family member within the previous 2 years significantly increased the risk of breast cancer. To summarize, misery will knock on the door when human connection is broken by death of a loved one, divorce, separation, or loneliness. Empathic engagement can dispel the misery of human disconnectedness.

Human Connections in Therapy

Human connection can generate an interpersonal dynamic that has a healing effect. For example, group therapy is a method of therapy conducted with a group of patients who often have similar problems. Support groups composed of patients or former patients who get together to discuss illness-related experiences represent another therapeutic approach. The unique elements of these types of therapies are interpersonal connection, mutual understanding, and sharing of experiences and concerns, all of which are elements of empathic engagement as well. Shamasundar (1999) postulated that participants in such groups experience relief from anxiety and distress through the process of diluting emotional states during empathic engagement that occurs while sharing of experiences with others. David Spiegel and colleagues (Spiegel, 1990, 1994; Spiegel & Bloom, 1983; Spiegel, Bloom, & Yalom, 1981) demonstrated that as a means of providing members with social support, group therapy and support groups lead to longevity for patients with cancer. In a series of articles, Spiegel and colleagues (Spiegel, 1993, 1994, 2004; Spiegel et al., 1989) demonstrated that the perception of belongingness associated with group membership could significantly increase the longevity of patients with metastatic breast cancer.

In one clinical study, patients with metastatic breast cancer were encouraged to express their feelings about their illness in a group (Spiegel et al., 1989). On the average, those patients lived approximately 18 months longer than did members of a control group. The researchers concluded that group support and expression of feelings can mobilize patients' vital resources more effectively. A similar phenomenon occurs during empathic clinician–patient engagement.

In a meta-analytic study, Bohart, Elliot, Greenberg, and Watson (2002) confirmed that group therapy led to slightly better patient outcomes than individual therapy did. A study with addicted physicians found that a peer-led self-help program similar to Alcoholics Anonymous was successful in treating the physicians' addiction (Galanter, Talbott, Gallegos, & Rubenstone, 1990). The authors identified three factors that contributed to the program's positive outcomes—shared beliefs, group cohesiveness, and mutual identification—all of which are elements of empathic engagement. Development of an empathic understanding among participants in group therapy or support groups as a result of sharing common goals and experiences could be a contributing factor to changes that occur in group behavior (Shamasundar, 1999). Feelings of being understood generate connectedness that diminishes patients' feelings of loneliness and perceptions of alienation that lead to the therapeutic alliance (Book, 1991).

The phenomenon known as mass psychogenic behavior often occurs at a group level among members of a network consisting of family members, friends, coworkers, and classmates who share similar experiences and concerns (Colligan, Pennebaker, & Murphy, 1982). The empathic relationship has been identified as a factor that contributes to the contagion of group psychogenic behavior (Colligan & Murphy, 1982). Also, contagious yawning triggered by seeing or imagining another person's yawning has been linked to the ability to empathize with others (Platek, Critton, Myers, & Gallup, 2003; Platek, Mohamed, & Gallup, 2005). For example, after-dinner yawning that triggers others at the dinner table to yawn may be akin to mass psychogenic behavior that is analogous to interpersonal mimicry or synchronized posture elicited by empathic engagement (Boruch, 1982). Platek and colleagues (2005) proposed that contagious yawning is an expression of cognitive processes involved in awareness of self and others and may be driven by the so-called mirror neuron system (see Chapter 3).

The Gift of Being Present in Patient Care

The human drive for connectedness increases during times of illness-related distress because illness often makes patients feel disconnected (Platt & Keller, 1994). Therefore, the availability of social support for patients is crucially important. As Morgan (2002) indicated, social support is synonymous with care in the context of health care. Being present when a person is in need of help is, in itself, a social support factor and is a therapeutic remedy described as the "gift of presence" (Nicholas, 2002). The clinician's presence is especially supportive when an empathic relationship is formed between clinician and patient.

The presence of a supportive ally, such as an empathic health care provider, serves as a buffer against the cardiovascular stress response (Christenfeld & Gerin, 2000). In particular, the presence of a woman who provides social support has been found to be more significant than the social support provided by a man (Christenfeld & Gerin, 2000). In an experiment on the influence of social support provided by men and women, study participants were assigned to deliver a short speech on euthanasia (Glynn et al., 1999). The researchers found that when the support was provided by women, who were in the audience and nodding in agreement, the magnitude of the systolic blood pressure was reduced in both male and female speakers. However, a cardiovascular effect of that magnitude was not observed in the speakers when men in the audience nodded in agreement. From the results of this experiment, the researchers concluded that the gift of the presence of supportive individuals, especially supportive women, would probably lead to fewer heart conditions (Glynn et al., 1999). (See Chapter 9 for a discussion of sex differences in the style of medical practice.) These findings also suggest the important role that nurses (most of whom are women) often play in providing care and support to the patients (e.g., the concept of caring versus curing described in Chapter 8).

The Empathic Clinician-Patient Relationships as the Epitome of Human Connection

The term social support applies to a broad range of conceptualizations of social network structures and their health-promoting function (Blumenthal et al., 1987; Cohen & Matthews, 1987). In that regard, the clinician–patient relationship can be conceptualized as a special kind of social support system. Cohen (2004) suggested that social support can provide the following three types of resources: (a) instrumental, involving the provision of material aids, (b) emotional, involving the expression of empathy, caring, and reassurance, and (c) informational, involving the provision of relevant information to help the individual understand the problem better and cope with difficulties. A cooperative clinician–patient relationship provides all of the aforementioned resources because research shows that mutual understanding of pain and suffering increases in cooperative as opposed to competitive relationships (Goubert et al., 2005).

The patient's perception of the clinician's support is a complex phenomenon that is a function of the nature of the patient's help-seeking behavior and desire for affiliation and the clinician's response through empathic communication. When a trusting relationship is established and is further reinforced by empathic engagement, constraints in the relationship vanish and a heart-to-heart human connection will form. This kind of human connection, characterized by full trust, can be formed between lovers as well as between clinicians and their patients.

The relevance and importance of the notion of social support in clinician–patient relationships becomes more evident, considering that patients exhibit an increased desire for affiliation that is naturally expected when people are in distress (Taylor, Klein, Gruenewald, Gurung, & Fernandes-Taylor, 2003). In his classical experiment, Stanley Schachter (1959) demonstrated that stress increases our desire to affiliate. In the experiment, participants in the high-stress condition (they were told they would receive painful shocks) were twice as likely as other participants to wait in the company of others than to wait alone to participate in the experiment. It has been shown that the presence of significant others can reduce the experience of pain and suffering (Romano, Jensen, Turner, Good, & Hops, 2000).

One plausible explanation is that human connectedness has a fear-reducing effect that contributes to positive health outcomes (House et al., 1988). It also has been demonstrated that an encounter between a clinician and a patient, in itself, has a potential healing power (Novack, 1987, Spiro,

1986). Because of this powerful impact, Balint (1957) described clinicians as the most frequently used therapeutic agents in the history of medicine.

The positive influence of clinician–patient encounters on patient outcomes has been called "Factor X", an unknown factor in healing human suffering (White, 1991). The patient's social support system in general and the nature and quality of the clinician–patient relationship in particular are among the components of the human factor in health and illness. In the process of interpersonal connection, empathy has a mediating role in improving the strength of the connections by increasing a sense of common identity and reducing prejudice (Stephan & Finlay, 1999). Thus, empathy paves the road to the interpersonal connection between clinicians and patients that is a special kind of social support system, with all of its beneficial healing powers.

Recapitulation

The human tendency to seek connections has an evolutionary root and a survival advantage. Abundant evidence indicates that satisfying the need for affiliation and human connectedness through marriage, family, peers, friends, community, and other social support networks leads to physical, mental, and social well-being. Conversely, breaking social connections leads to loneliness and its detrimental health outcomes. The opportunity for empathic engagement is one underlying reason for the health-promoting outcomes of human connections. Because the drive for human connection increases during times of distress and illness, the presence of an empathic clinician is a gift of social support for the patient and epitomizes the human connection, with all of its beneficial effects.

3

An Evolutionary Perspective, Psycho-Socio-Physiology, Neuroanatomy, and Heritability

Empathy can lead to the evolution of fairness

—(Karen Page & Martin Novak, 2002, p. 1101)

Empathy is a biological concept par excellence

—(Leslie Brothers, 1989, p. 17)

Preamble

For a better understanding of empathy, we need to understand its evolutionary roots, its psycho-socio-physiological function, and its neuroanatomy. During the course of evolution, human beings have been endowed with an innate capacity to express and understand emotions from nonverbal cues that has survival advantage and is conceptualized as primitive empathy. Different regions of the brain have been implicated in empathy—sometimes the neocortical areas, other times the limbic system probably because of a different conceptualization of empathy as either a cognitive or an emotional attribute. Neuroimaging technology, neurological impairment studies, and discovery of the mirror neuron system support the notions of neuroanatomy and brain function of empathy. Twin studies suggest that heritability is a significant component of empathy more often when a measure of emotional empathy is used.

Introduction

In Chapter 2, I described human beings as social creatures that evolved to be connected with other human beings because social groupings provided increased defense against predators (Plutchik, 1987). Empathic engagement, particularly at the time of distress, was viewed in that chapter as a special kind of social support system. In this chapter, I discuss empathy as having an evolutionary root with a psycho-socio-physiological function, a neuroanatomical structure, and a heritability component.

Long before they developed the capacity for verbal communication and invented language, our ancestors could relay their feelings, intentions, and expectations by nonverbal means, such as facial expressions, imitation, motor mimicry, and bodily postures. Nonverbal empathic communication has a longer history in the course of human evolution than does verbal communication. Thus, if the brain has areas for verbal communication and language (e.g., Broca and Wernik areas), it must have areas for nonverbal communication and understanding of emotions. Because empathy implies understanding of feelings, emotions, and inner experiences, any means of communicating these entities would be of interest in studies of the capacity for empathy.

Empathic exchanges, according to Buck and Ginsburg (1997a, p. 481) involve communication genes, "a genetically based, spontaneous communication process that is fundamental to all living things and that includes innate sending and receiving mechanisms (visual, auditory, or chemical displays and pre-attunements to such displays, respectively); empathy involves communicative genes." If one assumes that empathy is based on an *innate* mechanism and involves "communicative genes," then it must have an evolutionary root, a neuroanatomical structure, and a psycho-socio-physiological function.

An Evolutionary Perspective

Evolution lays out the historical path along which humankind has traveled to reach the present point. To understand human behavior, we must understand its evolution. According to the notion of evolution espoused by Charles Darwin (1965, 1981) human beings have evolved during a long evolutionary history of struggle for existence that resulted in the survival of the fittest. During that long history, emotions and their expressions and social cognition evolved for their adaptive advantages in dealing with the fundamental task of survival (Ekman, 1992).

Allport (1924) suggested that the expression of emotion originated from learning experiences *common* to all human beings. Similarly, Ekman (1992) proposed that our cognitive appraisal of situations that evoke emotions (e.g., those that threaten our survival) is primarily determined by our ancestral past. Carl Gustav Jung (1964) proposed the notion of "collective unconscious" as a transpersonal residue of experiences inherited from one generation to the next. These views imply the existence of a common evolutionary root in the expression of emotion and in cognitive appraisal that are vehicles of empathic communication.

In her thought-provoking article on the biological perspective of empathy, Leslie Brothers (1989) proposed that the capacity for empathy improves fitness for survival. The capacities our ancestors developed to read emotions from nonverbal clues (e.g., facial expression, bodily movement, tone of voice) provided a means of distinguishing foes from friends and danger from safety. The ability to understand social signals conveyed by facial expressions and bodily movements provides a competitive advantage over adversaries and protects against being deceived by them (Brothers, 1989).

Obviously, people who were armed with the capacity to understand other people's state of mind could escape danger more easily than could others who lacked that skill; thus, they were more fit for survival. People who failed to develop the capacity for empathy because of inappropriate psychosocial experiences, a nonfacilitative rearing environment, or arrested neurological development were less likely to survive. Natural selection, therefore, favored empathy (Humphrey, 1983; Ridley & Dawkins, 1981). Parallel to sensitivity in detecting social signals, human beings developed the skills of deception and manipulation to conceal their emotions and intentions from predators. These evolutionary adapted skills have implications for the study of empathy.

Evolutionary adaptation has contributed not only to the physical and anatomical changes but also to such social behaviors as mate selection (Buss, 2003), reproductive strategies (Buss, 1995; Buss & Schmitt, 1993), parental investment (Trivers, 1972), and prosocial behavior, altruism, and empathy (Buck & Ginsburg, 1997a; Ridley & Dawkins, 1981). During the long history of evolution, capacities have gradually evolved to achieve the ultimate purpose of life—preservation of genes. Dawkins (1999) proposed that the engine of the survival machine is driven by the "selfish gene," which determines whether to protect, fight, or flee to increase the probability of survival. However, Buck and Ginsburg (1997b, p. 19) argued that "some genes are selfish, and function to support the survival of the individual organism, but other genes are social functioning to support the survival of species."

Buck and Ginsburg's notion was supported by Hamilton (1964), who, in discussing the evolutionary concept of exclusive fitness, proposed that human beings are not programmed exclusively and egoistically to protect their own individual genes but are programmed inclusively and altruistically to protect the survival of others who share similar characteristics.

In support of this notion, de Quervain and colleagues (2004) used positron emission tomography (PET) to study the neural basis of *the social brain* with regard to intrinsic rewards for prosocial behaviors (e.g., cooperation and observing social norms) and punishment for violating them. The researchers found that people derive intrinsic satisfaction from punishing norm violators, which suggests that such altruistic punishment for the sake of the group's survival has been a decisive force in the evolution of human social behavior. A reward-related region of the brain, the dorsal striatum, has been implicated in the processing of rewards that accrue for socially desirable behavior (de Quervain et al., 2004).

The idea of a "non-selfish" gene that supports the survival of the group suggests that the unit of observation for the purpose of survival may be the group of individuals with common characteristics, rather than the individual. The chance of group survival increases with prosocial and altruistically motivated behaviors. The evolutionary basis of empathy, according to Hoffman (1978), can be linked to altruistic behavior in helping others in distress, sometimes even at a cost to the self.

Altruistic behaviors have puzzled evolutionary scholars who believe that the purpose of the struggle for existence is preservation of the individual's genes. However, the notion of a "non-selfish" gene can explain the underlying motivation for altruism. For example, sacrificing one's own life for the good of the country (patriotic behavior) was dramatically illustrated by Japan's kamikaze pilots during World War II. Political suicidal missions also can be explained by the concept of a "non-selfish" gene aiming at group rather than individual survival. Empathy may have a role in such self-sacrificing behaviors, rooted in the understanding of others' suffering.

The issue of whether unconscious (or conscious) efforts to survive are selfishly and egoistically directed toward the preservation of individual genes or are unselfishly and altruistically directed toward maintaining the group's genes has been hotly debated by evolutionary scholars. Although the details of such a debate are beyond the intended scope of this book, we should always remember that we are the product of millions of years of evolutionary adaptation for the purpose of either individual or group survival. Empathy is a by-product of this evolutionary adaptation.

Nonverbal Means of Empathic Communication

Through the process of evolution, the human brain has evolved to send and receive messages through nonverbal cues, such as facial expressions, motor mimicry, bodily gestures, change of facial skin color, sweating, and trembling as well as through vocal sounds, such as voice pitch, crying, and laughter, so that happiness, friendliness, and well-intended behaviors could be distinguished from sadness, disagreement, and hostile intent (Adolphs, Tranel, Damasio, & Damasio, 1994; Siegel, 1999). As a result of this evolutionary process, according to Darwin (1965), basic affects, such as happiness, sadness, anger, fear, and disgust, and the nonverbal means of expressing them can be understood and communicated easily regardless of language or cultural barriers.

In interpersonal behavior, as "a person's contributions to doing something with other people" defined by Westerman (2005, p. 22), expression of emotions plays a major role. The ability to send and receive communicative signals in interpersonal encounters is a means of survival. The ability to understand other people's emotions from external signals, such as facial expressions and bodily gestures, also is a core ingredient for forming an empathic relationship (Ekman & Friesen, 1974; Zahn-Waxler, Robinson, &

Emde, 1992). Empathy can be conveyed through lexical as well as kinetic means of communication (Mayerson, 1976). It has been suggested that behavioral or nonverbal cues may be even more effective in conveying emotional messages than lexical or verbal communication (Bayes, 1972).

Mimicry and Facial Expression

The human face presents fascinating and meaningful clues about a person's physical and mental status. The facial muscles, controlled by the central nervous system, have the unique ability to produce a wide variety of expressions (Dawson, 1994; Siegel, 1999). Because facial expressions and bodily postures are the external manifestation of the internal world, they facilitate empathic communication, especially in clinician–patient encounters. For example, the degree of rapport between clinician and patient, according to Goldstein and Michaels (1985, p. 107), is correlated with the occurrence of "shared posture."

Another nonverbal means of communicating experiences is mimicry, which occurs when one observes another person's expression and responds with a similar motor representation (Hess, Blairy, & Phillippot, 1999). For example, we all tend to assume the postural strains of athletes or dancers during moments when we are absorbed in observing their actions (Davis, 1985). Furthermore, most of us have either experienced or observed that while spoon-feeding their infants, mothers often open their own mouth *as if* they are spoon-feeding themselves. These examples suggest that mimicry is a nondeliberate imitation that serves the function of communication (Schaflen, 1964).

Because mimicry and its associated somatosensory outcomes can help us to understand another person's experiences (Wicker et al., 2003), its relevance to empathy is evident (Chartrand & Bargh, 1999). According to Davis (1985), appraising the concept of mimicry is important when analyzing the component of empathy. Mimicry and facial expression generate changes in the autonomic nervous system associated with feelings that correspond to the facial expression (Decety & Jackson, 2004). Basch (1983) proposed that unconscious, automatic imitation of another person's facial expressions (facial mimicry) and bodily gestures (motor mimicry) generates an automatic and synchronized response in the observer that leads to better understanding of experiences identical to those experienced by the observed individual.

Carr and colleagues (2003) proposed that individuals with a high degree of empathy compared with others exhibit more unconscious mimicry of other people's facial expressions and bodily postures. Chartrand and Bargh (1999) described this phenomenon as the "chameleon effect"—the mere perception of another person's behavior can automatically increase the likelihood of imitating the perceived behavior. Chartrand and Bargh suggested that the chameleon effect is the mechanism behind motor mimicry that satisfies the human need for connection and affiliation. Furthermore, they reported that individuals with high empathy scores on the Interpersonal Reactivity Index (Davis, 1983) (see Chapter 5) exhibited the chameleon effect to a greater degree than others with low empathy scores.

Experimental evidence suggests that the human brain is designed to be attentive to emotional signals emitted via facial expressions. For example, using the "still-face" procedure, Tronick, Als, Adamson, Wise, and Brazelton (1978) found that young children become distressed and withdrawn when their mothers assume an emotionless face, rather than reveal their emotions (see Chapter 4). Evidence also indicates that infants can imitate human facial gestures, such as sticking out the tongue, protruding the lips, and opening the mouth (Meltzoff & Moore, 1977, 1983). Mimicry and the ability to imitate facial gestures and to understand facial expressions has been conceptualized as a type of primitive empathy (Bavelas, Black, Lemery, & Mullett, 1986).

In addition, newly born infants will cry in response to the sound of another infant's cry (Sagi & Hoffman, 1976; Simner, 1971). This reactive crying does not occur in response to either a loud sound or a vocal sound that lacks the affective components of the other infant's cry, or even to the recorded crying of the newborn infant itself. According to Hoffman (1978), the human infant's reactive crying is based on a built-in mechanism that is an early precursor of empathic understanding.

Psycho-Socio-Physiology

The link between human physiology and social interaction has attracted the attention of scholars for a long time. For example, half a century ago, Boyd and DiMascio (1957) studied the concept of the "sociophysiology" of social behavior and found a relationship between emotions expressed in clinical interviews and autonomic physiologic responses, such as heart rate, skin resistance, and facial temperature. The notion of "interpersonal physiology" in clinician–patient interactions was first introduced in a study by DiMascio, Boyd, and Greenblatt (1957), who found that patients' and therapists' heart rates and skin temperatures were synchronized during clinical interviews. Goldstein and Michaels (1985, p. 68) reported that synchronization typically occurs between individuals who have "good rapport" with one another. Accuracy in perception of negative emotions was found to be a function of physiological synchrony between the perceiver and the target person (Levenson & Ruef, 1992). It is suggested that empathy can emerge as a result of the autonomic nervous system, which tends to simulate another person's physiological state (Ax, 1964). In other words, an empathic engagement reflected in good interpersonal rapport facilitates physiological synchronization during clinical interviews.

In another early experiment, investigators noticed that the physiological responses of healthy young soldiers were different when interacting with an officer (who was a psychiatrist) and with a person who was an enlisted man (Reiser, Reeves, & Armington, 1955). The researchers concluded that the psycho-socio-physiology of the relationship in clinician–patient encounters could be a function of the client's view regarding the care provider's prestige or status (Reiser et al., 1955).

In a recent review article, Adler (2002) proposed that the experience of an empathic relationship in clinical encounters reduces the secretion of stress hormones and concluded that "the immediate effect of a caring relationship flows from the physiologic consequences of feeling cared about, because the neurobiology of such a relationship promotes an endocrine response pattern that favors homeostasis and is the antithesis of the fight–flight response (p. 878)".

A physiological feedback loop is set in motion during clinical interviews that is a symbolic reflection of mutual understanding. Observing emotion in another person has been reported to result in a similar display of emotion in the observer (Lanzetta & Englis, 1989). Similarly, emotional distress in one person can automatically trigger similar distress in another person when the two are interacting (Eisenberg, 1989). A study of physiological changes, such as heart rate, during interpersonal interactions revealed that a clinician's interpersonal style (e.g., praising or criticizing) can influence the patient's physiological reaction (Malno, Boag, & Smith, 1957). For example, these investigators observed that patients' heart rates rose significantly more when the clinician had had a "bad" day. The results of a recent study indicate that physiological synchronicity (e.g., in heart rate and muscle activity) between people can lead to more accurate perceptions of their feelings (Decety & Jackson, 2006).

Kaplan and Bloom (1960, p. 133) proposed the idea that the empathic process involves not only placing oneself in another person's "psychological" shoes but placing oneself in that person's "physiological" shoes as well. However, Szalita (1976, p. 145) suggested that in empathic engagement with patients, "it is good to be able to put yourself into someone else's shoes, but you have to remember that you don't wear them." In a recent study of couples examined by using magnetic resonance imaging (MRI), Singer and colleagues (2004) found that couples who scored higher on the Empathy Scale (Hogan, 1969) (Chapter 5) and the Empathic Concern subscale of the Interpersonal Reactivity Index showed more intense brain activity when they observed their partner experiencing pain.

These findings suggest that empathic resonance involves shared physiological–neurological activities between people who are interacting. The notion of shared physiology between interacting people is intriguing (Ax, 1964; Kaplan & Bloom, 1960; Levenson & Ruef, 1992), and it opens up a window for studying the "physiological dance" that takes place in empathic engagement. More research is needed to investigate the underlying mechanisms involved in the psycho-socio-physiology of social behavior and the relevance of shared physiologic responses to empathic understanding and sympathetic feelings.

Neuroanatomy

According to Brothers (1989, p. 11) empathy as a social behavior is a concept that "appears to have a great potential utility in bringing together neural and psychological data." To achieve a better understanding of empathy, we must expand our knowledge about the cellular mechanisms involved in interpersonal relationships and the neuroanatomy of empathy. In a thoughtful article on a new intellectual framework for psychiatry, Eric Kandel (1998) proposed a basic principle that all mental, cognitive, and emotional processes, without exception, derive from neurophysiological operations of the brain. He further suggested that this principle applies to both individual behaviors and social interactions. Thus, empathy falls well within the scope of the brain's neurophysiological operations.

The human brain is a complex command-and-control center for cognition and emotions. Although the three divisions of the brain (brainstem, limbic system, and cerebral cortex) are structurally and evolutionarily distinct, they are closely interconnected through a complex neurological network. The brainstem (reptilian brain), phylogenetically the oldest section of the brain, controls the physiology of survival (e.g., heartbeat, breathing). The next oldest section, the limbic system, wraps around the brainstem and functions as the primary center for emotion and social behavior (MacLean, 1990). The limbic brain has an abundance of opiate receptors that not only can reduce physical pain but also can diminish the excruciating psychological pain arising from a broken interpersonal relationship (Lewis, Amini, & Lannon, 2000).

Included in the limbic system are a number of interconnected substructures, such as the amygdala, hippocampus, hypothalamus, and cingulate gyrus. Among the substructures of the limbic system, the role of the amygdala is important in understanding the neuroanatomy of social behavior because of its contribution to detecting social signals. The amygdala is an almond-shaped structure consisting of a highly interconnected cluster of neurons situated deep in the medial temporal lobes. It is implicated in producing emotional reactions, expressions of emotion (Milner, Squire, & Kanel, 1998), and responses to social signals. The amygdala is a gateway to a person's view of the social environment (Nauta & Feirtag, 1986) and plays a crucial role in the fight-or-flight response (Siegel, 1999). Empathy, when conceptualized by some researchers as an emotional attribute, could be linked to the amygdala.

The newest component of the brain, the cerebral cortex, which is largest in humans, has a great deal to do with complex cognitive behavior, abstract thinking, reasoning, language, and other high-level activities of the human brain. One striking change that occurred in the course of the brain's evolution is the tremendous increase in the complexity and size of the cerebral cortex in vertebrates in general and in human beings in particular (Nolte, 1993). The newest layers of the cerebral cortex, the neocortex, stem from complex social living (Keverne, Nevison, & Martel, 1997). These layers allow engagement in voluntary social behavior based on cognitive understanding (akin to empathy).

It appears that cognition is more likely to be a cortical activity, whereas emotion is more likely to be a subcortical activity (Nathanson, 1996). Most cognition occurs in the thalamic–neocortical axis (the thinking brain), whereas primary emotions are largely registered within the hypothalamic–limbic axis (the feeling brain) (Moore, 1996). Thus, one can speculate that the limbic system is more relevant to sympathy, whereas the neocortex is more relevant to empathy. (The differences between empathy and sympathy were discussed in Chapter 1, and their implications for patient care will be discussed in Chapter 6.)

A long evolutionary path that resulted in the development of the capacity for bonding and interpersonal relationships must have left durable footprints in the human central nervous system. It is now beyond dualistic dispute that our cognition and emotions are inextricably woven into the structure and function of the human brain (Damasio, 2003).

Behavioral scholars benefiting from the advanced technology of brain imaging are beginning to position themselves to view social and interpersonal behaviors from a neurobiological perspective (Bennett, 2001). Using advanced biomedical technology, such as functional brain imaging, a new and interesting line of research is shedding light on the uncharted territory of the empathic brain. New technologies, such as PET and, in particular, functional magnetic resonance imaging (fMRI), allow noninvasive exploration of the human brain at a high level of resolution that helps investigators understand not only the structural aspects but also the functional activities of the brain that are related to empathy. However, we currently have only a hint of what the neuroanatomical basis of empathy might be, despite all of the biotechnological advances.

Different areas of the brain have been implicated in studies on the neuroanatomy of empathy. Understanding the mental state of others, which is the backbone of empathic engagement, appears to be localized to areas of the frontal cortex (Platek, Keenan, Gallup, & Mohamed, 2004), especially the right frontal lobe (Stuss, 2001). Eslinger (1998) reported that the prefrontal cortex is particularly vital to empathic engagement and suggested that the dorsolateral region of the frontal cortex and its function could be linked to people's ability to understand other people's experiences and that the orbitofrontal region of the brain could be related to people's emotional responsiveness and sensitivity to the emotional states of others. Also, de Quervain and colleagues (2004) believe that both the prefrontal and orbitofrontal cortex are involved in integrating cognitive operations in interpersonal relationships and decision making. It is reported that dorsolateral lesions were associated with deficit in empathy as well as impaired cognitive flexibility, whereas patients with orbitofrontal cortex lesions were more impaired in empathy than in cognitive flexibility (Decety & Jackson, 2004). In addition, the orbitofrontal cortex has been implicated in the regulation of emotion that contributes to empathic engagement (Cahill, 2005). Singer and Frith (2005) reported that seeing pictures of unknown people getting hurt (e.g., a hand strapped in a car door, or someone's hand being pierced by a needle) elicited brain activities in the cognitive–affective section (anterior cingulate cortex), not in the sensory components of the brain. In their discussion of the "painful side of empathy," these authors suggested that mental activities are elicited even when people think about the pain of others. In another study using fMRI, Jackson, Meltzoff, and Decety (2005) concluded that assessing pain of others was associated with significant bilateral changes in activities in the anterior cingulated, the anterior insula, and the cerebellum that are known for their roles in the processing of pain. These authors concluded that their findings help to understand the neurological mechanisms that are implicated in human empathy. In a recent review of "The Functional Architecture of Human Empathy," Decety and Jackson (2004, p. 80) concluded that "part of the neural network mediating pain experiences is shared when empathizing with pain in others."

The right hemisphere seems to have an important role in the capacity for empathy. Interpersonal signals, such as facial expressions of emotion, are recognized best in the right cerebral hemisphere, and most mechanisms associated with regulating emotions are activated in the right hemisphere as well. The ability to recognize emotions conveyed by facial expressions is impaired in patients whose right hemisphere has been damaged (Kolb & Taylor, 1981) and recognition of facial expressions and empathic understanding were impaired in patients with atrophy of the right temporal lobe (Perry et al., 2001).

Expression and perception of nonverbal communication appear to be mediated by the right hemisphere, whereas verbal communication is mediated predominantly by the left hemisphere (Siegel, 1999). It is generally believed that the posterior region of the right hemisphere plays a special role in perceptions of emotion and recognition of emotional clues (Buck & Ginsberg, 1997a, 1997b). Cognitive aspects of empathy (mutual understanding), such as perspective-taking and role-taking skills, are linked to functions of the frontal lobe, whereas the emotional aspects of empathy (shared emotions) have been hypothesized to be associated with the orbitofrontal areas (Eslinger, 1998). Spinella (2002) reported that the emotional components of empathy (more akin to sympathy than to empathy), measured by the Emotional Empathy Scale (Mehrabian & Epstein, 1972) (see Chapter 5) correlated with smells identified by the right nostril, whereas the cognitive component of empathy did not. One explanation could be that the olfactory sense is closely linked to the limbic system, the brain's emotion processing center.

Carr and colleagues (2003) used fMRI with human subjects to confirm that to form empathic relationships, people need to invoke the representation of actions in the brain associated with the emotions they observe in others. The limbic system is crucially important for emotional processing through the circuit of the frontoparietal network, which interacts with the superior temporal cortex for manifestation of behaviors or representation of actions (Carr et al., 2003). The same circuit is crucial for activation of the mirror neuron system that will be described later in this chapter.

Neurological Impairment and Empathy

If we assumed that empathy is a function of cellular activities in the brain, it would be reasonable to expect that neurological damage in the brain could impair empathic capacity. This assumption is supported by studies of patients with brain lesions or certain neurological problems. The well-known case of Phineas Gage is a classic example of impaired social skills associated with lesions of the frontal lobe (Benton, 1991; Damasio, Grabowski, Frank, Galaburda, & Damasio, 1994; Hamilton, 1984). Gage was the foreman of a railroad construction company. In 1848, as a result of an accidental explosion, an iron bar was propelled completely through his skull and landed some 25–30 yards behind him (Macmillan, 2000). Although he recovered physically after treatment and survived for $11^1/_2$ years after the injury, he never regained his capacity for forming empathic relationships.

Eslinger (1998) reported that more than half of the neurologically damaged patients he tested scored more than two standard deviations below the mean on a measure of empathy. In a study involving patients with neurological damage caused by closed head injuries, ischemic hemispheric strokes, encephalitis, or multiple sclerosis, Eslinger, Satish, and Grattan (1996) found that both the cognitive aspect of empathy (measured with Hogan's Empathy Scale), and its emotional aspect (measured with the Mehrabian and Epstein's Emotional Empathy Scale) were impaired by the neurological damage. Brothers (1989) hypothesized that the impairment of empathy observed in certain neurological conditions, such as autism, or in certain lesions of the cortex in the right cerebral hemisphere suggested that empathy has a neurophysiological origin.

Of all the developmental disorders, autism is among the best clinical examples for studying the neurological determinants of empathy. Poor social skills are among the core features of autistic individuals, and the central pathology of autism is an impaired capacity for empathy (Brothers, 1989). The fourth edition of the *Diagnostic and Statistical Manual of Mental Disorders* (DSM-IV) states that a defect in social interaction is a primary criterion for the diagnosis of autism (Frances, First, & Pincus, 1995). It has been observed that autistic children never respond to their mother's smile, indicating that they do not exhibit a capacity to respond empathically to others (Decety & Jackson, 2004). In other words, empirical and clinical evidence suggests that compared to the general population, autistic individuals obtain lower scores on tests measuring the ability to understand facial expressions displayed in photographs of people with a happy, sad, or fearful face and display a seriously impaired capacity for empathy (Baron-Cohen, 2003).

In addition to autism, other pervasive developmental disorders (e.g., Asperger's syndrome) and some personality disorders (e.g., elective mutism, Tourette's syndrome, anorexia nervosa, and obsessive-compulsive disorder) have been linked to a deficit in empathy. Gillberg (1992, 1996) grouped these conditions in a category labeled "disorders of empathy." Gillberg (1996) assumed that humans have an "empathy quotient" that, like the intelligence quotient (IQ), has a normal distribution in the general population (a bell-shaped curve with a mean of 100 and a standard deviation of 15). Accordingly, Gillberg (1996) said that similar to the classification of intellectual capacity, autism could be arbitrarily classified as an empathic deficiency equivalent to a quotient below 50 (people with an IQ below 50 are classified as either moderately, severely, or profoundly retarded), and Asperger's syndrome (a milder form of autism) would be equivalent to a quotient in the range of 50–70 (people with an IQ between 50 and 70 are classified as mildly retarded).

Other neurological impairments also have been reported to influence the capacity for empathy. For example, in a study of character changes in patients with multiple sclerosis, decline in empathy (measured by the Hogan Empathy Scale) was observed that was attributed to a neurogenic frontal lobe syndrome (Benedict, Priore, Miller, Munschauser, & Jacobs, 2001). In another study, it is reported that affective agnosia in patients with lesions in the right temporoparietal area renders patients unable to understand emotions conveyed by vocal quality (Heilman, Scholes, & Watson, 1975). Another condition, aprosodic-agestural syndrome, caused by lesions in the right hemisphere, makes patients unable to express themselves through gestures (Ross & Mesulam, 1979). Yet another group of patients includes those with lesions in the left hemisphere that impair their ability for symbolic communication and make them unable to pantomime.

Alexithymia is a condition that impairs patients' perception of other people's affective status. Sufferers usually have difficulty recognizing and labeling emotions and feelings, which has been associated with impairment in empathic capacity (Mann, Wise, Trinidad, & Kohanski, 1994). Alexithymia was found to be inversely related to empathy measured by the Interpersonal Reactivity Index (Guttman & Laporte, 2002). Although no specific brain lesion has been identified as the cause of alexithymia, case studies of the patients with the condition should be of interest to empathy researchers because it may allow them to examine possible underlying mechanisms involved in the ability to recognize emotions that is needed to form empathic relationships.

It has been reported that acquired cerebral damage, such as focal damage to the prefrontal cortex in adulthood and damage to the frontal lobe in early childhood, can disturb social behavior, including the capacity for empathy (Eslinger, 1998). Research showed that empathic understanding was impaired subsequent to focal lesions of the prefrontal cortex (Decety & Jackson, 2004; Eslinger, 1998). Some research findings concerning the neuroanatomical basis of social behavior indicate that after damage to the frontal lobe, patients become profoundly inept in their social behavior in general (Grattan & Eslinger, 1989) and in their capacity for empathy in particular (Eslinger, 1998).

When brain damage impairs a person's emotional and cognitive capacities, the person obviously is at a great disadvantage, not only in adapting to the external environment appropriately, but also in managing the internal body mechanisms that facilitate such adaptation (Bennett, 2001). The inability to adapt to changes in the environment and an impaired ability to recognize one's own emotions and the emotions of others are among the underlying reasons for an impaired capacity for empathy in patients with certain neurological damage. This presumption was supported in a study in which it was reported that empathic change (measured by Hogan's Empathy Scale) after a brain injury could be a result of acquired disabilities, including cognitive inflexibility (Grattan & Eslinger, 1989).

Rankin, Kramer, and Miller (2005) reported that patients with semantic dementia showed low levels of both cognitive and emotional empathy, whereas patients with frontotemporal dementia showed deficits only in cognitive empathy measured by the Interpersonal Reactivity Index. In a study by Shamay-Tsoory, Tomer, Goldsher, Berger, and Aharon-Peretz (2004), impairment in cognitive empathy (measured by the Interpersonal Reactivity Index) and affective empathy (measured by Mehrabian and Epstein's Emotional Empathy Scale) was examined in patients with brain lesions. It was found that patients with prefrontal lesions (especially those with lesions involving orbitoprefrontal and medial regions) were significantly impaired in both cognitive and affective empathy. Also, patients with lesions in prefrontal cortex had significantly low empathy scores. Damage to the right hemisphere resulted in greater impairment in cognitive empathy, whereas damage to the right prefrontal cortex did not exert significant impairment on affective empathy (Shamay-Tsoory, 2004). It is important to note that, with the exception of the aforementioned study, no differentiation has been made between cognitive and emotional empathy (or between empathy and sympathy) in neuroanatomical studies on empathy. This lack of conceptual clarity can explain the mixed results regarding areas of the brain related to empathy and neurological impairment. My speculation is that the neocortical areas are often implicated as the key processing center in cognitive empathy. However, the limbic system is mostly implicated as the primary area of brain activities for emotional empathy or sympathy.

The Mirror Neuron System

An interesting phenomenon that connects social cognition and brain activity was discovered in the mid-1990s by a group of researchers using advanced neuroimaging technology (Gallese, Fadiga, Fogassi, & Rizzolatti, 1996; Keysers & Perrett, 2004; Rizzolatti, Fadiga, Gallese, & Fogassi, 1996). Neuroscientist Giacomo Rizzolatti and his colleagues at the University of Parma, Italy, discovered the mirror neuron system in monkeys in the early 1990s (Gallese et al., 1996; Rizzolatti et al., 1996). The group found that a specific set of neurons in the ventral premotor cortex of the monkey's brain (known as the F5 area) discharged when the monkey observed another monkey performing hand actions, such as grasping, tearing, and holding or manipulating an object. Furthermore, the same set of neurons discharged when the monkey actually performed the hand action it had observed. Vittorio Gallese and colleagues (Gallese, Keysers, & Rizzolatti, 2004, p. 396) concluded that "the observation of an action leads to the activation of parts of the *same* cortical neural network that is active during its execution" (emphasis added). This brain mechanism, known as the "mirror neuron system," serves as a bridge that correlates with the understanding of other's action and is considered as the neural basis of social cognition (Gallese et al., 2004).

Other studies led by Marco Iacoboni at the University of California at Los Angeles and other neuroscientists demonstrated the existence of a similar system of mirror neurons in humans (Buccino et al., 2001; Gallese, 2003; Hari et al., 1998; Iacoboni et al., 1999). The results of these studies led to the assumption that a region of the human brain, analogous to the F5 area of monkey's brain, is activated when we observe actions performed by others *as if* we were performing the actions ourselves.

Brain-imaging studies in humans have shown that the mirror neurons matching the hand action fire in the following sectors of the cortical network: Broca's region, premotor cortex, and posterior parietal cortex (Buccino et al., 2001; Gallese, 2003). Considering the homology between the F5 area of the monkey's brain and Broca's region in the inferior frontal lobe (involved in speech control) of the human brain (Hari et al., 1998; Kohler et al., 2002), one can find similarities in the mirror neuron matching system between monkeys and humans.

Furthermore, research has demonstrated that the "audiovisual" mirror neurons are activated whether the observer actually performs the observed act, or simply observes or hears about the act (Kohler et al., 2002; Keysers et al., 2003). Moreover, Wicker and colleagues (2003) discovered not only that observing another person's hand action activated the observer's mirror neuron system but that observing other people's expression of such emotions as disgust produced by unpleasant odors could activate the neural representation of such emotion, as well. By using fMRI, Wicker and colleagues concluded that anatomical and functional data provided evidence that the insula was the common neural basis of seeing and feeling disgust, a pathway to empathic understanding. Umilta and colleagues (2001) showed that when an action was observed in part (e.g., a hand reaching an object for grasping, but actual grasping was not observed) the monkey's mirror neuron system was activated suggesting that the complete act of grasping could be inferred. The mirror neuron system is believed to be the key neurophysiological indicator in gestural communication (Kohler et al., 2002)—another key ingredient of empathy.

According to Carr and colleagues (2003), the insula is a plausible candidate for relaying information about action representation to the area of the limbic system that processes emotional content. Lesions in this circuit can lead to impaired understanding of other people's emotions, thus blocking the pathway to empathic understanding.

The aforementioned studies support the notion that the neural structure implicated in the execution of an action or in the perception of an emotion is also active when those actions and sensations are observed. Thus, it makes intuitive sense that the observer and the observed person experience similar sensations that can lead to a common understanding (Goubert et al., 2005). Watching a spider crawling on another person's face can make the observer shiver as if the spider were crawling on his or her own face. By using brain imaging, Keysers and colleagues (2004) attributed this "tactile empathy" to brain activities in the secondary somatosensory cortex. Gallese (2003, p. 176) proposed that "sensations and emotions by others can also be 'empathized', and therefore *implicitly* understood, through a mirror matching mechanism." No wonder, when describing the meaning of *Einfühlung* (see Chapter 1), Lipps said that when he watched an acrobat walking on a hanging wire, he felt that he was inside the performing acrobat (Carr et al., 2003; Gallese, 2003). The notion that perception of a behavior in another person can activate one's own representation of that behavior is not new (Decety & Jackson, 2004); however, providing objective neuroimaging evidence for the notion and linking it to the neuroanatomy of empathy are new. The mirror neuron system plays an important role in understanding the experiences of others. And because the system enables humans to develop rich and diversified intersubjective experiences, it is hoped that it will lead to new discoveries about the neuroanatomical structure of the brain and its relationship to empathy.

Heritability

Mumford (1967) regarded empathy as a genetically determined quality that is enhanced or inhibited by positive or negative life experiences, respectively (cited in Szalita, 1976). A standard approach to research on heritability is the "twin study." In this research design, genetically identical, or monozygotic (MZ) twins (who share 100% common genes), are compared with fraternal, or dizygotic (DZ) twins, who share approximately 50% of their genes. Heritability can be determined with regard to a particular trait when MZ twins are more highly correlated than DZ twins are, assuming a similar rearing environment. In a sample of 278 MZ and 378 DZ twins, strong genetic influences were found in 78% of the twins younger than 11 years of age and in 66% of those aged 11 years or older concerning the heritability of social cognitive skills relevant to empathy (Scourfield, Martin, Lewis, & McGuffin, 1999).

In another study involving 114 MZ and 116 DZ twins, the researchers found a significant heritability component of 72% on a derived index of empathic concern (Matthews, Batson, Horn, & Rosenman, 1981). In yet another study involving 94 MZ and 90 DZ twins, the investigators found modest evidence of heritability in empathy (Zahn-Waxler et al., 1992).

Finally, in a study of 573 adult twin pairs of both sexes, empathy, as measured by the Emotional Empathy Scale had a relatively high heritability index (an intraclass correlation) of 0.53 (Rushton, Fulker, Neale, Nias, & Eysenck, 1986). The results of another study using the Interpersonal Reactivity Index showed evidence of significant heritability for the scales of Empathic Concern and Personal Distress but not for the Perspective Taking Scale (Davis, Luce, & Kraus, 1994). These findings generally suggest that indicators of so-called emotional empathy (e.g., Personal Distress), which is more akin to sympathy, are likely to have a higher heritability component than the cognitive measures of empathy are (e.g., Perspective Taking).

Recapitulation

The evolutionary roots of social behaviors, expression of emotion through nonverbal communication, the psycho-socio-physiology of social interactions, research findings on the neuroanatomy of empathy, the link between neurological impairment and deficiencies in empathic understanding, the results of heritability research, and the recent discovery of the brain's mirror neuron system suggest that the foundation of empathic function is hard-wired. However, the manifestation of empathy depends on experiential and environmental factors that will be described in Chapter 4.

4 Psychodynamics and Development

Love, and lack of it, changes the young brain forever.

—(Thomas Lewis, Fari Amini, & Richard Lannon, 2000, p. 89)

The key to the heaven is under mother's footsteps.

—(A popular Persian saying)

The hand that rocks the cradle rules the world.

—(A popular cliché)

Preamble

Empathy is nurtured in a facilitative early rearing environment, particularly in relation to the quality of relationship with the mother or a primary caregiver. Evidence regarding the newborn's preference for its mother's voice; maternal investment in child rearing; lactation and breast-feeding; and attachment relationships suggest that nature has endowed the mother with the innate ability to be the most adequate guardian of the development of the child's capacity for empathy. Experimental findings obtained by using the "still-face" and "visual cliff" paradigms indicate that infants can understand and react to their primary caregiver's emotional behavior. The foundation for the child's mental representation (internal working models) of the world is the early relationship with the mother that becomes an influential force in the regulation of emotions and empathic behavior throughout life.

Introduction

The search for the roots of the capacity for empathy is of paramount importance in understanding the course of its optimal development or the arrest of its development. In this chapter, I describe some of the factors that contribute to the nourishment of empathy. The central notion emphasized throughout the chapter is that empathy is nurtured in the early rearing environment in relation to the quality of the early attachment relationships with a primary caregiver (Henderson, 1974; Schaflen, 1964).

The Nature–Nurture Debate

The issue of whether nature or nurture contributes more to prosocial behavior has been debated for a long time. Proponents of nature place great emphasis on the notion that genetic makeup has an undeniable role in the development of human behavior. Recent developments in the Human Genome Project have provided more fuel in support of their argument (Collins, 1999).

However, proponents of nurture use Watsonian and Skinnerian approaches to classical conditioning and operant learning as evidence that human behavior can be molded according to the principles of behavior modification, and they believe that environmental and experiential factors have a more prominent role than genes do in the development of prosocial or antisocial behavior. The often-cited statement made by John Brutus Watson (1924, p. 82), the founder of the school of behaviorism in psychology, supports the nurture notion:

> *Give me a dozen healthy infants, well formed, and my own special world to bring them up, and I will guarantee to take any one at random and train him to become any type of specialist I might select—doctor, lawyer, artist, merchant-chief, and yes, even beggar and thief, regardless of his talents, penchants, tendencies, abilities, vocations, and race of his ancestors.*

Although some authors still believe that nurture matters more than nature does in determining human behavior (Hoover, 2000), most scholars nowadays are of the opinion that it is the interaction of nature and nurture that contributes to the development of social behavior. Human beings are born with a potential for "engageability," which is triggered to a certain degree by, and will develop to a certain extent depending on, environmental and experiential factors (Neubauer & Neubauer, 1990).

Although many genetics-oriented scientists were excited about the discoveries of the Human Genome Project (Collins, 1999), determining the basis of human behavior proved to be a more complicated matter than simply mapping the human genome. For example, findings in a study of 44,788 sets of twins indicated that environmental and life-style factors as well as inherited genes make significant contributions in the development of different types of cancers (Lichtenstein et al., 2000). Abundant research evidence has accumulated in support of the proposition that the family environment and parental care play an important role in the development of adults' prosocial behavior, including the propensity for empathic relationships.

The Family Environment

The family is the oldest and the most important social institution in the history of human civilization. It is "the seedbed of commitment, love, character, and social as well as personal responsibility" (Ashcroft & Straus, 1993, p. 1). The United Nations Convention on the Rights of the Child, adopted unanimously by the General Assembly, recognized that for full and harmonious development, children must grow up in a facilitative family environment in an atmosphere of happiness and love provided by their parents (Grant, 1991; Hojat, 1993, 1997). The calming experience of feeling felt and the echoes of love spring to life in the family first, then expand to embrace a broader social network, even the entire human race (Eibel-Eibesfeldt, 1979).

The family environment early in life not only shapes the quality of later interpersonal relationships (Fonagy, 2001) but also sows the seed for the growth of the capacity for empathic engagement. The way we are brought up in the early periods of our lives influences "all our later relationships, all our later days" (Neubauer & Neubauer, 1990, p. 81). The child whose emotional needs are unmet or denied in the family will not develop a sense of trust, a problem that will have a lasting negative influence on later social relationships (Rempel, Holmes, & Zanna, 1985). The capacity for empathy also can be negatively influenced by unmet emotional needs in the family (Eisenberg & Strayer, 1987b; Perry et al., 2001) because, as Guzzetta (1976) proposed, empathy springs from interpersonal relationships within the family. Development of empathy, according to Barnett (1987), occurs in a family environment in which parental warmth and responsiveness satisfy the child's emotional needs and provide opportunities for the child to observe and experience warm interpersonal responses in a variety of situations.

It is the family's importance in the development of the capacity for empathy that has led to health care researchers' apt description of the clinician's family of origin as the bedrock for the development of interpersonal skills in patient care (Farber, Novack, & O'Brien, 1997; Mengel, 1987).

The Parents

Empathy has a rich and complex developmental history (Shapiro, 1974). It arises from early sensory and tactile communication between mother and child (Schwaber, 1981). In a review of the literature on parental behavior that contributes to the development of empathy in children, Mehrabian et al. (1988) concluded that the parents of children with a strong capacity for empathy were more verbally explicit about their feelings, offered more emotional support, and were more tolerant. Early interactions with parents, according to Roe (1957), determine the child's future vocational choice in people-oriented versus other occupations.

Human beings differ from all other animals in the length of their dependency on a caregiver for survival and protection. This period of dependency is crucial for neurological development (e.g., the process of myelination) (Davison & Peters, 1970) and social growth. The critical period of susceptibility opens a window of opportunity during which activation of specific brain functions are essential for ongoing development of different areas of the brain related to social behavior (Siegel, 1999). That window will close after a certain period of time.

The importance of the critical period of neurological development was first noticed by Hubel and Wiesel, who found that suturing one eye closed in kittens during the first few weeks after birth caused a sharp decline in the number of cells in the visual cortex (Hubel, 1967; Hubel & Wiesel, 1963). The authors found that up to 5 years after the eye was opened, only a minimal amount of the visual cortex had recovered (Hubel & Weisel, 1970). In 1967, Hubel noticed that when kittens were not exposed to horizontal lines during a certain critical period of development, their visual cortex was unable to process horizontal input later in life.

Abundant evidence supports the existence of a critical period of neurological development. For example, baby chimpanzees reared in darkness during that period will be blind for the rest of their lives (Chow, Riesen, & Newell, 1957). MacLean (1967) found that if certain neural circuits were not formed during a crucially receptive period in the brain's development, the circuits were unlikely ever to be fully developed. The assumption is that the repeated activation of specific neuronal pathways as a result of early experiences reinforces the strength of connections between groups of neurons. The neurons that create interconnections through early experiences, according to Hebbian Association Theory (Hebb, 1946; Keysers & Perrett, 2004), will fire together later in life, so to speak, because neurons that fire together wire together.

In addition to physical stimulation, emotionally rich interactions in early life contribute to neurological development. One early experiment on the importance of early life experiences to human survival was conducted in the thirteenth century by Emperor Frederick II, who wanted to know what language children would speak if no one talked with them. Thus, "he bade foster mothers and nurses to suckle the children, to bathe and wash them, but in no way to prattle with them.... But he labored in vain, because the children died" (Ross & McLaughlin, 1949, pp. 366–367).

Parental warmth has been hypothesized to promote children's capacity for empathy and prosocial behavior (Hoffman, 1982; Janssens & Gerris, 1992). Children of empathic parents reacted vicariously to others' negative emotions (Robinson, Zahn-Waxler, & Emde, 1994; Trommsdorff, 1995). Cross-sectional and longitudinal research, using structural equation modeling, have confirmed that parents' (particularly mothers') expression of positive emotions is the mechanism that mediates a causal relationship between parental warmth and children's empathic capacity (Zhou et al., 2002).

The Hand That Sows the Seeds

Parents usually provide the love and affection their children need for healthy development. Research has shown that a supportive relationship with both the parents is predictive of high empathy scores as well as social sensitivity in children (Adams, Jones, Schvaneveldt, & Jenson, 1982). However, although both parents must share child-care responsibilities for their children to achieve ideal social development, some findings suggest that the mother's role may be more crucial than that of any other caregiver, including the father.

For example, in a study of Harvard University graduates who were followed up for 35 years, Russek and Schwartz (1997) found that 91% of the graduates who retrospectively perceived the lack of a warm and friendly relationship with their mother had serious health problems in midlife (e.g., coronary artery disease, high blood pressure, alcoholism) compared with 45% of the graduates who retrospectively perceived their relationship with their mother as having been warm and friendly. The corresponding figures for their perceived relationship with their father were 82% and 50%, respectively. Consistent with these findings, we found that medical students who perceived a satisfactory childhood relationship with their mother rated their general health more positively and reported more resilience in appraising stressful life events (Hojat, 1996).

Individuals' perceptions of their early relationships with parents generally are positively associated with personality attributes that contribute to interpersonal relationships (Hojat, Borenstein, & Shapurian, 1990). In our study of 422 medical students, we examined the differential effects of satisfactory early relationships with the mother and father and found that higher scores on the Jefferson Scale of Physician Empathy (see Chapter 7) were significantly associated with students' retrospective reports concerning the level of satisfaction with the early relationship with their mother (Hojat et al., 2005b). Such an association was not found regarding the students' perceived relationship with their father.

These findings are consistent with those in another study in which undergraduates reported that their mothers spent more time with them than their fathers did, were more affectionate with them, and expressed more empathy toward them (Barett, Howard, King, & Dino, 1980). The undergraduates' scores on Mehrabian and Epstein's Emotional Empathy Scale (1972) (see Chapter 5) were more related to their interactions with their mothers than with their fathers.

In another study, medical students' retrospective perceptions of a satisfactory relationship with the mother were significantly associated with a positive personality profile, such as higher self-esteem and more satisfactory relationships with peers (Hojat, 1998). In the same study, perceptions of satisfactory relationships with the mother were inversely associated with negative aspects of personality, such as depression, anxiety, and loneliness.

Such patterns of significant associations were not observed for students' perceptions of their early relationships with the father. Also, the students' perceptions of the availability of the mother in childhood were significantly associated with higher scores on self-esteem and lower scores on depression and loneliness (Hojat, 1996).

In a study with kindergarten children and their mothers, a substantial correlation was observed in the empathy between mother and child (Trommsdorff, 1991). One explanation is that empathic mothers are likely to engage in empathic exchanges with their children, and empirical research supports this speculation. For example, Wiesenfeld, Whitman, and Malatesta (1984) observed that the mothers' scores on Mehrabian and Epstein's Emotional Empathy Scale predicted their emotional responses to their infant's emotional distress and their desire to pick up the infant.Other researchers found that mothers with high scores on the Emotional Empathy Scale were less disturbed by their infant's cry and rated the crying as less irritating than low-empathy mothers did (Lounsburg & Bates, 1982). Conversely, a link was reported between mothers' low levels of empathy and maternal child abuse. For example, Letourneau (1981) reported that scores on Hogan's Empathy Scale and Mehrabian and Epstein's Emotional Empathy Scale could differentiate abusive and nonabusive mothers better than could a measure of stressful life events.

Why do mothers have a more crucial role in the development of their children's prosocial and empathic behavior? Nature has bestowed them with some unique privileges that enable them to perform their caregiving role. Some of these privileges are described here.

The Infant's Preference for the Mother's Voice and Face

Under normal circumstances, the voice the developing fetus hears most often is the voice of the expectant mother, who talks, may sing, and shouts, laughs, and cries. Thus, the onset of interpersonal connection is with the mother's voice. Although the fetus is unable to respond, it is able to hear the mother's voice again, again, and again. Her voice is different from the low-frequency rhythmic sound of her heartbeat, which probably has a calming effect.

Because the mother's voice is the most intense acoustical signal in the amniotic environment of the uterus, the newborn infant shows a clear preference for the sound of her voice within the first 3 days after birth (DeCasper & Fifer, 1980; Fifer & Moon, 1994). Fifer and Moon (1994) suggested that early experiences with voices have an enduring influence on the development of the infant's brain. The specific tone and range of pitch that mothers use to get the attention of preverbal infants have been described as the universal "maternal melodies" that serve as a potent mediator of affective communication (Papousek, Papousek, & Symmes, 1991).

By using a non-nutritive nipple attached to an electronic recorder that monitors the rate and amplitude of the infant's sucking pattern, DeCasper and Fifer (1980) found that newborn infants changed their sucking pattern when they heard a recording of their own mother's voice, but no such change was recorded for other female voices. Their sucking pattern also did not change when they heard a recording of their own father's voice (DeCasper & Prescott, 1984). DeCasper and Fifer (1980) suggested that the infant's preference for its mother's voice is important for initiating bonding with the mother. Thus, it appears that the biological mother has a unique advantage that is not shared by any other caregiver—the ability to establish the early attachment relationship with her newborn infant through the newborn's recognition of her voice. The onset of empathy can be traced back to this kind of early exchange between mother and child (Burlingham, 1967).

Preference for the maternal voice can lead the child to prefer the mother's face. Indeed, empirical data suggest that neonates quickly learn to recognize their mother's face. The infant not only shows a preference for her voice but pays particular attention to her varying facial expressions as well. Pascalis, DeSchonen, Morton, Deruella, and Fabre-Grenet (1995) reported that the 4-day-old neonate looks longer at its mother's face than at a stranger's face.

The Mother's Investment in Child Rearing

Trivers (1972) pointed out that in all mammalian species, the mother is usually more involved in the child-rearing endeavor than is any other caregiver, including the father. The following factors contribute to greater investment on the mother's part: scarcity of gametes and maternal certainty, the psychology of pregnancy, the neurochemistry of motherhood, lactation and breast-feeding, and the mother–child attachment.

The Scarcity of Gametes and Maternal Certainty

Evolutionary scholars have proposed two reasons for more maternal than paternal investment in child care. First, women have far fewer gametes than men do—usually one ovum every 4 weeks during the limited period of fertility versus millions of sperm per ejaculation. This scarcity of gametes leads to the mother's greater protection of offspring and consequently to her greater investment in their care (Bjorklund & Kipp, 1996; Buss & Schmitt, 1993). Second, because of internal gestation and childbirth, maternal certainty (the mother's confidence that she is the biological mother) has historically been much greater than paternal certainty (the father's confidence that he is the biological father), which has resulted in greater maternal investment in preserving one's own genes (Bjorklund & Kipp, 1996; Buss, 2003; Buss & Schmitt, 1993; Trivers, 1972).

The Psychology of Pregnancy and the Neurochemistry of Motherhood

The psychology of internal gestation leads to a fundamentally unique maternal experience of bringing new life into the world (Ballou, 1978). Early in her pregnancy, the mother perceives the child as a developing part of herself. The initial attachment begins to develop at this stage. Nine months of carrying the fetus, the subsequent experience of childbirth, and a long period of breast-feeding and nourishing the infant provide a sense of emotional investment that is a unique experience for the expectant mother and for no one else.

The neurochemistry of motherhood, including hormonal changes during pregnancy, after birth, and during lactation, is unique to the biological mother. For example, levels of oxytocin increase drastically in human mothers around the time of childbirth. These high concentrations of oxytocin are believed to serve as the thread that weaves the ties between mother and child (Lewis et al., 2000), ties that Freud (1964, p. 188) described as "unique, without parallel, established unalterably for a whole lifetime as the first and the strongest love-object and as the prototype of all later love relations—for both sexes."

Oxytocin can influence the activation of dopamine-producing neurons (Insel, 2000; Oliver, 1939), which makes motherhood more pleasurable under normal circumstances. Studies have shown that increased oxytocin can induce maternal behavior in nonpregnant rats (Pedersen & Prange, 1979; Pedersen, Ascher, Monroe, & Prange, 1982). Conversely, other studies have shown that reduced binding of oxytocin in the brain inhibits the onset of maternal behavior (Fahrbach, Morrell, & Pfaff, 1985; Insel, 2000).

Lactation and Breast-Feeding

Oxytocin prepares the biological mother to feed her newborn by stimulating the release of prolactin and thus lactation (Mori, Vigh, Miayata, & Yoshihara, 1990). Breast-feeding is another physiological privilege that nature has bestowed only on the biological mother. In addition to the nutritious quality of mother's milk, which contributes to the enhancement of the infant's immunocompetence and neurological development, breast-feeding is the first human interactive experience that satisfies the newborn's physiological and psychological needs. Winnicott (1987, p. 79) described the infant's breast-feeding experience as a means of communication that "sings a song without words." It paves the road to empathy.

The sequence of breast-feeding activities, such as proximity seeking toward the nipple; rhythmic movement of the head, mouth, and tongue; sucking that stimulates secretion of milk; ingestion of milk; and withdrawal and disengagement from the nipple, provides a unique opportunity for the behavioral and physiological regulation that develops in the mother–infant dyad (Smotherman & Robinson, 1994). Nursing at the breast is physiologically pleasurable for both mother and infant. The female physiological responses during coitus and lactation have been reported to be similar. For example, uterine contractions, nipple erection, and ejection of milk can occur during both sexual intercourse and breast-feeding (Newton & Newton, 1967). Breast-feeding not only has a calming effect on the human infant, mediated by activation of the opioid system (Smotherman & Robinson, 1994) but also serves as a thermoregulatory mechanism for the exchange of body warmth between mother and infant. During sucking, uterine contractions and increased skin temperature occur that are pleasurable to the lactating mother (Newton, Feeler, & Rawlins, 1968). The gratifying sensation mothers experience when breast-feeding their infants serves as a positive reinforcement of mother–child bonding. The seeds of empathy grow in the ecstasy of such loving interactions.

The universal synchronicity observed between mother and infant during breast-feeding (e.g., the holding position, visual gazes, and vocal exchanges) is, in itself, a unique model of human communication. According to Schore (1996), empathy is rooted in this early psychobiological attunement between mother and child. Isabella and Belsky (1991) reported that synchronous interactions between mother and infant open the highway to a secure attachment between them. All these early experiences affect the infant's growing brain by altering the strength of the synaptic connections that contribute to affective and cognitive behavior later in life.

It is these early physiological and psychological exchanges between the newborn child and the lactating mother that can alter the trajectories of neural development and later interpersonal behavior. The attachment between mother and child that is strengthened by these exchanges between the two can be viewed as a prototypical example of an empathic engagement.

The Attachment Relationship

The bonding between a mother and her child strengthens at the moment of birth during skin-to-skin contact between the mother and her newborn baby (Klaus & Kennell, 1970; Klaus et al., 1972). John Bowlby (1973, 1980, 1982) elegantly described the dynamics and consequences involved in the infant's repeated encounters with the primary caregiver in his attachment theory, which he systematically formulated, advanced, and elaborated in the widely cited trilogy of books.

The theory not only was conceived as a general theory of psychosocial development but also was viewed specifically as a framework for later interpersonal and social relationships. According to the tenets of the theory, a lovingly responsive mother serves as a secure base that allows the child to explore the world comfortably.

The mother's presence (or absence), her attentiveness and loving responses (or her inattentiveness or lack of responses) to her baby's signals, and her provision (or lack of provision) of physical and emotional nourishment gradually become a fact of life for the growing child. The formation of a secure mother–child attachment is most likely to occur in the presence of a lovingly responsive mother, whereas the opposite (an insecure attachment) is likely to occur if the mother is physically or emotionally unavailable (Bowlby, 1988). (For a review, see Hojat, 1995, 1996, 1998.) A strong mother–child attachment is a major antecedent of early interest in others and is a necessary condition for the development of the capacity for empathy (Mussen & Eisenberg-Berg, 1977).

The quality of the mother–child attachment relationship is assessed by the Strange Situation Procedures, a frequently used test developed by Ainsworth and associates (Ainsworth, Blehar, Waters, & Wall, 1978). Individual differences among infants and toddlers concerning the quality of attachment with their primary caregiver can be measured with this controlled laboratory procedure, which takes approximately 20 minutes and includes the following seven episodes, each lasting 3 minutes or less: (1) an infant or a toddler (usually aged 12–18 months) and its mother are brought into a laboratory room containing some toys; (2) a stranger (usually a woman) enters the room, sits down, and talks to the mother and child; (3) the mother then leaves the room while stranger stays in the room; (4) the mother then returns and the stranger leaves the room; (5) again, the mother leaves the room, leaving the child alone; (6) the stranger returns; (7) finally the mother returns.

According to Ainsworth and her colleagues, the reaction of the child, particularly in the two episodes of mother–child reunion in this procedure (Episodes 4 and 7) reflected the nature and quality of the mother–child attachment. Originally, the researchers identified three types of mother–child attachment. Briefly, if the child explored and played with the toys when the mother was present, expressed less interest in the toys when she left the room, and sought to be near her and initiate positive expression with her when she returned, the attachment was classified as a *secure* attachment (Ainsworth, 1985b). However, if the child continued to explore the toys during all seven episodes, exhibited no distress when the mother left the room, and avoided her when she returned, the child's attachment was classified as *avoidant*. Finally, if the child tended to be wary of the stranger, became intensely upset when the mother left, and exhibited ambivalent behavior when she returned (wanting to approach her and simultaneously being angry and avoiding being near her, thus difficult to soothe), attachment was classified as *ambivalent*. Main and Solomon (1990) introduced a new category of attachment, the "disorganized attachment," in an attempt to explain the situation when none of the other three patterns of attachment applies.

The type of attachment developed in early childhood is likely to endure throughout life (Ainsworth, 1985a, 1985b). Research has shown that securely attached children develop a sense of trust with caregivers who respond to them empathically and therefore develop the capacity to respond sensitively and empathically toward others in later relationships (Kestenbaum et al.,

1989). Furthermore, research has shown that the lack of a secure attachment with the mother can result in aggressive and noncompliant behaviors in later years that are not conducive to empathic engagement (Belsky, 1988; Karen, 1994). (For a review, see Hojat, 1995.)

In a study of preschool children, Kestenbaum et al. (1989) observed a continuity between the quality of a child's early relationship with the primary caregiver and the child's capacity to respond empathically later. This observation confirmed the notion that "it is with the aid of modified mother–child signals that we establish and maintain friendly contact with our fellow men" (Eibel-Eibesfeldt, 1979, p. 230). Severe abnormalities in interpersonal relationships have been observed in infants, such as Romanian orphans, who have been deprived of maternal love (Konner, 2004). The abnormality in connecting to others known as "reactive attachment disorder" is another testimony to the importance of the quality of early attachment to later empathic behavior or the lack thereof.

According to Bowlby (1988, p. 82), the need for a secure attachment remains "from cradle to grave." More important, as Bowlby pointed out, the quality of the child's early relationship with the mother will lead to the development of cognitive schemata regarding the world that reside deep in the child's mind and "tend to persist and are so taken for granted that they come to operate at an unconscious level" (p. 130). In other words, the prototypical model of the world as friendly and caring or as hostile and uncaring becomes an influential property of the child's cognitive structure, serving primarily as an unconscious motivational force that significantly influences the adult's interpersonal relationships and the capacity for empathic engagement (Ainsworth, 1985a, 1985b).

The nature and quality of the child's early interpersonal experiences with the primary caregiver and the positive or negative outcomes engrave relatively permanent cognitive images on the mind that attachment scholars describe as "internal working models" (Bretherton, 1987). This mental representation of the world, or the psychological "script," becomes a major motivational factor in empathic relationships later in life (Nathanson, 1996; Tomkins, 1987). The assertion that attachment relationships in childhood can influence interpersonal behavior across the life-span has broad implications for developmental, social, and clinical psychology. Also, it has been reported that relationships with family members, peers, and others are influenced by early attachment experiences (Bartholomew & Horowitz, 1991). Shaver and Hazan (1989) reported that adult love relationships share similarities with, and are rooted in, the early attachment experiences with a primary caregiver. It also been reported that attachment history can predict medical students' specialty preferences. For example, students with a secure attachment history are more likely to choose specialties that require more interaction with patients (Ciechanowski, Russo, Katon, & Walker, 2004). Early attachment experiences also can influence the style of clinical practice. For example, clinical psychologists with an insecure attachment history who reported less empathic parental responses, were more in need of support, and were more vulnerable to work stress (Leiper & Casares, 2000).

The child's attachment behavior in all cultures becomes extremely strong in the second year of life, when major pathways of the limbic system become encased in myelin. According to Konner (2004), the aforementioned phenomenon improves the function of the subcortical circuits that process emotions and social behavior. Therefore, the quality of the mother–child attachment exerts a lasting influence on the development of the brain and prosocial behavior as well.

Because the capacity for empathy is deeply rooted in the early attachment relationship with a primary caregiver, a number of empirical studies have addressed the link between empathy and relationships with one's parents. The outcomes of these studies generally confirm a significant relationship between scores on empathy and the nature and quality of the early relationship with the primary caregiver and the rearing environment.

Kestenbaum et al. (1989) reported that children aged 12–18 months with a secure attachment to their mothers grew up to be more empathic to others and exhibited more prosocial behavior. Zahn-Waxler, Radke-Yarrow, and King (1979) reported that empathic caregiving (determined by whether mothers responded promptly to their child's hurts, anticipated dangers, and provided nurturant caregiving) was significantly associated with greater prosocial and altruistic behavior in the children. The aforementioned theoretical perspectives and empirical findings suggest that the seeds of empathy are sowed by the same hand that rocks the cradle. Because of the importance of the mother–child relationship in the development of children's capacity for empathy, Goldstein and Michaels (1985) proposed a series of training programs to enhance empathic communication between mothers and their children.

There are resemblances between the mother–child attachment and the clinician–patient relationship. The child needs the mother's help and protection to survive, and the attachment behavior (e.g., proximity seeking) intensifies when the child is in distress or pain. Similarly, patients have a natural tendency to bond with a caring figure (the clinician) to maintain their health during a time of pain and suffering. Therefore, clinician–patient bonding is associated, though unconsciously, with the early attachment relationship. One can speculate that people with a history of a secure attachment are more likely to form stronger empathic relationships quickly than are those with a history of an ambivalent or avoidant attachment. This behavioral tendency also should be true for both clinician and patient.

Other Paths to the Development of Empathy in Childhood

The following factors feed the development of empathy and social behavior in children.

Facial Imitation and Motor Mimicry

Nature has bestowed human infants with the gift of an imitative brain, which allows them not only to understand others' affective state of mind but to learn from the emotions of others as well. As was mentioned in Chapter 3, Meltzoff and Moore (1977, 1983) found that young infants only 12–21 days old could imitate human facial gestures, such as protruding their tongue or lips and opening their mouth—an ability conceptualized as a type of primitive empathy (Bavelas et al., 1986). Early in life, the infant pays attention to expressions of emotion on the human face. The infant's attention to facial expressions and its apparent responses are described as "telepathic" exchanges that lay the foundation for empathic communications (Burlingham, 1967). Understanding one's own emotions and those of others emerges from these exchanges (Ickes, 1997). According to Decety and Jackson (2004), one adaptive advantage of mimicry is that it connects people together and fosters empathy.

Motor mimicry (e.g., wincing when a person or an animal is injured, mimicking a facial expression similar to the expression of another person who is in pain) is indeed a nonverbal mode of communication based on observing another person's affect. This phenomenon, which has been observed in children and adults alike, supports the notion that individuals are intricately and visibly connected in their interpersonal interactions (Bavelas et al., 1986). According to Decety and Jackson (2006), people can "catch" the emptional states of others as a result of motor mimicry. Bush, Barr, McHugo, and Lanzetta (1989) suggested that an observer's mimetic facial responses may play an important role in the development of empathic responses.

Theory of Mind

The capacity to represent the mental states of others is described in theory of mind (Fonagy & Target, 1996; Wellman, 1991) as part of the human being's cognitive-emotional development. According to this theoretical perspective, empathy is the capacity to stand in another person's *mental shoes* (Gallese, 2001). In contrast to Jean Piaget's proposition (1967) that children between the ages of 2 and 7 years are primarily egocentric and unable to stand in another person's shoes, subsequent research demonstrated that young children are aware of other people's emotions and therefore are capable of responding empathically to other people's feelings (Borke, 1971). The mechanisms involved in the human neonate's ability to understand and imitate facial gestures provide the foundation for understanding other people that is a key ingredient in the conceptualization of empathy (see Chapter 1).

The "Still-Face" Experiments

Additional evidence supporting the infant's capacity to understand other people's emotions is provided by the "still-face" procedure developed by

Tronick et al. (1978). In this procedure, the mother is instructed to distort her affective feedback to her infant by assuming an expressionless face (a still face) after a period of normal playful exchanges with her child. The child first becomes unpleasantly surprised to observe the mother's emotionless expression; the child then attempts to get her attention in an effort to restore affect to her emotionally blank face. When these efforts fail, the child becomes overtly uncomfortable, distressed, and anxious. Finally, when the mother's face does not change, the child becomes indifferent, detached, and apathetic. Most infants react physiologically to the mother's still face with an increased heart rate, which Weinberg and Tronick (1996) attributed to disruption of the infant's goal of relating to others. The still-face experiments with infants indicate that although the infant has not developed language to facilitate verbal communication, the face-to-face interactions between a mother and her child is a goal-directed, reciprocal system of communication that serves as a regulator of emotions in social relationships and a primary step toward the development of empathic capacity.

The "Visual Cliff" Experiments

Young children's understanding of others' emotions was also demonstrated in experiments involving the "visual cliff" apparatus (Gibson & Walk, 1960). This apparatus consisted of a sheet of heavy glass supported approximately one foot off the floor by a tablelike frame. Patterned material in the open space under the glass looked to the infant like a bottomless crevasse. The baby was placed on one side of the frame and the mother stood on the other side and encouraged the child to come to her by crawling over the glass. Human infants can recognize depth as soon as they are old enough to crawl; the infants refused to crawl over the glass.

Sorce, Emde, Campos, and Klinnert (1985) demonstrated that by 12 months of age, children were more likely to feel confident enough to cross over the visual abyss when their mothers looked joyful or assumed a positive facial expression. However, when the mother adopted a negative facial expression, such as fear or anger, the children hesitated to cross over the glass. These findings suggest that young children not only can recognize the mother's emotional expressions but also can be encouraged by her positive look to risk crossing the cliff. The relevance of these findings to empathy was described by Campos and Sternberg (1981), who suggested that one developmental root of empathic understanding is a form of emotional communication known as "social referencing," through which children attempt to infer emotional information from interactions with others to adjust their own behavior accordingly.

Infants' ability to imitate facial expressions and mimic motor activities and to understand emotions indicates that infants possess a remarkable innate ability to establish social connections in the early days of life. Nurturing this ability lays the foundation for the development of a capacity to understand other people's positive and negative emotional states (Stern, 1985). Such understanding is the royal road to empathy.

Regulation of Emotions

According to Marx, Heidt, and Gold (2005), regulation of emotions is defined as the process that enables individuals to control the quality, frequency, intensity, or duration of their emotional responses. It is reported that regulation of emotion is positively linked to an important aspect of empathy: namely, being concerned for others (Decety et al., 2004). One mechanism for linking caregivers' behavior to the development of empathy in children can be explained by the process of regulation of emotions, which plays an important role in organizing, motivating, and sustaining social behavior and attributing meaning to experiences (Nathanson, 1996). Human infants are well-equipped for socialization because they are endowed with a system of affect that can be regulated and therefore lays the foundation for a key ingredient in the development of interpersonal relationships.

Some developmental scholars have proposed that regulation of emotions begins extremely early—from the face-to-face interactions with the primary caregiver (as attested to by infants' reactions in the "still-face" and "visual cliff" experiments) and from the quality of the mother–child attachment (as attested to by the experiments regarding secure and insecure attachment).

Regulation of emotions develops as a result of emotional attunement between mother and child (Black, 2004) and involves a process in which people recognize and express their emotions (Archer, 2004). Regulation of emotions is a necessary condition for demonstrating prosocial behavior, and it functions as a mechanism to achieve an internal state that is optimal for social relationships. Regulation of emotion plays an important role in maintaining a boundary between self and others (Decety & Jackson, 2006) that is an important aspect of empathic engagement in patient care.

Although emotions play an important role in social behavior, their regulation also is believed to play an essential role in empathic relationships (Demos, 1988). The infant's emotional response depends on his or her regulatory capacities and the regulatory scaffolding provided by the mother (Weinberg, Tronick, & Cohn, 1999). Thus, the mother is the most important first regulator of emotions because she provides a supplementary context for the development of her infant's social behavior (Lott, 1998). The self-regulated behavior is a function of the quality of interactions with a primary caregiver during the formative period of brain development (Nathanson, 1996). Together, the mother and infant are a regulatory unit, and the mother's role in the regulatory exchanges is influenced by her own early attachment relationships (Mays, Carter, Eggar, & Pajer, 1991).

The nature and quality of the neonate, infant, or young child's interaction with the mother sets the stage for the development of a psychological script (Nathanson, 1996; Tomkins, 1962, 1963), an internal working model (Ainsworth, 1985a, 1985b; Bretherton, 1987), and an emotional regulatory system (Lott, 1998; Weinberg et al., 1999) that will serve as a guiding force for empathic behavior during the rest of one's life. The implicit memories of the early warm relationship with the primary caregiver lead to the development of an enduring neural structure that influences self-regulatory behavior reflected in interpersonal relationships (Amini et al., 1996). The emotional arousal generated by feelings of other people's pain and suffering needs regulation and control for empathic understanding (Decety et al., 2004). According to Watson (2002), a propensity to regulate emotions in clinical encounters can enhance empathic engagement and improve patient outcomes.

Recapitulation

Evidence suggests that infants are endowed with a capacity to understand and respond to emotions. Empathy is nurtured in a facilitative family environment where opportunities are provided for forming secure attachment relationships with a primary caregiver (usually the mother). The motivation for prosocial behavior and the capacity for empathic relationships are the outcomes of early social–emotional exchanges that lead to the development of an internal working model, a mental script, and an emotional regulatory system that guide interpersonal responses from the cradle to the grave.

5

Measurement of Empathy in the General Population

If a thing exists, it exists in some amount.
If it exists in some amount, it can be measured.

—(E. L. Thorndike, cited in Issac & Michael, 1981, p. 101)

Preamble

Some of the instruments that have been developed to measure empathy in children and adults are briefly described in this chapter. The three that have been used most often in medical education and health care research are Hogan's Empathy Scale, Mehrabian and Epstein's Emotional Empathy Scale, and Davis's Interpersonal Reactivity Index. Although these instruments are useful for some applications in the general population, their relevance in the context of patient care is limited for two reasons. First, as the content of the items in the three instruments implies, none is framed in the context of physician–patient (clinician–client) relationships. Thus, the validity of their use in that context is questionable. Second, the three instruments were not developed specifically to address the cognitively defined concept of empathy, a conceptualization that is more desirable in the context of patient care. Researchers have raised concerns about the validity of instruments that attempt to measure empathy. The biotechnological advancements in functional brain imaging and the recent discovery of the mirror neuron system have opened up a new window for measuring empathy that is extremely promising. In an era of changes in the health care system that interfere with the physician–patient relationship, a psychometrically sound instrument for measuring empathy and studying its antecedents, development, and outcomes is in high demand.

Introduction

In Chapter 1, I indicated that one reason for the dearth of empirical research on empathy in the health professions is the lack of a psychometrically sound instrument that can be used to measure the concept in the context of medical care. This chapter briefly describes some of the instruments that have been used most often to measure empathy in the general population and presents sample items enabling us to judge their *face validity* in the context of patient care. Although a detailed analysis of the psychometric properties of these scales can be informative, such a technical discussion is beyond the scope of this book. However, in Chapter 7, I will describe in detail the development and psychometric properties of the Jefferson Scale of Physician Empathy, which was specifically designed to measure empathy among medical students, practicing physicians, and other health professionals.

In general, an instrument serves not only as a device for measurement but also as the basis of a common language that researchers use to communicate their empirical findings. Therefore, familiarity with the instruments and the scores they generate is necessary to comprehend the results of research. For that purpose, I have selected a few research instruments designed to measure empathy in child and adult populations that are described in the following sections.

Measurement of Empathy in Children and Adolescents

The section describes representative methods that have been used to measure empathy in children.

Reflexive or Reactive Crying

Simner (1971) systematically investigated newborn infants' reactive crying and reported that newborns who heard another newborn crying cried significantly more often in response (reflexive crying) than they did to any other nonstartling noise. These findings were later replicated in other studies (Martin & Clark, 1982; Sagi & Hoffman, 1976). It is interesting to note that the newborns did not respond to their own cries (Martin & Clark, 1982) suggesting that infants are capable of distinguishing between self and others early in life (Decety et al., 2004). The reaction of one infant to another infant's crying has been used as an indicator of empathy in infants based on the assumption that an infant crying in response to another infant's distress is a reflection of an empathic response (Eisenberg & Lennon, 1983). Eisenberg (1989) suggested that the capacity to respond to cues of another person's distress in childhood is a primitive precursor of more mature empathic abilities that develop later. However, the assumption that reactive crying in infants is an indicator of empathy needs to be verified empirically in longitudinal studies.

The following findings raise questions about the validity of reflexive crying as an indicator of empathic capacity. Martin and Clark (1982) reported that children of both sexes cried more in response to a male newborn's crying than to a female newborn's crying. According to Eisenberg and Lennon

(1983), no convincing evidence is available to confirm that reflexive crying necessarily implies an empathic response.

The Picture or Story Methods

One popular method of measuring empathy in young children, developed by Eisenberg and Lennon (1983), has been to expose children to another person's distress by showing them pictures or telling them stories depicting hypothetical situations. The children are subsequently asked to describe their own feelings about the story's protagonist either verbally or by choosing a picture from a set of pictures representing a variety of faces exhibiting various expressions, such as a happy or sad face. A match between the child's feelings and the protagonist's feelings is considered to be an indication of empathic understanding. The difficulty of differentiating empathy from sympathy when using picture or story methods of assessment raised concern about the validity of this method. Also, the predictive validity of this method awaits empirical verification.

The Feshbach Affective Situations Test of Empathy

The Feshbach Affective Situations Test of Empathy (FASTE), published by Feshbach and Roe (1968), is a widely used variation of the picture or story method of measuring empathy in children. Children (usually aged 6 or 7 years) are shown cartoons on a series of slides accompanied by hypothetical stories depicting children in different affectively charged conditions (happiness, sadness, fear, and anger). The children are then asked to describe their own feelings and emotions about the picture or story either verbally or by choosing a response from a set of facial expressions depicting different emotions. For example, a theme for happiness is a picture of a birthday party, a theme for sadness is a lost dog, a theme for fear is a frightening dog, and a theme for anger is a false accusation. The child's capacity for empathy is determined by a match between the child's expressed feeling and the theme depicted in the picture or story. The FASTE has been modified to accommodate studies by different researchers (Zhou et al., 2003).

Some have criticized the FASTE because of its weak psychometric support, its suggestive test instructions (e.g., instructions designed in a way that elicits the desired behavior), and a lack of clarity in scoring (Eisenberg-Berg & Lennon, 1980; Eisenberg & Lennon, 1983; Hoffman, 1982; Zhou et al., 2003). Concern also has been raised about the confounding effect of the "demand characteristic" in children's responses (Goldstein & Michaels, 1985). This phenomenon makes the respondents modify their responses to what they believe the testing situation demands. The demand characteristic (e.g., a tendency to respond in a certain way that can undermine the validity of the results) is inherent in children's self-reports when an adult constantly asks them about their feelings. Another concern is the confounding effect of the experimenter's sex on the results of the FASTE because research indicated that when the experimenter was a woman, girls scored higher than boys did (Levine & Hoffman, 1975; Roe, 1977).

The Index of Empathy

The self-report Index of Empathy, developed by Bryant in (1982) consists of 22 items designed to measure empathy in children and adolescents. The measure is comparable to Mehrabian and Epstein's Emotional Empathy Scale, which was developed to measure empathy in the adult population (this scale will be described later in this chapter). The author of the Index of Empathy indicated that these comparable instruments can be useful for exploring changes in empathy at different ages. A sample item is "I really like to watch people open presents, even when I don't get a present myself." The internal consistency reliability coefficients of this measure were reported to be 0.54 for first graders, 0.68 for fourth graders, and 0.79 for seventh graders (Bryant, 1982; Zhou et al., 2003).

Although the above-mentioned methods of measuring empathy in children and adolescents seem to be useful for measuring reactions to affective situations, no convincing evidence is available in support of the instrument's predictive validity as indicators of the capacity for empathy.

Measurement of Empathy in Adults

The Most Frequently Used Instruments

The first three self-report measures of empathy discussed in this section—Hogan's Empathy Scale, Mehrabian and Epstein's Emotional Empathy Scale, and Davis's Interpersonal Reactivity Index—have been the most frequently used instruments in empathy research. Although they were developed for use in the general population, rather than with health care professionals, they have been used often in health care research. These measures are briefly described in the order in which they were originally published. Although other instruments have been designed to measure empathy, they have not received widespread attention. Some of them will be briefly described later in this chapter.

The Empathy Scale

Published by Robert Hogan (1969) and based on his doctoral dissertation at the University of California at Berkeley, the Empathy Scale includes 64 true–false items adopted from the California Psychological Inventory (CPI), the Minnesota Multiphasic Personality Inventory (MMPI), and other tests used at the Institute of Personality Assessment and Research. The scale was developed within the framework of the theory of moral development. A typical item is "I have seen some things so sad that I almost felt like crying."

Evidence in support of the scale's validity was provided by showing that high scorers were more likely than low scorers to be socially acute and sensitive to nuances in interpersonal relationships, and low scorers were more likely to be hostile, cold, and insensitive to the feelings of others (Hogan, 1969). Also, in a group of medical students, Hogan found a significant and positive correlation between scores on this scale and a criterion measure of sociability on the CPI ($r = 0.58$) and a significant negative correlation with social introversion on the MMPI ($r = -0.65$) (Hogan, 1969). Factor analysis of the Empathy Scale across different studies resulted in an inconsistent factor structure. For example, Greif and Hogan (1973) reported the following factors: "even-tempered disposition," "social ascendancy," and "humanistic sociopolitical attitudes," and Johnson, Cheek, and Smither (1983) reported "social self-confidence," "even temperedness," "sensitivity," and "nonconformity." These inconsistent findings raised questions about the scale's construct validity. Based on the factor analytic findings, it is suggested that the entire scale may not capture the essence of empathy (Baron-Cohen & Wheelwright, 2004). The scale's reliability also has been questioned (Cross & Sharpley, 1982). A computer on-line search conducted in September 2005 using "Hogan" and "Empathy Scale" as keywords resulted in 41 entries in the PsycInfo database and 8 entries in the Medline database.

The Emotional Empathy Scale

This instrument was developed by Albert Mehrabian and Norman Epstein (1972) and includes 33 items intended to measure emotional empathy. "It makes me sad to see a lonely stranger in a group" is a typical item. The title of the measure and the contents of the items pertain to susceptibility to emotional contagion (Zhou et al., 2003), indicating that the authors used an affective conceptualization of empathy when developing the scale (Davis, 1994). This conceptualization conflicts with the definition of empathy as a primarily cognitive concept in the context of patient care that was adopted in this book (see Chapter 6).

Items are answered on a 9-point Likert-type scale (Very Strongly Agree = +4, Very Strongly Disagree = −4). The split-half reliability of this scale was reported to be 0.84, and the internal consistency reliability was 0.79 (Zhou et al., 2003). The validity of this scale was determined by using an experimental paradigm similar to Milgram's experiments (1963, 1968) in which high scorers on this scale were less likely than low scores to administer electric shocks to the experimental subjects (Mehrabian & Epstein, 1972) (see Chapter 8 for a description of Milgram's experimental paradigm). On the basis of their subjective view, Mehrabian and Epstein reported that the scale included the following components and identified the items that measured each of these components: extreme emotional responsiveness, appreciation of the feelings of unfamiliar and distant others, tendency to be moved by others' emotional experiences, and tendency to be sympathetic. A study by Dillard and Hunter (1989) failed to support the aforementioned multidimensional components. Later, Mehrabian et al. (1988) changed the scale's name to the Emotional Empathic Tendency Scale. A computer online search conducted in September 2005 using "Mehrabian and Epstein" and "Emotional Empathy" as keywords resulted in 54 entries in the PsycInfo database and 18 entries in the Medline database.

The Interpersonal Reactivity Index

As part of his doctoral dissertation at the University of Texas at Austin, Mark Davis developed the Interpersonal Reactivity Index (IRI) (Davis, 1983) to measure individual differences in empathy. The instrument includes 28 items tapping four components of empathy in the cognitive and emotional domains. These four components are reflected in four subscales (Perspective Taking, Empathic Concern, Fantasy, and Personal Distress), each of which includes seven items answered on a 5-point scale ranging from 0 (Does not describe me well) to 4 (Describes me very well). These components were originally determined by subjective judgment without statistical support. However, confirmatory factor analysis provided mixed results concerning the existence of the four subscales (Cliffordson, 2002; Litvack-Miller, McDougall, & Romney, 1997).

The Perspective Taking subscale measures the tendency to adopt the views of others spontaneously. "I sometimes try to understand my friends better by imagining how things look from their perspective" is a typical item. The Empathic Concern subscale measures a tendency to experience the feelings of others and to feel sympathy and compassion for unfortunate people. A typical item is "I often have tender, concerned feelings for people less fortunate than me." The Fantasy subscale measures a tendency to imagine oneself in a fictional situation. A typical item is "After seeing a play or movie, I have felt as though I were one of the characters." The Personal Distress subscale taps a tendency to experience distress in others. "When I see someone who badly needs help in an emergency, I go to pieces" is a representative item. According to Davis, the Perspective Taking subscale is more likely to measure cognitive empathy, whereas the other three subscales are more likely to measure emotional empathy.

The internal consistency reliability coefficients ranged from 0.71 to 0.77 for the four subscales, and their test–retest reliabilities ranged from 0.62

to 0.71 (Davis, 1983). The test–retest reliabilities in an adolescent sample over a 2-year period ranged from 0.50 to 0.62 (Davis & Franzoi, 1991; Zhou et al., 2003). In correlating the IRI subscale scores with scores on Hogan's Empathy Scale, the highest positive correlation was found for the Perspective Taking subscale ($r = 0.40$) and the highest negative correlation was found for the Personal Distress subscale ($r = -0.33$) (Davis, 1983). The Perspective Taking subscale of the IRI yielded the lowest correlation with the scores of Mehrabian and Epstein's Emotional Empathy Scale ($r = 0.24$), and the Fantasy and Empathic Concern subscales yielded the highest correlations (0.52 and 0.60, respectively) (Davis, 1983). This pattern of correlations confirms Davis's claim about the cognitive nature of the Perspective Taking subscale.

In 1994, Davis stated that convincing evidence existed in support of some psychometric aspects of the IRI, although no satisfactory statistical evidence has been presented to confirm the stability of the four components of the index. In a study with physicians and undergraduate psychology students, Yarnold, Bryant, Nightingale, and Martin (1996) discovered an additional component called "involvement" in their statistical analysis of the IRI. The findings that scores on the Personal Distress subscale of the IRI were negatively correlated with scores on the Perspective Taking subscale raise a serious question about the validity of scoring the IRI by summing up the scores of all its subscales, including the Personal Distress subscale. According to D'Orazio (2004), because of the negative correlation between the Personal Distress and Perspective Taking subscales and because high scores on Personal Distress are associated with dysfunctional interpersonal relationships, summing up the scores of all four subscales of the IRI would not be meaningful. A computer on-line search conducted in September 2005 using "Interpersonal Reactivity Index" as the keyword resulted in 154 entries in the PsycInfo database and 28 entries in the Medline database.

Other Instruments

Several other instruments for measuring empathy in the adult population are described here in chronological order.

Kerr developed a test of empathy with the intention of measuring respondents' ability to "anticipate" certain typical reactions, feelings, and behavior of other people (Kerr, 1947). The test consists of three sections, which require respondents to rank the popularity of 15 types of music, the national circulation of 15 magazines, and the prevalence of 10 types of annoyances for a particular group of people (Chlopan, McCain, Carbonell, & Hagen, 1985). The respondent's rankings are compared to the empirical data to assess the accuracy of the respondent's rankings. This test seems to be a measure of general information, rather than a measure of empathy. Nevertheless, Kerr and Speroff (1954) claimed that the test was an indicator of empathic understanding and that it could predict a person's popularity, feelings for others, leadership, and sales records.

A measure of insight and empathy was introduced by Dymond (1949, 1950). This measure was based on the conceptualization of empathy as the imaginative transposing of oneself into another person's thinking, feeling, and acting. In Dymond's Rating Test (of empathic ability), respondents rate themselves and one another on a 5-point scale on six attributes such as "superior–inferior," "friendly–unfriendly," "leader–follower," "self-confidence," "selfish–unselfish," and "sense of humor." The concordance between individual's ratings of himself or herself and the individual's predictions of how others would rate him or her was considered as a measure of empathic ability. High scorers on the Dymond's Rating Test were classified as empathizers by analyses of their responses to the Thematic Apperception Test (TAT) (Dymond, 1949). Although no satisfactory evidence is available to confirm the instrument's validity as a measure of empathy, some preliminary data on its psychometric characteristics were presented by Chlopan et al. (1985). However, those investigators raised concerns about the measure's lack of easy administration and scoring procedures.

Barrett-Lennard (1962) developed an instrument called the Relationship Inventory, which was designed to investigate changes in the clinician–client relationship in the psychotherapeutic context. The instrument can be completed by either the clinician or the client.

The original inventory included 92 items. However, one revised version consists of 64 items divided into four subjectively determined subtests of interpersonal relationships: (1) Empathic Understanding, described as the extent to which one person is conscious of the awareness of another person, (2) Level of Regard, the affective aspect of one person's response to another, (3) Unconditionality of Regard, the degree of constancy of regard one person feels for another person, and (4) Congruence, the degree to which one person is functionally integrated in the context of his or her relationship with another person (Barrett-Lennard, 1986). The "Willingness To Be Known" subtest included in the original version of the Relationship Inventory was defined as the degree to which a person wants to be known as a person by another person. This subtest was dropped in the revised version because of its nonsignificant predictive validity concerning therapeutic outcomes (Barrett-Lennard, 1986). Subsequent versions of the Relationship Inventory have been developed for use in nonclinical situations involving family, friendship, coworker, and teacher–pupil relationships (Bennett, 1995).

A 16-item subtest of this instrument called Empathic Understanding contains such items as "He [clinician/client] understands me." Items are answered on a Likert-type scale ranging from −3 ("No," as strongly felt disagreement) to +3 ("Yes," as strongly felt agreement). A negligible clinician–client correlation of 0.09 was reported for the Empathic Understanding subtest (Barrett-Lennard, 1962).

Truax and Carkhuff (1967) developed the 141-item Relationship Questionnaire to measure clients' perceptions of psychologists or counselors in psychological counseling and psychotherapy. Forty-six of the 141 items of the Relationship Questionnaire form a subscale called the Accurate Empathy Scale, which consists of such items as "He sometimes completely understands me so that he knows what I am feeling even when I am hiding my feelings." A number of questions have been raised about the validity, reliability, and score stability of the Accurate Empathy Scale (Beutler, Johnson, Neville, & Workman, 1973; Blass & Hech, 1975; Chinsky & Rappaport, 1970).

Carkhuff (1969) developed the Empathic Understanding in Interpersonal Processes Scale. This single-item instrument gives clinicians an overall empathy score based on five levels of empathic behavior, as judged by observers. Clinicians who score at Level 1 are judged as unable to express any awareness of even the most obvious of a client's feelings, whereas those who score at Level 5 are judged to be fully aware of and able to respond accurately to all of the client's feelings. Because an observer rates clinicians' empathic global behavior on a single item, the validity of this instrument is questionable (LaMonica, 1981).

The Fantasy–Empathy (F-E) Scale developed by Stotland et al. (1978) measures the tendency to respond emotionally to situations. The scale contains three items answered on a 5-point scale: for example, "When I watch a good movie, I can very easily put myself in the place of a leading character." Some psychometric data on this brief scale have been reported (Stotland, 1978). For instance, a correlation of 0.44 was reported between the F-E Scale and Mehrabian and Epstein's Emotional Empathy Scale (Williams, 1989).

Layton (1979) developed the Empathy Test, a two-part 48-item instrument, as part of a research project designed to teach empathy to nursing students. The purpose of this measure was to evaluate whether empathy can be learned by observing models of empathic behavior. Each part of the Empathy Test consists of 12 true–false items and 12 multiple-choice items. According to Layton's reports, the reliability coefficients for the measure are unacceptably low (in the 0.20s), and no significant correlations were found between this measure and the Empathic Understanding subtest of Barrett-Lennard's Relationship Inventory and Carkhuff's Empathic Understanding in Interpersonal Processes Scale (Carkhuff, 1969).

Another instrument for measuring empathy is the Empathy Construct Rating Scale developed by LaMonica (1981). The instrument consists of 84 items about the respondent's feelings or actions toward another person, answered on a 6-point Likert-type scale (−3, Extremely Unlike; +3, Extremely Like). A typical item is "Seems to understand another person's state of being." The bipolar grand factor of this scale includes the notion of "well-developed empathy" (e.g., "Shows consideration for a person's feelings and reactions") at one pole and "lack of empathy" (e.g., "Does not listen to what the other person is saying") at the opposite pole.

Recently, a new measuring instrument—Empathy Quotient (EQ)—was developed in England by Baron-Cohen, Lawrence, and colleagues that contains 40 empathy items plus 20 filler items to distract the participants from relentless focus on empathy (Baron-Cohen & Wheelwright, 2004; Lawrence, Shaw, Baker, Baron-Cohen, & David, 2004). Each item is answered on a 4-point Likert-type scale from Strongly Agree to Strongly Disagree. Although the authors claim that the EQ was explicitly designed to have clinical applications, the contents of most of the items do not support such an application. Sample items are "I really enjoy caring for other people" and "I tend to get emotionally involved with a friend's problems." A test–retest reliability of 0.83 is reported for the EQ. Three factors, Cognitive Empathy, Emotional Reactivity, and Social Skills, emerged from factor analyses of the EQ. With the exception of the Cognitive Empathy factor, which was not correlated with any subscales of the IRI, the EQ yielded moderate correlations with the Empathic Concern and Perspective Taking subscales of the IRI and a negligible negative correlation with the Personal Distress subscale (Lawrence et al., 2004).

Physiological and Neurological Indicators of Empathy

Some social psychologists have studied empathy by using physiological measures, such as heart rate, skin conductance, palmar sweating, and vasoconstriction, as indicators of understanding other people's distress (Goldstein & Michaels, 1985; Stotland et al., 1978). Although most of these physiological measures are likely to be free of a social desirability response set, they seem to be indicative of a person's emotional reaction to another person's distress. Such physiological reactions are more likely to be akin to sympathy than to empathy, as was discussed in Chapter 1. Correspondingly, they may not be appropriate for the measurement of cognitively defined empathy in patient care.

Recently, functional brain-imaging methods (e.g., fMRIs and PET scans) have been used as indicators of brain activity in individuals experiencing empathy (Carr et al., 2003; Wicker et al., 2003). In addition to advancements in functional brain imaging, the recent discovery of the mirror neuron system activated by observing another person perform an act (see Chapter 3) is, I believe, the beginning of a promising approach to quantifying neurophysiological manifestations of empathy in future research.

Relationships Among Measures of Empathy

The results of studies attempting to determine correlations among different measures of empathy have not been encouraging. For example, Jarski, Gjerde, Bratton, Brown, and Matthes (1985) tested a group of medical students and found no significant correlations among the Empathy Scale

(Hogan, 1969), the Empathic Understanding subtest of the Relationship Inventory (Barrett-Lennard, 1962), and the Empathic Understanding in Interpersonal Processes Scale (Carkhuff, 1969).

Another study with registered nurses examined correlations among four measures of empathy (Layton & Wykle, 1990). The results showed that Carkhuff's Empathic Understanding in Interpersonal Processes Scale was moderately correlated ($r = 0.25$) with Layton's Empathy Test but was not correlated with the Empathic Understanding subtest of Barrett-Lennard's Relationship Inventory. In addition, LaMonica's Empathy Construct Rating Scale was not correlated with Layton's Empathy Test but was moderately correlated ($r = 0.37$) with Carkhuff's Empathic Understanding in Interpersonal Processes Scale and highly correlated ($r = 0.78$) with the Barrett-Lennard's Empathic Understanding subtest of the Relationship Inventory.

In a review article, Chlopan and associates (1985) reported the findings of studies on the validity and reliability of several measures of empathy, including Mehrabian and Epstein's Emotional Empathy Scale and Hogan's Empathy Scale. Chlopan and associates argued that both scales seem to measure two different aspects of empathy. As its name indicates, the Emotional Empathy Scale is more likely to measure the affective aspects of empathy, or general emotional arousability (Mehrabian et al., 1988), whereas the Empathy Scale is more likely to measure role-taking ability, a cognitive aspect of empathy. Chlopan and colleagues also indicated that the subscales of the IRI seem to tap both the emotional (e.g., Personal Distress subscale) and the cognitive (Perspective Taking subscale) aspects of empathy.

The intercorrelations among these empathy measures are often weak and inconsistent and, in most cases, nonsignificant or negligible (Bohart et al., 2002; Gladstein et al., 1987). One reason for these inconsistent findings is that different instruments tap different aspects of empathy based on different definitions of the concept. Although these instruments can have potential value in particular situations, none can be recommended as the best for all patient-care situations (Bennett, 1995). With the exception of the Perspective Taking subscale of the IRI, the contents of the other instruments described in this chapter do not reflect the cognitive conceptualization of empathy adopted in this book (see Chapter 6). Thus, their face validity (and content validity) would be questionable when empathy is conceptualized as a predominantly cognitive attribute in the context of patient care advocated in this book.

A Measure Specifically Designed for the Patient-Care Context

A measure that assesses empathy in patient care—particularly in medical treatment—needs to be more specific than the instruments I have discussed in this chapter so far. Because of the changes evolving in the American health care system and the expansion of market-driven managed-care delivery systems that hamper physician–patient relationships (see Chapter 9), the empirical study of empathy in health care education and practice is both important and timely. Empathy in patient-care education and practice needs an operational definition and a psychometrically sound measure. In 2000, in response to this need, our research team in the Center for Research in Medical Education and Health Care at Jefferson Medical College began developing a scale specifically designed to measure empathy among students and practitioners in the health care professions. This scale will be described in detail in Chapter 7.

Recapitulation

Several instruments exist that claim to measure empathy in children and adults. Questions have been raised about the validity of physiological measures that may reflect affective arousability or emotional reactions to another person's distress, rather than empathy. Recently, functional brain-imaging technology that has been used to address brain activities in interpersonal relationships has emerged as a promising path for measuring empathic engagement in the future. The three frequently used instruments intended to measure empathy in adults—Hogan's Empathy Scale, Mehrabian and Epstein's Emotional Empathy Scale, and Davis's IRI—were developed for testing in the general population, and the examination of their contents suggests that they do not tap the essence of empathy in the context of patient care. Thus, there was a need for an instrument specifically developed to measure empathy in the context of patient care.

Part II

Empathy in Patient Care

6

A Definition and Key Features of Empathy in Patient Care

Clinical study amounts to the study of one person by another, and dialogue and relationship are its indispensable tools.

—(George L. Engel, 1990, p. 15)

Preamble

Empathy in patient care is addressed in this chapter in the context of the World Health Organization's (WHO) definition of health and with regard to the notion of a biopsychosocial paradigm of illness. I define empathy in the context of patient care as a predominantly cognitive attribute that involves an understanding of the patient's experiences, concerns, and perspectives, combined with a capacity to communicate this understanding. I then elaborate on the importance of the three key features (cognition, understanding, and communication) used in the definition of empathy and suggest that in the context of patient care, it is important to distinguish between cognition and emotion, between understanding and feeling, and between empathy and sympathy because of their different effects in patient outcomes. An abundance of empathic engagement, I suggest, is always beneficial in the context of patient care, whereas excessive sympathetic involvement can be detrimental to both the physician and the patient. I also maintain that to achieve positive patient outcomes, communication of understanding in empathic engagement between physician and patient must be reciprocal, confirming the patient's significant role in the outcome of patient care.

Introduction

We cannot scientifically study empathy in patient care unless an agreement exists concerning its definition and unless a psychometrically sound instrument is available to measure the defined concept. The definitions and descriptions of empathy presented in Chapter 1 provide a framework for the definition and conceptualization of empathy in the context of patient care. I begin in this chapter by describing the definition of health proposed by the WHO and briefly describe the biopsychosocial paradigm of illness. Then I offer a definition of empathy in patient care and elaborate on the definition's key features and their implications for patient outcomes.

The World Health Organization's Definition of Health and a Biopsychosocial Paradigm

The constitution of the WHO (1948, p. 1) defines health as "a state of complete physical, mental, and social well-being, and not merely an absence of disease or infirmity." This definition is consistent with the biopsychosocial paradigm of illness in medicine (Engel, 1977, 1990; Hojat, Samuel, & Thompson, 1995). Generally, human infirmity can be viewed from two different perspectives: biomedical and biopsychosocial.

The *biomedical* paradigm of disease postulated by the German physician Robert Koch and the French scholar Louis Pasteur, although still valid for some diseases, presents an incomplete picture of infirmity suffered by humankind. This "microbe hunting" model of disease (DeKruif, 1926) has a more limited scope than the triangular *biopsychosocial* paradigm of illness (Engel, 1977, 1990; Hojat et al., 1995; Ray, 2004). In the biopsychosocial paradigm, the targeted treatment of an affected organ is replaced by curing the whole patient, who is viewed as a system of being, always in relation to the biological, psychological, and social elements interacting closely with one another (see Chapter 12 for a discussion of the systems theory). Because of its limited scope, the biomedical model can neither describe the underlying interpersonal reasons for the victories in overcoming human illnesses (Frenk, 1998; McKinlay & McKinlay, 1981) nor explain the health-promoting effects of human connections, including empathic physician–patient engagement in health and illness.

In addition to the importance of pathophysiological determinants of infirmity, in the biopsychosocial paradigm of health and illness, psychological, social, and interpersonal factors are taken into consideration as well (Engel, 1977, 1990). This paradigm of health and illness attests that curing occurs when the science of medicine (the biomedical and pathophysiological aspects of disease) and the art of medicine (the psychological, social, and interpersonal aspects of illness) merge into one unified holistic approach to patient care. Empathy is a key element in this holistic approach.

The art of medicine, according to Blumgart (1964), consists of skillfully applying the science of medicine in the context of human relationships to maintain health and ameliorate illness. The unit of observation in the art of medicine is the individual person in relation to social and cultural factors, whereas the unit of observation in the science of medicine is the affected organ or the pathophysiology of disease. The science of medicine in the treatment of diseases and the art of medicine in the curing of illnesses are not independent entities; they supplement one another (Peabody, 1984). As Peabody (1984, p. 814) pointed out, "Treatment of disease may be entirely impersonal, but the care of the patient must be completely personal." Considering that the physician–patient relationship is an indispensable tool in clinical situations to achieve better patient outcomes (Engel, 1990), health care professionals should pay attention not only to the biomedical aspects of disease but to the psychosocial factors of illness as well (Spiro, 1992). Treating a pathophysiological disease may not require as much empathy as is required in curing the patient's illness (Novack, 1987; Novack, Epstein, & Paulsen, 1999).

Definition and Key Features of Empathy in Patient Care

Empathy in patient care has been characterized as arising "out of a natural desire to care about others" (Baron-Cohen, 2003, p. 2). Gianakos (1996, p. 135) referred to empathy in patient care as "the ability of physicians to imagine that they are the patient who has come to them for help." Greenson (1967, p. 367) described empathy in patient care as follows: "I have to let a part of me become the patient, and I have to go through her experience *as if* I were the patient." (Remember the "as if" condition in Rogers's definition of empathy described in Chapter 1.)

The notion of an empathic relationship with the patient was elegantly described in a statement attributed to Sir William Osler (1932): "It is as important to know what kind of man [sic] has the disease, as it is to know what kind of disease has the man." (This quotation is often attributed to Osler, as cited in White, 1991, p. 74; it also is attributed to Hippocrates, as cited by Ray, 2004, p. 30.) In any case, this statement best describes the biopsychosocial paradigm in which science and the art of medicine are complementary. To Larson and Yao (2005, p. 1105) empathy is the royal road to treatment and "a symbol of the health care profession." Engaging in empathic relationships makes physicians more effective healers and makes their careers more satisfying. Freud (1958a) suggested that empathy is not only a factor in enhancing the physician–patient relationship; it also provides a condition for correct interpretation of the patient's problems. Therefore, empathy is valuable both in making accurate diagnoses and in achieving more desirable treatment outcomes. Both the patient and the physician benefit from empathic engagement. This topic will be discussed in more detail in Chapter 8.

Definitions of the key concepts in research serve as a common language to understand the nature of the concepts under study. Although not all experts may agree on all aspects of any definition, at least some agreement should exist on the key features of a definition; otherwise, research based on a vague concept obviously will prove to be fruitless. By considering the various descriptions and features of empathy that were described in Chapter 1 and by taking into account the specific nature of empathy in patient care and its implications for positive patient outcomes, our research team at Jefferson Medical College proposed the following definition of empathy in the context of patient care (Hojat et al., 2002b, 2002d, 2003b):

> Empathy is a predominantly *cognitive* (rather than an emotional) attribute that involves an *understanding* (rather than feeling) of experiences, concerns and perspectives of the patient, combined with a capacity to *communicate* this understanding.

The three key terms in this definition are printed in italics to underscore their significance in the construct of empathy in the context of patient care. We developed this definition after a comprehensive review of the literature (Hojat et al., 2001b; Hojat et al., 2003b) and a careful consideration of the factors that contribute to positive patient outcomes. Our original intention was to present a working definition that would clarify the key ingredients our research team believed were conceptually relevant to empathy in patient care and to provide a framework for quantifying the defined concept by developing an instrument with which to measure empathy in the context of patient care (the instrument will be described in detail in the next chapter). Our choice of the three key ingredients in the definition of empathy—*cognition*, *understanding*, and *communication*—needs some elaboration.

Cognition

Our research team viewed empathy as a predominantly cognitive (rather than an emotional) attribute based on a belief that in patient-care situations, empathy emerges as a result of mental activities described in Chapter 1 as facets of cognitive information processing. Such facets include reasoning and appraisal, which are the basis of clinical judgment. Although cognitive mental processing (a key feature of empathy) can lead to positive patient outcomes, overwhelming emotion (a key feature of sympathy) can impede the optimal outcomes by obscuring objectivity in clinical judgments.

Cognition and emotion, although seemingly related, have different qualities independent of their joint appearance (Lazarus, 1982). Experienced therapists tend to respond to patients' distress with cognitive, rather than emotional, feedback. For example, an analysis of the interpersonal responses between Carl Rogers and his patients showed that approximately two-thirds of his responses were referred to as cognitive reactions (Tausch, 1988).

The distinction between cognition and emotion (and correspondingly, between empathy and sympathy) may not seem as important in situations where patient care is not a primary consideration. In the context of patient care, however, such a distinction must be made because of the different implications regarding patient outcomes. Physicians should feel their patients' feelings only to the extent necessary to improve their understanding of the patients without impeding their professional judgment (Starcevic & Piontek, 1997). It is not essential for physicians to feel their patients' feelings to an overwhelming degree. Emotional overinvolvement is a feature of sympathy, not empathy (Olinick, 1984). However, for the purpose of more accurate diagnoses, it is essential for physicians to understand, as much as possible, their patients' feelings and concerns.

The notions of "detached concern," "compassionate detachment," and "affective distance" have been used to describe the limits of emotional engagement in the physician–patient relationship (Blumgart, 1964; Halpern, 2001; Jensen, 1994; Lief, Lief, & Lief, 1963). Ayra (1993) suggested that physicians' dissociation from patients' emotions can help them to retain their mental balance. Farber and associates (1997) reported that although medicine is a profession characterized by caring and empathy, it also has been characterized throughout history as aspiring to "objective detachment." This is possible when emotional involvement in physician–patient encounters is restrained. Despite this restraint, however, *complete* emotional detachment has its own perils in the context of patient care (Friedman, 1990). As I described in Chapter 1, emotion is acceptable to some extent, and sometimes it is difficult to distinguish when emotion ends and cognition begins in the context of patient care. I believe the controversy about detached concern in physician–patient encounters arises from confusion about the nature and meaning of empathy and sympathy. Maintaining an affective distance to avoid emotional overinvolvement (a feature of sympathy) makes the physician's clinical judgment more objective, but cognitive overindulgence (a feature of empathy) can always lead to a more accurate judgment. Objectivity when making clinical decisions can be better achieved by avoiding emotional overinvolvement, which clouds medical judgment (Koenig, 2002).

It is difficult to be highly emotional and objective at the same time (Wispe, 1986) because excessive emotion in patient care can interfere with the principle of objectivity when making diagnostic decisions and choosing treatments (Blumgart, 1964; Gladstein, 1977; Spiro, 1992). Perhaps one reason why physicians are advised not to treat close family members who have serious health problems is the notion that excessively sympathetic feelings toward close family members can impede clinical objectivity (Aring, 1958). Indeed, the professional guidelines on the treatment of immediate family members in the American Medical Association's Code of Ethics (Section E-8.19) states that "Professional objectivity may be compromised when an immediate family member or the physician is the patient; the physician's personal feelings may unduly influence his or her professional medical judgment, thereby interfering with the care being delivered." (Retrieved March, 2005, from http://www.ama-assn.org/pub/category/print/8510.html.)

Borgenicht (1984) suggested that in performing certain procedures, physicians must maintain a certain degree of emotional distance from the patient because overwhelming emotional involvement may prevent them from making objective decisions at times of crisis. Too much affect impedes effective communication between physician and patient, whereas an abundance of understanding facilitates it. Brody (1997) suggested that the real danger to the physician's effectiveness lies in sympathetic overengagement with the patient. Leif and Fox (1963) introduced the concept of "detached concern" in the medical education literature to prevent emotional overengagement between physicians and patients. In contrast, no one has ever expressed concern about excess in understanding. An "affective distance" between physician and patient is desirable not only to avoid an intense emotional involvement, which can jeopardize the principle of clinical neutrality, but also to maintain the physician's personal durability (Jensen, 1994). Because excessive emotions can obscure the physician's judgment concerning the patient's predicament, Freud (1958b) proposed that to achieve better therapeutic outcomes, clinicians must put aside all of their human sympathies!

For practical reasons, a distinction between cognition and emotion is important because of its implications with regard to determining the contents of the items in instruments intended to measure empathy (see Chapter 7), developing educational programs to enhance empathy, and assessing patient outcomes. The amenability to change will vary for cognitive and emotional behaviors. Cognitive attributes are more prone to change as a result of educational programs than are emotional responses (see Chapter 11).

Understanding

Understanding others' feelings and behaviors is central to human survival (Keysers & Perrett, 2004). Understanding is also a key ingredient of empathic engagement in the physician–patient relationship (Levinson, 1994). Patients' perception of being understood, according to Suchman, Markakis, Beckman, and Frankel (1997), is intrinsically therapeutic because it helps to restore a sense of connectedness and support. Empathy in patient care is built on the central notion of connection and understanding (Hudson, 1993; Sutherland, 1993). Because being understood is a basic human need, the physician's understanding of the patient's physical, mental, and social needs is, in itself, relevant to the fulfillment of a basic human need. Accordingly, our research team proposed elsewhere that "when an empathic relationship is established, a basic human need is fulfilled" (Hojat et al., 2003b, p. 27).

According to Schneiderman (2002, p. 627), "the better we understand them [the patients], the closer we come to discovering the true state of affairs, and the more likely we will be able to diagnose and treat correctly." Understanding of the patient's perspective was considered as an essential element of physician–patient communication by a group of medical education experts in the Kalamazoo, Michigan, conference held in 1999 (Makoul, 2001). A specific feature of understanding in the physician–patient relationship is the ability to stand in a patient's shoes without leaving one's own personal space and to view the world from the patient's perspective without losing sight of one's own personal role and professional responsibilities. With this background in mind, our research team decided to consider "understanding" (rather than "feeling") as a keyword in the definition of empathy in the context of patient care.

Accuracy of understanding is another topic of discussion in empathy research. As Rogers (1975, p. 4) advised clinicians, "perhaps if we wish to become a better therapist, we should let our clients tell us whether we are understanding them accurately." In general, the accuracy of understanding depends on the strength of the empathic relationship and the feedback mechanisms. Because the accuracy of understanding is an issue that may be a subject of debate, physicians should occasionally verify the degree to which their understanding is accurate by *communicating* with the patent—another essential ingredient of empathy in patient care that will be discussed in the following section.

Communication of Understanding

According to Carkhuff (1969) and Chessick (1992), the central curative aspect of clinician–patient relationships rests not only on the clinician's ability to understand the patient but also on his or her ability to communicate this understanding back to the patient. Reynolds (2000) and Diseker and Michielutte (1981) included communication of understanding as a feature of empathy in physician–patient relationships. For example, Carkhuff (1969, p. 315) indicated that "[empathy is] the ability to recognize, sense, and understand the feelings that another person has associated with his (her) behavioral and verbal expressions and to accurately communicate this understanding to him or her." Similarly, Reynolds (2000, p. 13) defined empathy as "an accurate perception of the client's world and an ability to communicate this understanding to the client."

Communication of understanding also is a key feature in LaMonica's description of empathy: "Empathy... involves accurate perception of the client's world by the helper, communicating of this understanding to the client, and the client's perception of the helper's understanding" (LaMonica, 1981, p. 398). Truax and Carkhuff (1967, p. 40) described empathy as involving the ability to sense the client's "private world" and to communicate this understanding in "a language attuned to the client's current feelings." A physician who has an empathic understanding of the patient but does not communicate such an understanding would not be perceived as an empathic physician (Bylund & Makoul, 2005). According to Branch and Malik (1993), there are windows of opportunities in clinical encounters for expressing mutual understanding when patients describe emotional, personal, and family concerns. Physicians must capture these moments of "potential empathic opportunities" (Suchman et al., 1997) to express their understanding of patients' concerns.

An important aspect of communication in patient care is the notion of "reciprocity" or "mutuality" (Makoul, 1998; Miller, 2002; Raudonis, 1993). Although the idea that empathy involves mutual understanding is not widely discussed in empathy research (Bennett, 2001), it must be regarded as an essential ingredient of empathic engagement in patient care. Mutual understanding generates a dynamic feedback loop that is helpful not only in strengthening empathic engagement but also in making a more accurate diagnosis and thus providing better treatment. It is important to note that mutual understanding and reciprocal feedback during verbal and nonverbal exchanges indicate that both physician and patient must play an active role to enhance empathic engagement. Without such features, empathic engagement cannot fully develop.

Physicians should let their patients know that their health problems and their psychosocial concerns are fully understood. It is also desirable for a patient to confirm the physician's understanding. By using a coding system (Empathic Communication Coding System), Bylund and Makoul (2005) reported that most patients do provide physicians with potential empathic opportunities. In their coding system, physicians' reactions to these potential opportunities were recorded on a 7-point scale (0 = physician ignores the empathic opportunity, 6 = physician makes an explicit statement to express understanding of the patient's concerns). They found that more than 80% of physicians could detect the opportunities and reacted either by confirmation, acknowledgment, and pursuing or elaborating the issues of concern. The patient's belief concerning the physician's understanding reinforces the empathic engagement between the two. The following statements represent some simple approaches to the communication of empathic understanding: "I understand your feelings. You have gone through a lot of difficulties", "I can see how being in a cast would make you helpless" (the expression of empathic understanding approach); "I can understand why this problem is so difficult for you" (the validation approach); "I understand your problem very well because I went through a similar situation" (the self-disclosure approach); "I want to make sure that I understand your concern. Let me rephrase it this way...." (the rephrasing approach); "It is saddening to have that kind of feeling" (sympathy); or "This reminds me of the story of...." (the metaphorical approach) (Matthews, Suchman, & Branch, 1993; Mayerson, 1976).

Mutuality generates a belief in the patient that not only enhances the empathic relationship but also has a mysterious beneficial effect on clinical outcomes (Hudson, 1993). Although the mechanism of the positive effect of mutuality in understanding is not well understood, one could speculate that the beneficial outcomes are attributable to greater satisfaction with the health care provider, to better compliance with treatment, or to such psychological factors as reduced anxiety, enhanced optimism, and perceptions of social support, which are activated in mutually understood interpersonal relationships. The reciprocal communication can help to remove the constraints of physician–patient relationships because, as a golden rule in interpersonal relationships, when constraints vanish, people begin to reveal their secrets.

Recapitulation

The triangular biopsychosocial paradigm of health and illness, consistent with the definition of health in the WHO's constitution, suggests that empathic engagement in physician–patient encounters should lead to enhanced physical as well as mental and social well-being. The definition of empathy discussed in this chapter emphasizes three specific features of empathy in the context of patient care: cognition, understanding, and communication. The requirement of mutual understanding and reciprocal feedback supports the notion that the patient's recognition of the physician's empathy through the physician's verbal and nonverbal communication plays a significant role in patient outcomes.

7 The Jefferson Scale of Physician Empathy

Science begins in the nothingness of ignorance
and moves toward truth
by gathering more and more information,
constructing theories as facts accumulate.

—(Stephen Jay Gould, 1981, p. 321)

Preamble

On the basis of the belief that measuring instruments that were developed for the general population did not tap the essence of empathy in the context of patient care, we developed an operational measure of empathy specifically applicable to medical care. This chapter describes the steps taken in the development and psychometric analyses of the *Jefferson Scale of Physician Empathy* (*JSPE*). The evidence presented in support of the JSPE's validity (face, content, construct, criterion-related, convergent, and discriminant validities) and reliability (coefficient alpha in support of internal consistency and test–retest reliability in support of score stability) can enhance the confidence of researchers who are searching for a psychometrically sound instrument developed specifically to study empathy in the context of patient care. The general findings on the JSPE's measurement properties suggest that the instrument can serve as an operational measure of empathy among students (S-Version) and practitioners in the health professions (HP-Version). Further research is needed to investigate the relationship between scores on the JSPE and clinical outcomes, such as accuracy of diagnosis, patient satisfaction, patient compliance, and reduced risk of malpractice claims.

Introduction

Empathy has been described in the literature as the most frequently mentioned attribute of the humanistic physician (Linn et al., 1987), yet empirical research on the topic is scarce because of the ambiguity of the term (see Chapter 1) and the lack of a psychometrically sound measure of empathy in the context of patient care. Some researchers believe that the instruments developed for the general population do not tap the essence of the construct of empathy in the context of patient care and are not adequate for that purpose (Evans, Stanley, & Burrows, 1993).

To the best of my knowledge, no psychometrically sound instrument was available to measure empathy among students and practitioners in the health professions until the JSPE was developed. None of the instruments described in Chapter 5 is specific enough to capture the essence of empathy in the context of patient care. In more technical terms, none of the instruments has "face" and "content" validity in patient-care situations.

Our research team at Jefferson Medical College recognized the need for an instrument that would enable researchers to conduct empirical investigations on the development of empathy among students and practitioners in the health professions, to study group differences, and to examine correlates, antecedents, and outcomes of empathy in different stages of training as well as in different types of practices. In response to this need, we developed the JSPE. Originally designed for medical students (Hojat et al., 2001b), the JSPE was subsequently modified to be applicable to practicing physicians and other health professionals (Hojat et al., 2002d). A brief history of JSPE's development and modifications is presented in the following sections.

Development of a Framework

Review of the Literature

To construct a test, one must develop a framework for understanding the concept and its related elements that one intends to measure. The journey begins with a comprehensive review of the literature to explore conceptual frameworks, theoretical views, and empirical research on the topic and to identify behaviors that are relevant to the concept in question. Accordingly, in 1999, we searched the Medline database for all studies published beginning in 1966 (the starting date in the Medline database) that would identify contexts and contents we could use as a guide while drafting items for the preliminary version of the instrument. Using "empathy" as a keyword in our search, we found 3,541 published sources in English. Cross-searching with the terms "empathy" and "physician/physicians" resulted in 107 published entries. A review of these and other relevant references, most of which were cited in the original 107 entries, provided us with some ideas about what the contents of items in the preliminary version of the instrument should be to measure empathy among medical students and physicians.

Examination of Face Validity

The second step, subsequent to the review of the literature, was to examine the face validity of the drafted items. Face validity involves subjective judgments, usually by nonexperts, about the relevance of the contents of the items to the concept being measured. Our research team drafted 90 items for the preliminary version of the JSPE that appeared to be relevant to empathy and, therefore, seemed to have face validity.

The items in the preliminary version covered broad areas, such as understanding subjective experiences of the patients and their families; interpersonal relationships with the patients; attention to verbal and nonverbal signals in physician–patient communications; humor; attention to art, poetry, literature, and narrative skills; absorption in stories, plays, and movies; cognitive and affective sensitivities; emotional closeness and distance between physician and patient; objectivity in clinical decision making; clinical neutrality; clinicians' emotional expression and control; sentiments; imagination; tactfulness; perspective taking; role playing; and cues in communication.

During the process of examining the face validity of the items, a particular item may seem, at first glance, to be irrelevant to the topic. Consequently, including such an item must be justified. A convincing argument should support the inclusion of every item in case a question is raised concerning the item's relevance to empathy. We used the rational scale method of theory-based item selection (Reiter-Palmon & Connelly, 2000) for that purpose. For example, we included items related to an interest in literature and the art based on the theoretical argument that studying literature and the art can improve a person's understanding of human pain and suffering (Herman, 2000; McLellan & Husdon Jones, 1996; Montgomery Hunter, Charon, & Coulehan, 1995). Therefore, such an interest would be relevant to the capacity for empathy (see Chapter 11). Another example was inclusion of an item about a sense of humor based on the assumption that a clinician's sense of humor can reduce the stress perceived by the patient, thus contributing to an improved clinician–patient relationship (Yates, 2001). Additional theoretical support for this proposition is based on observations that humor can reduce the restraints in clinician–patient relationships by relieving tension and reducing inhibitions (Lief & Fox, 1963). Also, a sense of humor has been listed as an element of professionalism in medicine (Duff, 2002). According to Golden (2002), humor is a "magical force" that detaches patients from their pain and suffering through the healing power of laughter. A recent movie based on a real story about the life of Doctor Patch Adams beautifully depicted the role of humor in medical care. Thus, we included an item about sense of humor in the instrument.

In addition, we made every effort to incorporate components that were consistent with our definition of empathy (see Chapter 6). For example, because "understanding" is a key component of our definition, the word appears in approximately one-third (7 items) of the items in the final scale.

Examination of Content Validity

Examining the content validity of a new instrument is another important step in its development. Content validity involves the systematic examination of the instrument's contents, usually by experts, to confirm the relevance and representativeness of the items in covering the domains of behavior the test intends to measure (Anastasi, 1976). We probed the JSPE's content validity to ensure that the instrument included a representative sample of the behaviors expected to fit within the concept of empathy, particularly in relation to patient-care situations.

To examine the content validity of the preliminary version of the JSPE, we used an abbreviated version of the Delphi technique (Cyphert & Gant, 1970), which is usually used to obtain systematic and independent judgments from a group of experts. We mailed the preliminary version of the instrument to 100 clinical and academic physicians. A cover letter described the purpose of our study as the development of an instrument to measure empathy among health professionals, such as physicians. The letter briefly described empathy as an understanding of patients' experiences, emotions, and feelings as opposed to sympathy, which was described as feeling emotions similar to the way patients feel them.

Respondents were asked to cross out any item they considered to be irrelevant to the measurement of empathy, as described in the brief definition. They were also asked to edit the remaining items for simplicity and clarity and to add new items they regarded as important to include in an instrument intended to measure empathy in patient-care situations. The 55 physicians who responded offered suggestions, made editorial improvements, and provided conceptual comments. They also made recommendations about revisions, additions, and deletions.

During this stage of the study, we excluded all items from the preliminary version that five or more physicians had crossed out. We also incorporated appropriate editorial suggestions the respondents had made. After several iterations and revisions to assure that the items reflected distinct and relevant aspects of empathy in patient-care situations, 45 of the original 90 items were retained (Hojat et al., 2001b). It was this 45-item version of the instrument that was used in the preliminary psychometric analyses.

Preliminary Psychometric Analyses

For the purpose of a preliminary psychometric study, the 45-item instrument was administered to 223 third-year students at Jefferson Medical College (193 completed the instrument, an 86% response rate). Also, a group of 41 residents in the internal medicine program at Thomas Jefferson University Hospital and its affiliated hospitals completed the instrument.

Likert-Type Scaling

A 7-point Likert-type scale (1 = Strongly disagree, 7 = Strongly agree) was used to respond to each item in the instrument (Likert, 1932). We chose a Likert-type scale rather than a simple, dichotomous (Agree/Disagree, Yes/No) response format because Likert-type scales provide a wider range of item scores, which allows for more variation and thus more precise discriminatory power (Oppenheim, 1992). Furthermore, a Likert scale usually yields a distribution that resembles a normal distribution (Likert, 1932) and results in numeric scores that can be treated as an interval scale of measurement. The underlying assumptions for using more powerful parametric statistical techniques would not be violated by the presence of a distribution approaching a normal distribution and an interval scale of measurement. We also chose a 7-point Likert-type scale, rather than the more common 5-point scale, because the two additional points could reduce respondents' tendency to use the extreme points of the scale consistently (Polgar & Thomas, 1988; Reynolds, 2000).

Factor Analysis to Retain the Best Items

Factor analysis is a statistical method used to examine the empirical relationships among a set of variables that can be efficiently summarized by a theoretical formulation (a confirmatory factor analysis) (Gorsuch, 1974). It also is a method of exploring the underlying constructs associated with a set of items (an exploratory factor analysis). The set of items that are highly correlated with one another would emerge under one factor (or a hypothetical construct). In addition, factor analysis is used to reduce the length of an instrument by retaining the items that have relatively high factor loadings (e.g., greater than |0.30|) under the important and meaningful factors (Gorsuch, 1974).

To screen for the best items to include in the next version and thus reduce the length of the preliminary instrument, we used factor analysis with the data collected from 193 medical students for the 45-item instrument. We used principal component factoring, followed by orthogonal varimax rotation. This type of mathematical rotation is frequently used to obtain a simpler factor structure and to produce independent (uncorrelated) factors.

On the basis of the results of the factor analysis, we retained 20 of the 45 items. Those 20 items had the highest factor structure coefficients (greater than 0.40) on the first extracted factor (grand factor). The eigenvalue (latent root) of this grand factor was 10.64, which was much higher than the eigenvalue for the next factor, 3.45. Eigenvalues indicate the importance of extracted factors in terms of the proportion of variance accounted for. A relatively large eigenvalue for the first factor is indicative of the factor's importance. A sudden drop in the magnitude of the eigenvalue and no significant decrease in the eigenvalues of subsequent factors is used to retain the substantial factors and disregard the trivial ones. This guideline is known as the "scree test" (Cattle, 1966).

The Generic Version of the Scale

The generic version of the JSPE contained 20 items (Hojat et al., 2001b). The item with the highest factor structure coefficient on the grand factor was "Empathy is an important therapeutic factor in medical and surgical treatment." This item was regarded as an "anchor" with which to evaluate the other items by examining the magnitude and direction of correlations between the anchor item and the other items. Because the sample size of 41 residents was insufficient (e.g., the ratio of the size of the sample of medical residents to the number of variables was less than 10; Baggaley, 1983), we did not perform a factor analysis for that sample. However, an examination of the patterns of interitem correlations showed considerable similarities between medical students and residents (Hojat et al., 2001b).

In the generic version of the JSPE, 17 items with positive factor structure coefficients and positive and statistically significant correlations with the "anchor" item were directly scored on the 7-point Likert-type scale (e.g., 1 = Strongly disagree; 7 = Strongly agree). The other 3 items, which had negative factor structure coefficients on the grand factor and also yielded negative correlations with the "anchor" item, were reverse scored (1 = Strongly agree, 7 = Strongly disagree). An example of a directly scored item in the final generic version is "Willingness to imagine oneself in another person's place contributes to providing quality care," and an example of a reverse scored item is "Emotion has no place in the treatment of medical illness." A higher score on the JSPE indicates a greater degree of empathy.

The descriptive statistics for the generic version of the JSPE from the two preliminary study samples of medical students and residents are reported in Table 7.1.

Construct Validity

Construct validity is the extent to which a test measures the theoretical constructs of the attribute that it purports to measure (Anastasi, 1976). Factor analysis helps to determine whether the scale's dimensions (underlying factors) are consistent with the theoretical constructs of the concept one intends to measure. Therefore, using factor analysis to examine construct validity can reveal the major dimensions that characterize the test scores (Anastasi, 1976).

To investigate the underlying structure of the generic version of the JSPE, data collected from the medical students were subjected to principal

Table 7.1 Descriptive statistics for the generic version of the JSPE

Statistics	Residents ($n = 41$)	Medical students ($n = 193$)
Mean	118	118
Standard deviation	12	11
Median (50th percentile)	119	117
Mode	119	112
25th percentile	110	111
75th percentile	126	126
Possible range[a]	20–140	20–140
Actual range[b]	88–140	87–139
Alpha reliability estimate	0.87	0.89

[a] The minimum and maximum possible scores.
[b] The lowest and highest scores obtained by the samples.
© Reproduced with permission from Hojat et al., 2001b.

component factoring with orthogonal varimax rotation. Four factors emerged, each with an eigenvalue greater than 1. An eigenvalue equal to or greater than 1 known as the Kaiser's criterion (Kaiser, 1960), which is often used to retain the most important factors. The four extracted factors accounted for 56% of the total variance. Ten items had factor coefficients greater than 0.40 on the first factor (eigenvalue = 7.56, accounting for 38% of the variance). We chose the magnitude of 0.40 as the minimum salient factor loading needed to assume a meaningful relationship between the item and the relevant factor (Gorsuch, 1974).

Assigning a title to a factor in factor analytic studies is a subjective judgment made according to the contents of the items with higher factor coefficients under the corresponding factor. Based on the contents of the 10 items with the highest factor coefficients, the first factor was called a construct of "the physician's view of what the patient's perspective is." The item with the highest factor coefficient under this factor was "A physician who is able to view things from another person's perspective can render better care."

Five items had a factor coefficient greater than 0.40 on the second factor, which accounted for 7% of the variance (eigenvalue = 1.30). Based on the contents of items with high factor coefficients, this factor was titled "Understanding patient's experiences, feelings, and clues." The item with the highest factor coefficient on this factor was "What is going on in a patient's mind can often be expressed by nonverbal cues such as facial expressions or body language that must be carefully observed by physicians."

Two reverse-scored items had factor coefficients greater than 0.40 on the third factor (eigenvalue = 1.14, accounting for 6% of the variance), which was titled "Ignoring emotions in patient care." The item with the highest coefficient on this factor was "Because people are different, it is almost impossible for physicians to see things from their patients' perspectives."

Finally, two items had factor coefficients greater than 0.40 on the fourth factor (eigenvalue = 1.01, accounting for 5% of the variance), which was titled "Thinking like the patient." The item with the highest coefficient on this factor was "The best way to take care of a patient is to think like a patient." According to Velicer and Fava (1998), a minimum number of three items per factor is required for a stable factor pattern. According to this criterion, the last two factors may not be as stable as the first two.

Also, a sudden drop in the magnitude of the prerotational eigenvalue after extracting the first factor suggests that the first factor is the most salient and reliable among all other extracted factors. The factor structure of the generic version of the JSPE is consistent with the multifaceted concept of empathy reported in the literature (Spiro, McCrea Curnen, Peschel, & St. James, 1993). Details regarding the factor analysis of the generic version of the JSPE and a table of factor structure coefficients are reported elsewhere (Hojat et al., 2001b).

Criterion-Related Validity

Criterion-related validity involves an examination of the correlations between the test scores and selected criterion measures. One approach to criterion-related validation is to demonstrate significant correlations between scores on the scale and conceptually relevant variables (convergent validity) accompanied by nonsignificant correlations with conceptually irrelevant measures (discriminant validity). Convergent and discriminant validities are concepts derived from the method of Campbell and Fiske (1959), initially used in their analysis of the multitrait–multimethod matrix of correlations to describe a pattern of higher relationships among conceptually more relevant variables (convergent validity) than among conceptually less relevant variables (discriminant validity) in different methods of assessment.

We included the criterion measures listed in Box 7.1 in a questionnaire to examine the criterion-related validity of the generic version of the JSPE. Measures 1–6 were available for both medical students and residents. The remaining 10 measures of personal attributes (Items 7–16) were defined on the questionnaire and were answered on a 100-point scale. Respondents were asked to place a mark on the scale to identify the extent to which they perceived themselves as having each particular personal attribute.

The Pearson correlation coefficients between the JSPE and all 16 criterion measures (in the box) are reported in Table 7.2. The correlations between the JSPE scores and the scores for the IRI's Empathic Concern subscale were

Box 7.1 Criterion measures used for the validity study

1. *Empathic concern.* A subscale of the Interpersonal Reactivity Index (IRI) (Davis, 1983) (see Chapter 5).
2. *Perspective taking.* A subscale of the IRI.
3. *Fantasy scale.* A subscale of the IRI.
4. *Warmth.* A facet of personality (8 items) from the revised version of the NEO Personality Inventory (NEO PI-R©), a widely used instrument measuring the big five personality factors and their facets (Costa & McCrea, 1992). The inventory has been used in the United States with samples of both physicians and members of the general population. Physicians scored higher than the general population on Warmth (Hojat et al., 1999a). Also, positive female role models in medicine scored higher than the general population on this facet of personality (Magee & Hojat, 1998).
5. *Dutifulness.* A facet of personality from the NEO PI-R © (8 items). Both male and female positive role models in medicine scored higher than the general population on this facet (Magee & Hojat, 1998).
6. *Faith-in-people scale.* This scale was developed by Rosenberg (1957, 1965) and contains 5 items measuring one's degree of confidence in the trustworthiness of people (Robinson, 1978). A typical item is "Most people are inclined to help others."
7. *Global empathy.* Defined as "Standing in the patient's shoes in the experience of the illness."
8. *Global sympathy.* Defined as "Developing feelings for the patient's sufferings."
9. *Global compassion.* Defined as "Sympathy for the patient combined with the intention of doing good and a desire to help."
10. *Trust.* Defined as "Belief that patients report their illness experience honestly."
11. *Tolerance.* Defined as "The ability to evaluate a patient who shows offensive and self-destructive behavior without becoming judgmental or losing interest in helping."
12. *Personal growth (through interaction with the patient).* Defined as "Learning and gaining reward through emotionally intense (either positive or negative) interactions with patients."
13. *Communication (of the understanding).* Defined as "The capacity to reflect patient's emotions by providing some statements which validate the patient's feelings."
14. *Self-protection.* Defined as "Protecting one's self from being overwhelmed by patients' emotions and/or suffering."
15. *Humor.* Defined as "Ability to laugh with the patients about human foibles and absurdities related to their illness and treatment, as well as to appropriate jokes and lighter topics unrelated to illness."
16. *Clinical neutrality.* Defined as "Controlling expressions of emotional reactions to patients, whether their reactions are positive or negative."

Table 7.2 Correlations of scores of the generic version of the JSPE with criterion measures

Criterion measures	Residents ($n = 41$)	Medical students ($n = 193$)
IRI scales[a]		
Empathic concern		0.41**
Perspective taking		0.29**
Fantasy		0.24**
Self-report (7-point scale)[b]		
Compassion	0.56**	0.48**
Sympathy	0.27***	0.33**
NEO PI-R personality facets[c]		
Warmth[c]	NA	0.33**
Dutifulness[c]	NA	0.24**
Faith-in-people (misanthropy)[d]	NA	0.12***
Self-report (100-point scale)[e]		
Empathy	NA	0.45**
Compassion	NA	0.31**
Trust	NA	0.27**
Sympathy	NA	0.26**
Tolerance	NA	0.25**
Personal growth	NA	0.15*
Communication	NA	0.13***
Self protection	NA	0.11
Humor	NA	0.05
Clinical neutrality	NA	−0.05

* $p < 0.05$. ** $p < 0.01$. *** $p < 0.10$.
[a] Scales from the Interpersonal Reactivity Index (Davis, 1983).
[b] Single items.
[c] Personality facets from the NEO PI-R © (Costa & McCrea, 1992).
[d] Faith-in-People Scale (Rosenberg, 1957, 1965).
[e] Self-reported personal attributes on a 100-point scale.
NA: Data were not available.

moderate. The correlations were lower, although statistically significant, for the other two IRI subscales: Perspective Taking and Fantasy (we did not use the IRI Personal Distress subscale for two reasons: We wanted to reduce the length of the questionnaire and increase the response rate, and we thought the subscale was less applicable to patient-care situations).

Although statistically significant, the correlations between the JSPE scores and conceptually relevant variables, such as compassion, warmth, dutifulness, faith-in-people, trust, tolerance, personal growth, and communication, were not large in magnitude—possibly the result of the low reliability of the single items used as criteria. However, the fact that all these conceptually relevant criteria yielded positive and statistically significant correlations with JSPE scores is consistent with our expectations, thus providing support for the scale's "convergent" validity. Conversely, a lack of significant relationships between scores on the JSPE and on personal attributes that seemed conceptually irrelevant to empathy (e.g., self-protection and clinical neutrality: Items 14 and 16) supports the scale's "discriminant" validity.

Sympathy (Item 8) overlapped with the JSPE scores to a limited degree, with correlations ranging from 0.26 to 0.33 (see Table 7.2). Self-reported empathy and compassion (Items 7 and 9) yielded the highest correlations with the JSPE scores, with correlations ranging from 0.31 to 0.56 (see Table 7.2). These correlations provide evidence supporting the criterion-related validity of the JSPE. (Details of these analyses are reported elsewhere; Hojat et al., 2001b.)

The moderate magnitude of the correlations with the criterion measures in our studies suggests that empathy can be regarded as a distinct personal attribute with a statistically significant but practically limited overlap with compassion, concern, sympathy, perspective taking, imagination, warmth, dutifulness, tolerance, personal growth, trust, and communication.

Internal Consistency Reliability

The reliability of an instrument is an indication of the precision and stability of responses in a single testing situation (internal consistency) or in multiple testing situations (score stability). We studied the internal consistency of the JSPE's reliability by calculating Cronbach's coefficient alpha (Cronbach, 1951). The coefficient obtained was 0.89 for the sample of medical students and 0.87 for the sample of residents (Hojat et al., 2001b). Reliability coefficients of this magnitude are desirable for educational and psychological instruments (Anastasi, 1976).

Revisions to Develop the Health Professional and Student Versions

Because the generic version of the JSPE was originally developed to measure medical students' orientations or attitudes toward empathic relationships in the context of patient care, our research team decided to modify the scale slightly so that two versions would be available: one version applicable to physicians and other health professionals (the HP-Version; see Appendix A); the other version applicable to students in medical and other health professions (the S-Version; see Appendix B).

The HP-Version was to be geared more to the clinician's empathic behavior in patient encounters, and the S-Version was to reflect students' orientation or attitudes toward empathy in patient care. For example, the item in the S-Version reading, "Because people are different, it is almost impossible for physicians to see things from their patients' perspectives," was modified as follows in the HP-Version: "Because people are different, it is almost impossible to see things from my patients' perspectives." The modifications also were intended to make the JSPE applicable to practitioners in other health professions as well as to physicians (Hojat et al., 2002e).

Revisions to Balance Positively and Negatively Worded Items

There were only three negatively worded items (reverse scored) in the generic version of the JSPE. Negatively worded items are usually used in psychological or personality tests to reduce the confounding effect of a response pattern known as the "acquiescence response style"—a tendency to agree or disagree constantly with the statements used as test items. (In the sociopolitical context, these people are called "yeasayers" or "naysayers.")

In the modified version, a balance was maintained by making 10 items positively worded and the other 10 negatively worded. The positively worded items were directly scored according to their Likert weights (1=Strongly disagree, 7= Strongly agree), whereas the negatively worded items were reverse scored (1=Strongly agree, 7=Strongly disagree).

Revisions to Improve Clarity for an International Audience

Minor revisions also were made in the wording of a few items to improve their clarity for international audiences. For example, while researchers in Italy and Mexico were translating the JSPE into Italian and Spanish, a question arose about the verbatim translation of the verb "touch" in the following item: "I do not allow myself to be touched by intense emotional relationships between my patients and their family members" (a negatively worded item). The symbolic meaning of "to be touched by" (to be affected or influenced by) was not apparent in the translated versions. Therefore, we revised this item by substituting "to be influenced" for "to be touched" to avoid confusion in translations into foreign languages.

Comparisons of the Generic, Health Professional, and Student Versions

To study the effects of our modifications and revisions on the JSPE, we administered the generic version and the HP-Version to a group of 42 residents in internal medicine by using a cross-over design so that half the residents completed the HP-Version first and then the generic version, and the other half completed the two versions in the reverse order. The correlation between scores on the two versions was 0.85 ($p < 0.01$). We noticed an extremely slight nonsignificant trend toward improvement in the Cronbach's coefficient alpha reliability estimate of the HP-Version (an increase from 0.81 to 0.85). No significant change occurred in the descriptive statistics of the two versions. For example, the mean score on the generic version was 120.9 (SD = 10.1), and it was 120.2 (SD = 10.7) for the HP-Version (Hojat et al., 2003b). Recently collected data on medical students using the S-Version showed descriptive statistics that were similar to those reported in Table 7.2 on medical students using the generic version.

Two studies were conducted to examine the descriptive statistics and psychometric characteristics of the HP- and S-Versions. In the first study, we examined the psychometric properties of the HP-Version; in the second study, we investigated the psychometric properties of the S-Version.

Psychometric Properties of the Health Professional Version

To study the psychometric and other aspects of the HP-Version, we mailed the scale to 1,007 physicians in the Jefferson Health System, affiliated with Thomas Jefferson University Hospital and Jefferson Medical College in the greater Philadelphia area (postage-paid return envelopes were provided). After two follow-up reminders, 704 physicians completed and returned the questionnaire, a response rate of 70% (Hojat et al., 2002e). A response rate of 70% is considerably higher than the typical rate of 52% reported for surveys mailed to physicians (Cummings, Savitz, & Konrad, 2001). However, some researchers have suggested that a response rate of at least 75% should be achieved for surveys mailed to professionals to ensure the representativeness of the sample (Gough & Hall, 1977). A comparison of respondents and nonrespondents failed to show any significant differences between the two groups with regard to the distribution of their specialties, providing support for the representativeness of the study sample (Hojat et al., 2002e).

To study the stability of scores on the HP-Version over time (test–retest reliability), 100 physicians who had completed the HP-Version were selected at random to receive a second copy of the scale plus a letter thanking them for their participation and requesting that they complete the second copy of the scale to help us establish the scale's reliability. Seventy-one physicians responded, and their scores on the two tests were correlated. The exact time interval between completion of the two tests could not be determined accurately because we did not ask physicians to specify the date on which they completed the survey. However, by examining the postmarks, we were able to reach a rough estimate of approximately 3–4 months as the testing interval. The test–retest reliability was 0.65 ($p < 0.01$) (Hojat et al., 2002e).

Underlying Components (Factors)

When we conducted an exploratory factor analysis to investigate the underlying components of the HP-Version, three factors with eigenvalues greater than 1 emerged (4.2, 1.5, and 1.3), accounting for 21, 8, and 7% of the total variance, respectively (Hojat et al., 2002e). The factor coefficients, the magnitudes of eigenvalues, and the proportions of variance are reported in Table 7.3. The 10 positively worded items had factor coefficients greater than 0.40 on Factor 1 (shown in bold). This factor can be regarded as the grand component of the JSPE, as the magnitude of its eigenvalue indicates. On the basis of the contents of items with high factor coefficients, the first factor can be titled "Perspective Taking," a component of the JSPE that has been described as the core cognitive ingredient of empathy (Davis, 1994; Spiro et al., 1993). This major component is similar to the grand factor of "Physician's View of What the Patient's Perspective Is" that emerged in the generic version.

Factor 2 included 8 of the negatively worded items with factor coefficients higher than 0.35. This factor can be regarded as a construct involving "Compassionate Care" according to the contents of the items (the positive pole of the contents of the items that were negatively worded but reverse scored). Conceptually, this construct is similar to the two factors that emerged in the generic version of the JSPE: "Emotions in Patient Care" and "Understanding Patient's Experiences, Feelings, and Clues."

Finally, Factor 3 included two other negatively worded items with high factor coefficients that can be called "Standing in the Patient's Shoes" (the positive pole of the contents of the negatively worded but reverse scored items). This is a trivial component that is similar to the factor "Thinking Like the Patient," which emerged in the generic version.

These findings suggest that the factor structure of the JSPE is consistent with the notion of the multidimensionality of empathy (Davis, 1983, 1994; Kunyk & Olson, 2001). In addition, the stability of the similarity between the factor structure and components across different samples (medical students and physicians) and across different versions (generic and revised) provides further support for the JSPE's construct validity (Hojat et al., 2002e).

Item Characteristics and the Item–Total Score Correlations

The mean item scores on the HP-Version ranged from a low of 4.8 to a high of 6.5 on the 7-point scale (Hojat et al., 2002c). This finding suggests that

Table 7.3 Rotated factor loadings of items in the HP-Version of the JSPE[a]

Items	Factors		
	1	2	3
1. An important component of the relationship with my patients is my understanding of the emotional status of the patients and their families.	**0.70**	0.21	−0.08
2. I try to understand what is going on in my patients' minds by paying attention to their nonverbal cues and body language.	**0.62**	0.06	0.23
3. I believe that empathy is an important therapeutic factor in medical treatment.	**0.60**	0.28	−0.25
4. Empathy is a therapeutic skill without which my success as a physician would be limited.	**0.58**	0.22	−0.16
5. My understanding of my patients' feelings gives them a sense of validation that is therapeutic in its own right.	**0.58**	0.32	0.03
6. My patients feel better when I understand their feelings.	**0.50**	−0.02	0.16
7. I consider understanding my patients' body language as important as verbal communication in physician–patient relationships.	**0.48**	−0.18	0.30
8. I try to imagine myself in my patients' shoes when providing care to them.	**0.46**	0.29	0.28
9. I have a good sense of humor, which I think contributes to a better clinical outcome.	**0.45**	−0.02	0.14
10. I try to think like my patients in order to render better care.	**0.46**	0.20	0.25
11. Patients' illnesses can be cured only by medical treatment; therefore, affectional ties to my patients cannot have a significant place in this endeavor.	0.17	**0.60**	−0.01
12. Attentiveness to my patients' personal experiences is irrelevant to treatment effectiveness.	0.07	**0.59**	0.07
13. I try not to pay attention to my patients' emotions in interviewing and history taking.	0.02	**0.54**	0.02
14. I believe that emotion has no place in the treatment of medical illness.	0.22	**0.50**	−0.03
15. I do not allow myself to be touched by intense emotional relationships between my patients and their family members.	0.13	**0.44**	0.26
16. My understanding of how my patients and their families feel is an irrelevant factor in medical treatment.	−0.03	**0.43**	0.14
17. I do not enjoy reading nonmedical literature and the arts.	0.05	**0.37**	0.13
18. I consider asking patients about what is happening in their lives as an unimportant factor in understanding their physical complaints.	0.10	**0.37**	−0.12

(*continued*)

Table 7.3 (*Continued*)

Items	Factors		
	1	2	3
19. It is difficult for me to view things from my patients' perspectives.	0.10	0.05	**0.74**
20. Because people are different, it is almost impossible for me to see things from my patients' perspectives.	0.17	0.20	**0.66**
Eigenvalues	4.2	1.5	1.3
Variance	21%	8%	7%

[a]Items are listed based on the descending order of the magnitude of the factor structure coefficients within each factor. Values greater than 0.35 are in boldface. Responses were based on a 7-point Likert-type scale. Responses were reverse scored on items 11–20 (Strongly agree = 1, Strongly disagree = 7); otherwise, items were directly scored (Strongly agree = 7, Strongly disagree = 1).

the physicians' responses to the items tended to be skewed toward the upper tail of the scale although the distribution of their responses showed that the physicians actually used the full range of possible responses on all items. The standard deviations for the items ranged from 0.9 to 1.6 (Hojat et al., 2002c).

The two items with the highest mean scores (6.5), both of them negatively worded and reverse scored, were "My understanding of how my patients and their families feel is an irrelevant factor in medical treatment" and "I believe that emotion has no place in the treatment of medical illness." The item with the lowest mean score (4.8) was "I try to think like my patient in order to render better care."

The item–total score correlations were all positive and statistically significant ($p < .01$), ranging from 0.30 to 0.60 with a median correlation of 0.43. Two items with the highest item-total score correlations ($r = 0.60$) were "I try to imagine myself in my patients' shoes when providing care to them" and "My understanding of my patients' feelings gives me a sense of validation that is therapeutic in its own right." Two items with the lowest item–total score correlations ($r = 0.30$) were "I do not enjoy reading nonmedical literature" (negatively worded, reverse-scored item) and "My understanding of how my patients and their families feel is an irrelevant factor in my medical treatment" (reverse scored) (Hojat et al., 2002c). The findings support the correct direction of scoring of the items and each item's significant contribution to the total JSPE score.

Descriptive Statistics and Reliability

The descriptive statistics and the distribution of scores for the HP-Version are reported in Table 7.4. Also, the internal consistency aspect of reliability (the coefficient alpha) was 0.81 for the sample of physicians, and the test–retest reliability coefficient was 0.65 (Hojat et al., 2002d). The reliability coefficients indicate that the HP-Version is internally consistent and its scores are relatively stable over time (see Table 7.4).

It would be desirable to develop norms based on representative national samples of physicians for comparative purposes or for evaluation of each individual physician's score (e.g., a female physician practicing family

Table 7.4 Score distributions, percentiles, and descriptive statistics for the HP-Version of the JSPE ($n = 704$ physicians)

Score interval	Frequency	Cumulative frequency	Cumulative percentage
≤ 75	3	3	<1
76–80	3	6	1
81–85	2	8	1
86–90	3	11	2
91–95	13	24	3
96–100	21	45	6
101–105	31	76	11
106–110	57	133	19
111–115	97	230	33
116–120	111	341	48
121–125	114	455	65
126–130	126	581	83
131–135	85	666	95
136–140	38	704	100
Mean		120	
Standard deviation		11.9	
25th percentile		113	
50th percentile (median)		121	
75th percentile		128	
Possible range		20–140	
Actual range		50–140	
Alpha reliability estimate		0.81	
Test–retest reliability[a]		0.65	

[a] Test–retest reliability is calculated for 71 physicians within an interval of approximately 3–4 months between testing.

medicine) against the norm (e.g., percentile ranks) derived from a corresponding national sample (e.g., a national sample of female physicians in family medicine). Obviously, the data reported in Table 7.4 cannot serve that purpose.

Psychometric Properties of the Student-Version

We collected data from 685 first-year students at Jefferson Medical College (those who had matriculated in 2002, 2003, or 2004). Because the patterns of statistical findings were similar when we analyzed the data for each class separately, the data for all three classes were combined for the final statistical analyses.

The mean item scores ranged from a low of 4.57 to a high of 6.63 on the 7-point scale, and the standard deviations ranged from 0.78 to 1.45. All the item–total score correlations were positive and statistically significant ($p < 0.01$), ranging from a low of 0.30 for "Because people are different, it is difficult to see things from patients' perspectives" to a high of 0.66 for "Physicians' understanding of the emotional status of their patients, as well as that of their families, is one important component of the physician–patient relationship." The median item–total score correlation was 0.50. Descriptive statistics and reliability coefficients for the S-Version are reported in Table 7.5.

It would be desirable to develop norm tables based on samples of medical students from different medical schools for comparative purposes or for evaluation of an individual student's score against a national norm (e.g., percentile rank). Needless to say, the data reported in Table 7.5 cannot serve that purpose.

Other Indicators of Validity

The "Contrasted Groups" Method

Other indicators that support the validity of both the S- and HP-Versions of the JSPE are based on the notion that a measuring instrument is valid when it can demonstrate group differences or relationships in the expected direction. The expectations are based on previous research, theories, and behavioral tendencies described in the literature. This approach, in which different groups are compared to examine whether the differences in their scores are in the expected direction, is known as validation by the method of "contrasted groups" (Anastasi, 1976). For example, in a majority of studies, women scored higher than men did on measures of empathy (see Chapter 9). Some authors have suggested that women's behavioral style is generally more

Table 7.5 Distributions, percentiles, and descriptive statistics for the S-Version of the JSPE ($N = 685$ medical students)

Score interval	Frequency	Cumulative frequency	Cumulative percentage
≤75	1	1	<1
76–80	1	2	<1
81–85	3	5	1
86–90	4	9	1
91–95	16	25	5
96–100	34	59	8
101–105	61	120	17
106–110	109	229	19
111–115	120	349	33
116–120	130	479	70
121–125	102	581	85
126–130	76	657	96
131–135	24	681	99
136–140	4	685	100
Mean		115	
Standard deviation		10	
25th percentile		108	
50th percentile (median)		115	
75th percentile		122	
Possible range		20–140	
Actual range		75–140	
Alpha reliability estimate		0.80	

"empathizing" than men's style is (Baron-Cohen, 2003). Thus, we expected to find a sex difference in favor of women in scores on both versions of the JSPE. Empirical confirmation of this expectation could be regarded as an indicator of the JSPE's validity. In our studies, female medical students and practicing physicians consistently obtained significantly higher mean scores than male students and physicians did (Hojat et al., 2001b, 2002c, 2002e).

In addition, we expected that physicians who chose to practice in people-oriented specialties, such as family medicine, internal medicine, and pediatrics, would score higher on the HP-Version than would physicians in technology- or procedure-oriented and hospital-based specialties, such as surgery, pathology, radiology, and anesthesiology. The results of our studies confirmed this expectation (Hojat et al., 2002c, 2002e) (sex, medical specialty, and empathy are discussed in more detail in Chapter 9).

In another study with the first-year medical students (Hojat et al., 2005b) we found that high scores on the JSPE were associated with students' plan to pursue people-oriented (as opposed to procedure-oriented) specialties after graduation from medical school. However, in his master's thesis, Smolarz (2005) did not find a significant difference in the JSPE scores between first-year medical students who majored science and non-science disciplines as undergraduates.

Relationships With Relevant Measures

In a study with medical students (Hojat et al., 2005b) we found that the scores on the JSPE were significantly and positively correlated with "Sociability" scores measured by the short form of the Zuckerman–Kuhlman Personality Questionnaire (ZKPQ) (Zuckerman, 2002). We also obtained a significant but negative correlation between the scores on the JSPE and the "Aggressive-Hostility" subscale of the ZKPQ. Furthermore, higher levels of self-reported satisfaction with the early maternal relationship were significantly associated with higher scores on the JSPE (Hojat et al., 2005b).

In a study of pharmacists that was the subject of his doctoral dissertation, Reisetter (2003) reported significant correlations between JSPE factor scores and subscale scores of the Physician Belief Scale (PBS) (Ashworth, Williamson, & Montano, 1984; McLellan, Jansen-McWilliams, Comer, Gardner, & Kelleher, 1999). For example, the correlation between the "Compassionate Care" factor scores of the JSPE and the "Belief and Feeling" subscale of the PBS (defined as the clinician's concern about his or her ability to address the client's psychosocial problems) was $r = 0.50$. A negative correlation ($r = -0.30$) was found between the JSPE "Standing in the Patient's Shoes" factor scores and the PBS "Burden" subscale (defined as the difficulties perceived by the clinician in addressing the client's psychosocial problems).

In a sample of dental students at the University of Washington School of Dentistry, Sherman and Cramer (2005) found positive and significant correlations between scores on the JSPE and 18 of 26 measures of attitudes toward clinical competencies. The highest correlation was found between JSPE scores and ratings of the following clinical competency: "application of the principles of behavioral sciences that pertain to patient-centered oral health care" ($r = 0.52$). The reliability coefficient alpha for the JSPE in Sherman and Cramer's study was 0.90, and the scale's factor structure was similar to that reported for medical students and physicians (Hojat et al., 2001b, 2002d).

Correlations Between Scores on the JSPE and the IRI

During the development of the generic version of the JSPE, we examined the correlations between scores on the JSPE and scores on the IRI, which has been widely used to measure empathy in the general population.

We obtained modest relationships between scores on the two instruments among medical students (Hojat et al., 2001b). In another study involving 93 residents in internal medicine at Thomas Jefferson University Hospital, we examined the relationships between total scores and factor scores (Perspective Taking, Compassionate Care, and Standing in the Patient's Shoes) on the HP-Version and the IRI total and subscale scores (Perspective Taking, Empathic Concern, Fantasy, and Personal Distress) (Hojat, Mangione, Kane, & Gonnella, 2005a). One study found that the Perspective Taking and Empathic Concern subscales of the IRI were likely to measure empathy, whereas the Personal Distress and Fantasy subscales were likely to measure sympathy (Yarnold, Bryant, Nightingale, & Martin, 1996). We assumed that the IRI's Perspective Taking and Empathic Concern subscales were more relevant to the clinician–patient relationship than were the Personal Distress and Fantasy subscales. Therefore, we expected significant but moderate correlations between the JSPE total and factor scores and scores on the IRI total and its Perspective Taking and Empathic Concern subscales. Conversely, we expected to obtain trivial correlations between scores on the JSPE (and its factors) and scores on the IRI's Personal Distress and Fantasy subscales. A summary of the results are reported in Table 7.6.

As expected, the correlations between scores on the IRI Personal Distress subscale and total and factor scores on the JSPE were all nonsignificant. Scores on the IRI Fantasy subscale yielded modest correlations with scores on the JSPE's Perspective Taking and Compassionate Care subscales ($r = 0.24$, $p < 0.05$, and $r = 0.37$, $p < 0.01$, respectively). The highest correlations were found between the scores on the IRI Empathic Concern subscale and the JSPE Compassionate Care and Perspective Taking factors ($r = 0.41$, $p < 0.01$, and $r = 0.40$, $p < 0.01$, respectively). The correlation between the scores on the perspective-taking dimensions of both instruments was

Table 7.6 Correlations between scores on the JSPE and the IRI ($N = 93$ first-year internal medicine residents)

IRI subscales	JSPE factors			
	Perspective taking	Compassionate care	Standing in patient's shoes	Total score
Perspective taking	0.35**	0.31**	0.17	0.40**
Empathic concern	0.40**	0.41**	0.16	0.48**
Fantasy	0.24*	0.37**	0.12	0.35**
Personal distress	0.01	0.02	0.13	0.02
Total score	0.34**	0.40**	0.22*	0.45**

*$p < 0.05$. **$p < 0.01$.

$r = 0.35$ ($p < 0.01$), and the correlation between the total scores on the two instruments was $r = 0.45$ ($p < 0.01$).

Therefore, our expectation was confirmed regarding significant correlations of moderate magnitude between total and factor scores on the JSPE and scores on the Perspective Taking and Empathic Concern subscales of the IRI. Our prediction concerning the relationship between JSPE factor scores and the IRI Fantasy subscale scores was partially confirmed. Furthermore, our prediction about the lack of relationship between the scores on the JSPE and the scores on the IRI Personal Distress subscale was correct (Hojat et al., 2005a). Perspective Taking and Empathic Concern seem to emerge from an altruistic motivation, whereas Personal Distress seems to emerge from an egoistic motivation to reduce one's own distress rather than to help others to reduce their stresses. These findings provide further evidence in support of the JSPE's validity.

Relationship Between Scores on JSPE and Academic Performance

We expected to find a positive and significant relationship between medical students' scores on the S-Version of the JSPE and global ratings of their clinical competence in core clinical clerkships. The reason for this expectation was that an ability to communicate with patients and understand their concerns is often considered when assessing global clinical competence. Our expectation was confirmed in a study with third-year medical students in which we found that students with higher scores on the S-Version obtained better ratings of clinical competence than did classmates with lower empathy scores (Hojat et al., 2002a).

The lack of convincing evidence precluded a hypothesis that performance on objective (multiple-choice) tests of academic knowledge should be associated with empathy scores. Therefore, we did not expect such an association and, indeed, did not find one (Hojat et al., 2002a). Our findings were consistent with those of other researchers (Diseker & Michielutte., 1981; Hornblow, Kidson, & Jones, 1977; Kupfer, Drew, Curtis, & Rubinstein, 1978).

Administration and Scoring

Both versions of the JSPE can be administered either individually or in groups. Half the items are directly scored according to their Likert weights (1 = Strongly disagree, 7 = Strongly agree) and the other half are reverse scored (1 = Strongly agree, 7 = Strongly disagree). We recommend that if a respondent fails to answer more than 20% of the items (4 items), the scale should be regarded as incomplete and be excluded from the data analysis. In the case of a respondent with four or fewer unanswered items, we recommend replacing each missing value with the mean score calculated from items completed by the respondent. The scale is "untimed" and takes approximately 5–10 minutes to complete. We do not recommend a time limit for completing the scale.

The HP-Version (Appendix A) and S-Version (Appendix B) can be administered to physicians and medical students, respectively, without any modifications. However, the word "physician" in 13 items of the S-Version (Items 1–5, 9–11, 13, and 15–18) must be replaced with an appropriate title (e.g., nurse or therapist) for students in other health professions. Such modification does not appear to be necessary in the HP-Version if used with health professionals other than physicians.

I must emphasize that the psychometric evidence reported in this chapter is based primarily on data obtained from medical students, practicing physicians, and a small sample of nurses. We plan to examine the JSPE's psychometric characteristics with a broader audience by conducting large-scale studies with representative samples of students and practitioners in other health professions. Although researchers are welcome to use the scale with students and practitioners in other health professions, they must be cautious when interpreting the results and be prudent when examining the psychometric characteristics of the instrument in their own research samples.

A Brief Scale to Measure Patients' Perceptions of Physicians' Empathy

To investigate the relationship between physicians' self-report scores on the JSPE and their patients' perceptions, we developed a brief scale to measure patients' perceptions of physicians' empathic behavior and concerns. Patients complete the Jefferson Scale of Patient's Perceptions of Physician Empathy (JSPPPE) (Appendix C) to assess their physician's empathy.

The patient's perception scale contains five brief items that patients can answer in a few minutes after the encounter with the physician. For example, a physician's concern regarding a patient and the patient's family is reflected in the following item: "This physician seems concerned about me and my family." The physician's perspective taking is reflected by the following item: "This physician can view things from my perspective (see things as I see them)." In a study conducted by Kane and colleagues with residents in an internal medicine program (Kane, Gotto, Mangione, West, & Hojat, 2005) and in another study by Glaser and colleagues with residents in a family medicine program (Glaser, Markham, Adler, McManus, & Hojat, 2005), scores on this scale correlated significantly with selected items from the Physicians' Humanistic Behaviors Questionnaire developed by Weaver, Ow, Walker, and Degenhardt (1993) and also with selected items from a questionnaire measuring patients' appraisal of physicians' performance developed by Matthews and Feinstein (1989).

In the two aforementioned preliminary studies of the JSPPPE conducted at Thomas Jefferson University Hospital, data for 225 encounters between patients and resident physicians in the internal medicine residency program (Kane et al., 2005) and 90 encounters between patients and residents in the family medicine residency program (Glaser et al., 2005) were used. Item–total score correlations were statistically significant in both departments (median correlations were 0.78 for family medicine and 0.81 for internal medicine study). The item and total scores on the JSPPPE in the Department of Internal Medicine study also yielded significant correlations with scores obtained from a rating form for patients developed by the American Board of Internal Medicine to assess physicians' communicative skills, humanistic qualities, and professionalism (Lipner, Blank, Leas, & Fortna, 2002). The median correlation between the two instruments was 0.64. The internal consistency reliabilities (coefficient alphas) of the patient perception scale were in the lower range (0.50s) probably because of the small number of items.

The correlation coefficient between patients' ratings of their physicians on the patient perception scale and the residents' self-ratings on the JSPE was 0.48 ($p < 0.05$) in the family medicine study, but it was only 0.24 (nonsignificant) in the internal medicine study. Further inspection of data for Department of Internal Medicine showed that the majority of patients (78%) gave the highest possible scores to the residents, leading to a highly skewed JSPPPE score distribution with a restricted range of scores. This serious "ceiling effect" would not allow the correlation between residents' self-reported empathy and patients' perceptions of residents' empathy to be fully captured. In another study, it also was found that although the relationship between physicians' self-report measures of empathy on Hogan's Empathy Scale and patients' evaluations was positive, it was statistically nonsignificant (Linn et al., 1987). A possibility exists that patients' views regarding their clinicians' empathic behavior may differ from the clinicians' views of their own empathy. Further research is needed to explore this possibility.

The link between physicians' self-reported empathy and patients' perceptions of their physicians' empathy could be strengthened by physicians' efforts to communicate their understanding to their patients (Free, Green, Grace, Chernus, & Whitman, 1985). Measuring patients' perceptions is important because research has shown that their perceptions of clinicians' empathy yield the highest correlations with clinical outcomes, followed by observers' ratings of clinicians' empathy and, finally, by clinicians' self-reported empathy (Bohart et al., 2002). Because other factors can contribute to patients' perceptions of clinicians' empathy, including the degree to which patients can cope with their illnesses (Mercer, Watt, & Reilly, 2001), more studies are needed to examine the complex reasons for patients' and clinicians' concordant and discordant views on empathic engagement in clinical encounters.

Broad National and International Attention

Subsequent to the publication of our studies using the JSPE, we received many requests from researchers in the United States and abroad for copies of the instrument and for permission to use it. As of this writing, we had received more than 200 such requests from the United States and 20 other countries. The JSPE has already been translated into 15 languages: Chilean, Dutch, German, Greek, Hebrew, Hungarian, Italian, Japanese, Korean, Norwegian, Persian, Polish, Portuguese, Spanish (Mexican), and Turkish. We strongly recommended using the back translation procedure (Brislin, 1970, 1980; Guillemin, Bombardier, & Beaton, 1993; Geisinger, 1994) in all translations to ensure that the contents of the translated versions closely match the original English version.

Interestingly, the patterns of findings we have received so far from researchers in five countries are similar to those we have reported for samples in the United States. These researchers are Adelina Alcortal Gonzalez, M.D., Ph.D., in Mexico; Americo Cicchetti, Ph.D., Alessandra LoScalzo, Ph.D., and Francesco Taroni, M.D., in Italy; Reza Shapurian, Ph.D., Roya Shapourian, M.D., and Reza Roshanpajouh, M.D., in Iran; Shmuel Eidelman, M.D., in Israel; Joanna Kliszez, Ph.D., in Poland; Gabi Stummer, Ph.D., in Germany; and Dr. Aysegul Yildirim and Dr. Olzem Malkondu in Turkey.

Because of the increasing national and international attention the JSPE is receiving, we decided to develop a data bank for occasional meta-analytic studies that would contain JSPE data collected by different researchers from different samples in different countries. Researchers who are willing to share their data with us will be included in the study and will receive credit for their participation. We hope that in the future, a large and valuable central data bank will be available for meta-analytic and comparative studies of empathy in patient care in the Center for Research in Medical Education and Health Care at Jefferson Medical College.

To assure integrity in scoring and statistical analyses, we have developed scannable forms of both versions of the JSPE that can be used by researchers and can be processed at our center for scoring and other statistical analyses and for possible inclusion in our empathy project data bank if the researchers involved give their permission (information is posted at http://www.tju.edu/jmc/crmehc/medu/oempathy.cfm). Web-based administration of the scale is also available.

Two Caveats

Attitudes, Orientation, Capacity, and Behavior

When we submitted manuscripts describing the results of our empathy studies to peer-reviewed journals, a few reviewers expressed a legitimate concern about the link between physicians' scores on the JSPE and their actual empathic behavior. If one assumes that the physicians' scores on the JSPE indeed reflect their own attitude or orientation toward empathy in physician–patient relationships, and not necessarily their empathic behavior, a convincing argument plus empirical data are needed to establish a link between attitudes and behavior.

Although social psychologists have long debated the link between attitude and behavior, the issue has not been completely settled yet (for a meta-analytic review, see Wallace, Paulson, Lord, & Bond, 2005). When people have formed an attitude or an orientation toward a subject, they are no longer neutral about that subject. In other words, they are likely to take a stand or develop a behavioral tendency consistent with their attitude or orientation (Sherif, Sherif, & Nebergall, 1965). Attitude, orientation, and perception share common cognitive and neural elements that can activate relevant behavior (Prinz, 1997; Vivian, 2002).

A concordance between an attitude and behavior is necessary to avoid an unpleasant psychological tension that resembles "cognitive dissonance" (Festinger, 1964), which occurs when a person is caught in a cognitive struggle between opposing motivational forces. Attitudes often generate strong emotions (affective components) and form a cognitive orientation (cognitive components) leading to preferences that ultimately elicit actions (behavioral components) (Rosenberg & Hovland, 1960). Therefore, attitudes, orientations, beliefs, and intentions are all motivating forces that can elicit corresponding behaviors (Fishbein & Ajzen, 1975). For example, acculturation studies have reported that attitudinal changes, even in relation to deeply rooted social institutions, such as marriage and the family, can lead to tangible behavioral changes, such as increased rates of marital discord and divorce (Hojat, Shapurian, Foroughi, Nayerahmadi, Farzaneh, et al., 2000; Hojat, Shapurian, Nayerahmadi, Farzaneh, Foroughi, et al., 1999). An abundance of empirical studies have been published about hostile or hateful behaviors resulting from prejudicial attitudes toward members of the opposite sex and toward racial, ethnic, and religious groups. For corroborative proof of such behaviors, one only needs to consult a daily newspaper.

In a recent meta-analysis of 797 studies (Wallace et al., 2005), it was found that the mean of attitude–behavior correlations was 0.41, but the magnitude of the relationship varied, depending on social pressure and perceived difficulty. Considering that the average effect of only 0.21 was found in an analysis of more than 33,000 studies in social psychology (Richard, Bond, & Stokes-Zoota, 2003), the aforementioned attitude–behavior correlation seems impressive. These findings suggest that forming an empathic attitude, possessing the capacity to understand others, or developing a tendency or an orientation toward empathic relationships do not necessarily ensure empathic behavior. What is certain, however, is that a higher degree of empathic attitude, tendency, orientation, or capacity will increase the likelihood that these qualities will be manifested as empathic behavior under certain conditions. All measures of empathy, including the JSPE, are at best a proxy of empathic behavior. Validity evidence would indicate the extent to which these measures are predictive of actual empathic behavior and positive clinical outcomes.

Transparency and Social Desirability Response Bias

Respondents can always manipulate their answers on self-report personality tests to produce a more socially desirable result. Edwards (1957), who was the first to systematically study the "social desirability phenomenon," believed that respondents were likely to be unaware of this tendency to show themselves in the most socially acceptable light.

Because some items in the JSPE are transparent and thus susceptible to social desirability response bias, they can be answered in a way that is recognized as more socially acceptable. Constructing socially neutral items that measure personal attributes, such as empathy, is difficult and raises questions about not only the face and content validities of such items but the empirical validity of the test as well. For example, the relevance to empathy of nontransparent items, such as those about an interest in literature and the arts or a sense of humor, is not necessarily apparent. Indeed, some peer reviewers who evaluated the manuscripts we submitted to professional journals questioned the reasons for including those items in the JSPE. (The reasons for including those items were discussed earlier in this chapter.)

The degree to which socially desirable responses to items have a confounding effect on test scores could be a function of the test taker's belief in testing outcomes. For example, when testing is used to screen applicants for employment or college admission, test takers may be more inclined to provide socially acceptable answers to test items that will increase their advantage.

In response to concerns about the possible effect of socially desirable responses in our empathy studies, we offer three explanations. First, the JSPE has been administered in "nonpenalizing" situations where the purpose was described as research, not college admission or employment. Respondents were assured that their responses would be confidential and would be used only for research purposes approved by the Institutional Review Board's Research Ethics Committee. This assurance, in itself, could reduce respondents' tendency to give socially desirable responses.

Second, the pattern of relationships in our validity studies, particularly the convergent and discriminant validities, suggests that social desirability response bias, even if operative, did not substantially distort the expected relationships. For example, we observed that the magnitude of the correlation between the JSPE scores and a more relevant concept, such as compassion, was twice the magnitude of the correlation between JSPE scores and a less relevant concept, such as personal growth (see Table 7.2). Such a correlational pattern would be unlikely to emerge in the presence of the significant confounding effect of social desirability response bias.

Third, we conducted an empirical study to investigate the influence of faking "good responses" on JSPE scores (Hojat et al., 2005b). In that study, we administered the JSPE and other personality tests, including the ZKPQ, to 422 first-year medical students who matriculated at Jefferson Medical College. The hypothesis that social desirability would not distort the validity of the JSPE scores in nonpenalizing testing situations was tested.

The ZKPQ includes an "Infrequency" subscale that was developed to detect intentionally false responses by identifying respondents with an invalid pattern of responses (Zuckerman, 2002). Scores on this subscale can be regarded as indicators of social desirability response bias. Attempts to give socially desirable responses were determined by a cutoff score of 3, which the test's authors suggested would identify respondents whose patterns of responses were of questionable validity. An examination of the distribution of scores on this subscale indicated that less than 5% of the respondents attempted to give false "good responses" or to respond carelessly without regard for the truth (Zuckerman, 2002).

We used two approaches to examine the possible effects of social desirability response bias on the outcomes of our research on the JSPE. First, analyses of data regarding the relationship between scores on the JSPE and on psychosocial or personality measures clearly demonstrated that research outcomes remain virtually unchanged whether or not respondents who respond carelessly to the instrument are included (determined by their scores on the "Infrequency" subscale that were above the cutoff point of 3). This finding was expected because of the small proportion of respondents (3%) who scored above the cutoff point. These results also suggest that the magnitude of such descriptive statistics as the mean and median are unlikely to be inflated as a result of respondents' possible faking in nonthreatening testing conditions because of the small proportion of those who score above the cutoff point.

Second, we used the analysis of covariance (ANCOVA) method to control the effect of giving false responses on the research outcomes by using the "Infrequency" score as a covariate. Again, we noted no substantial change in the general pattern of results. These findings suggest that social desirability response bias does not distort the validity of the JSPE scores.

Our findings were consistent with the results of an earlier study on the heritability of empathy by Matthews et al. (1981), who reported that their derived index of empathy was not affected by social desirability response bias or by scores on a "good impression" scale. Two other studies reported no significant correlations between empathy scores obtained on the Emotional Empathy Scale and social desirability response bias (Mehrabian & Epstein, 1972; Mehrabian & O'Reilly, 1980). Despite these findings, the confounding effects of giving false "good responses" and attempting to present a socially acceptable image in penalizing testing situations (e.g., by applicants for college admission or employment) need to be addressed in further studies.

Recapitulation

The JSPE was developed in response to a need for a psychometrically sound instrument specifically designed to measure empathy in the context of patient care. Evidence in support of the validity and reliability of the two versions of the JSPE (student and practicing health professional versions) can add to our confidence in using this scale in studies on empathy among students and practitioners in the health professions.

8

The Interpersonal Dynamics in Clinician–Patient Relationships

It is difficult to hate the people with whom you empathize.

—(Walter Stephan & Krystina Finlay, 1999, p. 736)

By far, the most frequently used drug in general practice was the doctor. It was not only the bottle of medicine or the box of pills that mattered, but the way doctor gave them.

—(Michael Balint, 1957, p. 1)

Preamble

In this chapter, I discuss factors that contribute to interpersonal dynamics in patient care and propose that clinicians as well as patients can benefit from empathic engagement. The curing versus caring paradigm and the concept of disease versus illness contribute to the development of attitudes that influence empathic behavior in clinical encounters. Findings regarding the tendency to bind with others for survival, comply with the orders of authority figures, and accept of authority figures uncritically; role expectations; and the effects of clinical environment on the behavior of clinicians and patients suggest that specific interpersonal dynamics operate in clinician–patient encounters. This chapter discusses important facets of interpersonal psychodynamics and their impact on empathic understanding in clinical encounters. The placebo effect of empathic relationships, cultural factors, personal space, and boundaries in clinician–patient encounters also are discussed. The chapter stresses how listening with the "third ear" and seeing with the "mind's eye" can enhance empathic understanding in the context of patient care.

Introduction

In Chapter 3, in the general context of human relationships, I described factors that contribute to the development of empathic understanding. This chapter describes the interpersonal dynamics specifically involved in clinical encounters. The way a clinician encounters patients can make a significant difference in patient outcomes. In support of this notion, Houston (1938) indicated that physicians are themselves therapeutic agents through which cures are effected. The "goodness of the physician" was viewed as a therapeutic agent by Hippocrates, who suggested in the 4th century B.C. that "the patient, though conscious that his condition is perilous, may recover his health simply through his contentment with the goodness of the physician." (cited in DiMatteo, 1979, p. 14).

The moments of understanding and connectedness in clinical encounters, according to Matthews et al. (1993, p. 973), "[are] often marked by physiological reactions such as gooseflesh or a chill; by an immediacy of awareness of the patient's situation (as if experiencing it from inside the patient's world), by a sense of being part of a larger whole; and by a lingering feeling of joy, peacefulness, or awe. Such moments seem to be therapeutic for the patient and the clinician alike."

Matthews and colleagues (1993) referred to this powerful interpersonal dynamic, which is beneficial for both clinician and patient, as a "connexion" ("co" for "being together" and "nexus" for "to form a whole") to indicate that the interpersonal dynamics in clinician–patient encounters generate a totality that is greater than the sum of its parts. The importance of empathic relationships in clinician–patient encounters has been discussed in the medical literature (Bylund & Makoul, 2002; Platt & Keller, 1994; Spiro et al., 1993; Squier, 1990; Winefield & Chur-Hansen, 2000), and the positive effect of empathy in patient outcomes has been confirmed (see Chapter 10).

In antiquity, medicine was primarily a "craft" (Lewis, 1998), and it was an art when practiced by Greek healers (many of whom were unable to read and write). Medicine was not based on the sciences (mathematics and philosophy in those days); it was based on observation, insight, tradition, and, most important, interpersonal relationships (Lewis, 1998).

As Rachel Lewinsohn (1998, p. 1268) rightly stated: "We cannot understand the disease without understanding the patient." The clinician cannot fully understand the patient without entering into the patient's world on the bridge of empathy. Empathy in patient care is bidirectional, affecting both the clinician and the patient. Because of the intrinsic reward associated with establishing a meaningful relationship with others, both clinician and patient can benefit from forming an empathic engagement. However, research attention on the beneficial effects of empathy has focused almost exclusively on the patient's side of the equation; the clinician's side has been the victim of benign neglect.

Benefits of Empathic Relationships for Clinicians

From the perspective of personal life, medicine and some other health care professions, although intrinsically self-rewarding, are stressful and often demand a life-style that restricts participation in social and family events. Such restrictions can contribute to the discontent of healers who themselves need to be healed. Despite these problems, the good news is that clinicians' satisfaction with their relationships with patients can serve as a buffer against the professional stress, burnout, substance abuse, and even suicide attempts that are reported to be unusually high among health professionals (Sullivan, 1990).

Physicians are not invincible, and research indicates that they are vulnerable to a number of psychosocial problems. For example, physicians are more than twice as likely as the general population to commit suicide (Miller & McGowen, 2000), and divorce rates also are higher among physicians than they are in the general population (Sotile & Sotile, 1996). Research indicates that physicians often do not practice what they preach to their own patients and sometimes are reluctant to seek medical help (Forsythe, Calnan, & Wall, 1999). It is important to note that Miller and McGowen (2000) found out that physicians who enjoyed the support of social networks (e.g., spouse, family, friends, and acquaintances) were less likely to abuse drugs or to suffer from burnout.

Because physicians often perceive empathic relationships with patients as meaningful interpersonal connections, those relationships can serve as a buffer against dissatisfaction with the health care system and professional burnout. Human life is lived in relationships (Lewis, 1998); thus, physician–patient relationships provide an intrinsically joyful reward that serves as a remedy for the stress of a demanding profession (Zuger, 2004). Empathy has been identified as a protective factor against the stress experienced by clinicians (Shamasundar, 1999) and as a potential factor for their well-being (Hyyppa, Kronholm, & Mattlar, 1991).

Executive physicians who treated patients expressed more satisfaction and happiness with their careers than did executive physicians who did not have an opportunity to treat patients (O'Conner, Nash, Buehler, & Bard, 2002). However, it should be mentioned that the relationship between physicians' satisfaction and number of encounters with patients is not linear after a certain saturation point; too large a patient load was likely to result in distress (Dunstone & Reames, 2001). Nonetheless, satisfactory physician–patient relationships, reinforced by empathy, can reduce professional stress and contribute positively to physicians' well-being.

Benefits of Empathic Relationships for Patients

Now let us shift our attention to the benefits that patients derive from empathic relationships with their clinicians. In clinical encounters, interpersonal communication is the primary tool for the exchange of information. A large volume of literature is devoted to the beneficial effects of clinician–patient relationships on patients' adherence to treatment regimens, satisfaction with the health care provider and the health care system, the recall and understanding of medical information, the ability to cope with the disease, improvement in quality of life, and physical, mental, and social well-being (see Chapter 10). Empirical research has shown that physicians' emotional demeanor when communicating with patients resulted in the patients' recalling less information and perceptions of more serious health condition (Shapiro, Boggs, Melamed, & Graham-Pole, 1992).

In the practice of medicine, an empathic physician–patient relationship is regarded as the royal road to optimal care. Illness cannot be understood without understanding the patient, and healing begins, not *when* medicine is administered, but *how* it is administered. In addition to a physician's knowledge and clinical skills, effective delivery of health care depends on other factors, such as the quality of clinician–patient interactions (Beisecker & Beisecker, 1990; Di Blasi, Harkness, Georgiou, & Kleijnen, 2001). It is obvious that the nature of the physician–patient relationship varies in different clinical encounters. For example, unlike chronic illnesses, which require continuous care, emergency surgical encounters are brief and thus preclude firm establishment of an empathic engagement. As indicated by Mayerson (1976), it might be difficult for a physician in an emergency room to feel empathy for an injured drunken driver who has killed a number of people in a car accident. However, by focusing on the patient's immediate needs and asking what would it be like to be in that situation, the physician may find it easier to make an empathic connection (Mayerson, 1976). Empathic understanding, however, is an important interpersonal capacity of physicians (Squier, 1990) regardless of the duration or nature of clinical encounters. Empathic engagement, according to Spiro (1998), helps healing and improves the medical practice.

Curing Versus Caring, Disease Versus Illness

In rendering treatment, two models of patient care—curing and caring—have been identified (Baumann, Deber, Silverman, & Mallette, 1998; DeValck, Bensing, Bruynooghe, & Batenburg, 2001; Spiro, 1986). In the "curing" model, the emphasis is placed on the biomedical paradigm of disease (see Chapter 6) in identifying the pathophysiology of the disease with the aim of treating the symptoms. In the "caring" model, the emphasis is placed on the biopsychosocial paradigm: The patient is viewed as a whole by focusing on the treatment of illness, not just on removal of the symptoms of disease. A disease can be detected by objective laboratory tests and microscopic examinations (as in the curing model), but detection of illness requires more than that. It is suggested that "cure is directed at disease, and care at patients" (Spiro, 1998, p. 2). The treatment of disease, according to Dr. Francis Peabody (1984), can be entirely impersonal, but the management of illness requires interpersonal attention and empathy.

Some investigators have argued that medical education and practice traditionally lean toward the curing model, whereas nursing education and practice emphasize the caring model (Baumann et al., 1998; Linn, 1974, 1975; Webb, 1996). Support for this argument is provided in a study in which nursing students were twice as likely as medical students (67% versus 33%) to agree that patients' recovery alone should not be the focal point of patient care. Significant differences in rates of agreement also were found between nursing and medical school faculty (89% and 51%, respectively) (Linn, 1975). Despite the heavy training of nurse practitioners in diagnostic and treatment procedures, their orientation toward care model was close to the nurses (Linn, 1974). It seems that in medical education more learning opportunities are provided for curing than the caring aspect of patient care. According to Spiro (1998, p. 2) "physicians learn how to *cure* but little about how to *care*."

The notion of professionalism in medical education and practice that places emphasis on the enhancement of empathy and compassionate care in the delivery of health care suggests that the curing and caring models must be integrated in the education of health professionals. Incorporating some of the educational concepts of the caring model from the nursing discipline into the curing model in medical education curricula could help to improve empathy in patient care.

For a better understanding of the nature of the curing and caring models, it is useful to distinguish between "disease" and "illness." A disease is a result of a malfunction or maladaptation of biological and pathophysiological processes that cause organ pathology, whereas an illness represents a personal reaction to the disease (Kleinman, Eisenberg, & Good, 1978; Spiro, 1986). Illness can be experienced in the absence of disease, as indicated by findings that approximately half of all visits to physicians are based on complaints that lack an ascertainable biological reason. These complaints are known as somatization disorders (Hojat et al., 1995; Kleinman et al., 1978), and patients with these disorders turn repeatedly to one physician after another, a phenomenon called "doctor shopping" (Ketterer & Buckholtz, 1989) or "doctor hopping" (Smith, 1991), because they do not experience empathic understanding from their physicians. In a survey of patients in California, 85% reported that they had changed their physicians in the past five years or were thinking of changing their physicians for reasons such as poor communication skills, the physician's inability to inspire confidence in the patient, and so forth (Moser, 1984).

It is argued that empathy in clinical encounters is cost effective because it leads to more accurate and early diagnosis, better compliance, and more efficient treatment planning, thereby avoiding doctor shopping and spiraling costs of unnecessary medical tests and hospitalizations (Bellet & Maloney, 1991; Book, 1991). In addition, a study of patients in primary care and surgical settings showed that the physician–patient visits tended to be more time consuming when physicians did not demonstrate understanding and empathy (Levinson, Gorawara-Bhat, & Lamb, 2000). Thus, an empathic physician–patient engagement can lead to the development of trust, which in turn will lead to better management of illness and containment of costs by preventing doctor shopping or hopping.

Uniqueness of Clinician–Patient Empathic Relationships

The encounter between clinician and patient is a purposeful interpersonal event, and its effectiveness in yielding positive clinical outcomes depends heavily on the clinician's skills in forming an empathic relationship, thus earning the patient's trust. A more positive patient outcome is achieved in a caring model in which clinician and patient establish a mutual understanding about the patient's health problem (Starfield et al., 1981), which has been identified as an important element of patient satisfaction with medical care (Kenny, 1995).

Being empathic is among the ingredients of the ethics of caring (Branch, 2000). The American Medical Association's first Code of Ethics, published in 1847, included the following: "The life of a sick person can be shortened not only by the acts, but also by the words or the manner of a physician. It is, therefore, a sacred duty to guard himself carefully in this respect, and to avoid all things which can have a tendency to discourage the patient and to depress his spirit" (cited in Katz, 1984, p. 20).

An empathic relationship develops when the clinician avoids being arrogant and curbs the sense of superiority and instead becomes friendly, confident, relaxed, unhurried, and capable of communicating his or her empathic understanding and genuine concerns to the patient as well as to the patient's family. Rosenow (1999) argued that physicians who are arrogant in interpersonal contacts are committing a sin that is worse than the sin of greed because arrogance interferes with the development of empathy.

The patient's need to survive, the unequal positions of the clinician and patient in clinical encounters, the atmosphere of patient care, the psychodynamics of interpersonal exchanges in seeking and giving help, and cultural factors and boundaries in patient care suggest that the clinician–patient relationship is unique compared to any other kind of human connection. The following studies provide support for the uniqueness of the clinician–patient relationship.

Bonding for Survival (the Stockholm Syndrome)

In 1973, during a bank robbery in Stockholm, Sweden, two robbers held four people hostage for 6 days. During the ordeal, the hostages developed an attachment to their captors, coming to believe that their captors were protecting them from harm by the police! After the hostages were released and the ordeal was over, one of the hostages began raising funds for the robbers' legal defense! The phenomenon of bonding with captors to reduce the fear of death is known as the "Stockholm Syndrome." Although this syndrome may seem to have no relevance to physician–patient encounters, some psychological factors are common to both situations.

First, bonding occurs in situations where a person's survival depends on the mercy of another person. Second, bonding occurs when a person perceives that the other person is not ignorant and therefore pays some attention to the person. Third, bonding occurs when a person feels isolated from other people. Fourth, bonding occurs when a person perceives that he or she is unable to escape without the help of another person.

Assuming that some or all of the psychological factors underlying the Stockholm Syndrome are present when a fearful patient consults a physician for treatment, possible hospitalization, and possible surgery, the similarity between psychological factors characterizing the syndrome and the physician–patient encounter becomes clearer.

The Clinician as an Authority Figure

In rendering help, the clinician is often perceived by the patient as an authority figure. This inequality in relation to power makes the patient more vulnerable to the clinician's influence (Koenig, 2002), which can be strengthened in the presence of empathic understanding.

Obedience to Authority (the Milgram Study)

In a well-known study of obedience conducted at Yale University, Stanley Milgram (1968) used an experimental paradigm to determine if people would be willing to comply with an authority figure's order even when compliance could have painful consequences. The study participants (who played the role of "teachers") were told they were participating in an experiment to improve learning and memory. Their task was to teach another group of participants (who played the role of "learners") a list of paired associations. The learners were supposed to recall the associated words. The teachers were instructed to administer an electric shock every time a learner made a mistake and were told the voltage would increase with each subsequent shock. The experimenter ordered the teachers to increase the intensity of the shock until a learner demanded to terminate the experiment or to continue delivering shocks as long as they liked regardless of the learner's protests. Therefore, the teachers could either comply with the experimenter's orders or refuse to comply and heed the learner's pleas. The experiment was carried out under three different conditions: (1) the teacher and learner were in adjacent rooms, and the teacher could not hear the learner's reactions to the shocks unless the learner expressed distress by pounding on the wall, (2) the teacher and learner were in adjacent rooms, but the teacher could hear the learner's reactions, and (3) the teacher and learner were in the same room. In reality, there were no actual electric shocks, and the experimenter had instructed the learners to pretend they were experiencing increased pain with each subsequent shock.

Milgram's results showed that approximately two-thirds of the teachers complied with the experimenter's orders and continued to deliver shocks up to the maximum levels although complying was stressful for them and seemingly painful for the learners! The results also indicated that teachers who could hear the learners' screams or see the learners' reactions, stopped delivering shocks earlier than did the teachers who were unaware of the learners' reactions. Milgram concluded that visual and auditory cues provided a more complete picture of another person's pain and suffering and thus could increase empathic responses. Although Milgram's research on obedience has been criticized on a number of ethical grounds, it continues to be viewed as a powerful demonstration of compliance with authority. Mehrabian and Epstein (1972) used Milgram's experimental paradigm to examine the construct validity of their Emotional Empathy Scale (see Chapter 5).

Assuming that the physician performs the role of the experimenter in Milgram's study and the patient performs the role of the research participant, the patient is psychologically set to comply with the physician's orders. As an authority figure, the physician has a profound influence on the patient's compliance with the treatment regimen even if the treatment is painful. More important, Milgram's finding that a suffering person's visual and auditory cues can enhance the empathic response in another person suggests that face-to-face clinician–patient encounters have an important advantage that cannot be replaced by any approach to patient care that precludes direct observation of the patient (e.g., computerized medical care, long-distance consultations, etc.).

Uncritical Acceptance of Authority (the Doctor Fox Lecture)

An experiment conducted by medical education researchers confirmed the influence that authority figures exerted, even on experts. Naftulin, Ware, and Donnelly (1973) hired a professional actor to deliver a lecture to an audience of 55 physicians, psychologists, social workers, educators, and medical school administrators attending a professional meeting. Introduced as "Dr. Myron L. Fox, a distinguished speaker and an authority on the application of mathematics to human performance," the actor delivered a lecture titled "Mathematical Game Theory as Applied to Physical Education."

The actor knew nothing about the subject. However, the researchers coached him on how to deliver the lecture and conduct the question-and-answer session with excessive use of double-talk, neologisms, and contradictory statements interspersed with humor and meaningless references to unrelated materials. When the researchers subsequently asked members of the audience to assess "Dr. Fox's" presentation, a large number of them highly praised the presentation!

This experiment has relevance to patients' adherence to physicians' orders and supports the notion that a physician's statements are likely to be accepted uncritically by patients, even by medically knowledgeable patients. Some have suggested that the experts' positive assessment of Dr. Fox's presentation was the result, in part, of the professional actor's nonverbal expressions when communicating information (Friedman, Prince, Riggio, & DiMatteo, 1980). This interpretation provides support for the importance of nonverbal communication in enhancing patients' trust in clinical encounters (see Chapter 3).

Role Expectations (the Stanford Prison Experiment)

The expectations of both clinician and patient can influence the process and outcome of their relationship to a significant degree. Role expectations, defined as "patterns of behavior viewed as appropriate or expected of a person who occupies a particular position" (Arnkoff, Glass, & Shapiro, 2002, p. 336), are a result of social learning and cultural factors. The interpersonal dynamics involved in role expectations were examined in a classical experiment conducted at Stanford University in the 1970s (Haney, Banks, & Zimbardo, 1973). Although the primary purpose of the experiment was to assess the power of social forces on individuals' behavior, the findings are relevant to clinician–patient encounters.

Twenty-one young healthy male college students were recruited to participate in the Stanford experiment in exchange for receiving money for each day they participated. Ten students were randomly assigned to play the role of prisoners and 11 were assigned the role of prison guards. The participants were told that the purpose was to study a simulated prison.

The mock prison was set up in a basement corridor in the university's psychology building. The prisoners and guards were dressed in different-colored uniforms to distinguish between the two groups. The researchers noticed immediately that the "prisoners" had adopted a generally passive role, and the "guards" had assumed an active role in their interactions with the prisoners.

Although it was made clear to the participants before the experiment began that no verbal abuse or physical violence would be allowed, the situation became so tense because of the guards' increasingly aggressive behavior and the prisoners' suffering that the experiment had to be terminated prematurely after only 6 days. Five prisoners suffered from extreme depression, crying, rage, or acute anxiety disorder. When the experiment had to be terminated prematurely because of the aforementioned problems, all the prisoners were delighted, but most of the guards seemed reluctant to give up their role of controlling prisoners. Although the researchers observed individual differences in the prisoners' coping behaviors and the guards' aggressive behavior, the findings generally suggest that role expectations were the determining factor in eliciting typical behaviors. An interesting observation was that the prisoners with higher empathy scores (a combined score on measures of helpfulness, sympathy, and generosity used in the study) were more resilient than other prisoners were during the adversity.

The relevance of the Stanford experiment to clinical encounters is that physicians and patients have different roles that lead to different behavioral manifestations. As an expert, the physician is often expected to play an active role, and the patient, as a person in need of help, usually plays a submissive role by complying with the physician's orders. It is interesting to note that even physicians who consult a colleague as patients are likely to adopt the patients' role by becoming more passive and less assertive. The role expectations in clinician–patient encounters are determining factors in patient outcomes (Shapiro & Shapiro, 1984; Turner, Deyo, Loeser, von Korff, & Fordyce, 1994). Needless to say, an empathic clinician–patient engagement can lead to more productive expectations.

The Effect of Environment (the Rosenhan Study)

The results of an experiment titled "On Being Sane in Insane Places" conducted by Rosenhan (1973) suggest that the environment in which a clinician encounters a patient creates specific expectations in the minds of both that influence their behavior. Rosenhan instructed a group of eight sane people (three psychologists, a psychiatrist, a pediatrician, a graduate student, a housewife, and a painter) to make appointments with physicians in different hospitals in five different states on the East and West coasts complaining that they were hearing unfamiliar voices in their heads.

All these "patients" used false names and were admitted to the hospitals' psychiatric wards. Upon admission, all the patients behaved normally but were diagnosed by hospital experts as schizophrenics "in remission" and were kept in the hospital for an average of 19 days. Interestingly, many of the hospitals' real patients were able to recognize that nothing was wrong with the study participants, telling them: "You are not crazy" or "You are a journalist or professor" (referring to the fact that the research participants were taking notes).

Rosenhan (1973) reported another experiment that was conducted at a research and teaching hospital whose staff had been aware of Rosenhan's original study and doubted that such an error could occur in their hospital. The hospital staff was informed that during the next 3 months, one or more pseudopatients would attempt to be admitted to the psychiatric ward. Staff members were asked to specify their level of confidence concerning their judgment regarding whether each patient admitted during the study period was one of the pseudopatients. Among 193 patients admitted during the period, 41 were judged to be pseudopatients with a high level of certainty by at least one staff member, and 23 patients were considered to be suspect by at least one psychiatrist. In reality, no pseudopatients were sent to the hospital during the study! Rosenhan's findings suggest that the patient-care environment creates specific expectations that may influence the dynamics of interpersonal relationships, leading to an exaggerated account of illness or an incorrect diagnosis. Needless to say, an empathic understanding is a useful defense against situational misunderstandings and can lead to more accurate diagnoses and to decisions more consistent with reality.

The Psychodynamics of Clinical Encounters

In addition to altruistic and egoistic motivational factors (Chapter 3), other psychological mechanisms can be involved in clinician–patient encounters. Because the psychological mechanisms involved in any interpersonal communication are complex, scrutinizing the psychodynamics involved in clinician–patient encounters is important to gain a better understanding of the underlying mechanisms that can enhance or impede the relationship. A few of the psychological mechanisms that function in clinical encounters are described in the following sections.

Identification

Among psychological defense mechanisms, identification is commonly associated with empathy (Berger, 1987). Freud (1955, p. 110) referred to the link "from identification by way of imitation to empathy" (cited in Szalita, 1976, p. 147). Identification is an unconscious mental process in which an individual attempts to satisfy some unmet needs by becoming like another person (Moore & Fine, 1968). To form an empathic relationship, the clinician should experience a sense of temporary oneness with the patient through a transient identification followed by a sense of separateness (Jaffe, 1986). In other words, the clinician should first think *with* the patient (identification, oneness) and then think *about* the patient (empathic separation) (Jaffe, 1986). According to Fenichel (1945), empathy consists of two acts: identification and awareness. Clinicians use the mechanism of identification to understand patients' concerns better while simultaneously becoming aware of both their own and their patients' feelings. Schwaber (1981) believed that identifying with the patient is a way of truly experiencing the patient's inner world and argued that empathy, although not equivalent to identification, occurs as an outcome of identification.

Identification may sometimes blur the boundaries between clinician and patient (Watson, 2002). Beres and Arlow (1974) proposed that empathy may involve a transient identification with another person's mental activities. In addition, they believed that empathy is mediated by communication of unconscious fantasies shared by the patient and the clinician through both verbal and nonverbal cues emanating from words, gestures, and behavior. The clinician's understanding of the mechanism of identification can facilitate forming empathic engagement with the patient.

The "Wounded Healer" Effect

Similar to the mechanism of identification, feeling similar to and sharing common characteristics with the patient can influence the empathic engagement between clinician and patient. Three decades ago, it was demonstrated that people who were led to believe that their personality and values were more like those of a "performer" empathized more with the performer who appeared to experience pleasure and pain (Krebs, 1975). According to Decety and Jackson (2004, p. 73), the sense of "self–other overlap" between the helper and the person in need of help can contribute to the enhancement of empathic understanding.

The tendency of health professionals to help those with whom they share common characteristics is described as the "wounded healer" effect (Jackson, 2001). For example, studies have shown that the therapists' own illness can constitute a source of cure for their patients (Cristy, 2001; Holmes, 1992). The notion is that a wounded healer can better understand the experiences of another wounded person by sharing common experiences, by reflection, and by validation of feelings (Laskowski & Pellicore, 2002).

Gustafson (1986) suggested that clinicians who have experienced pain are better able to understand the pain of others and to respond more appropriately. The successful resolution of psychological pain, according to Fussel and Bonney (1990), engenders empathy in the psychotherapist and influences the therapeutic process in a positive manner. Common wounds, according to Means (2002), provide a foundation for shared life experience and contribute to better understanding of patient's concerns, thus connecting clinicians with their patients. The philosophy underlying self-help programs, such as Alcoholics Anonymous, is based on the wounded healer concept. It is interesting to note that although perceived similarities between clinician and patient promote empathic understanding, patients' familiarity with their physicians does not predict empathic engagement (Makoul & Strauss, 2003). The fact that familiarity is not an important factor in empathic engagement in clinical situations suggests the unique nature of empathy in clinical encounters.

Transference

In his analysis of psychological illness, Sigmund Freud (1958a) noticed that two psychological phenomena could occur during clinician–patient encounters. One occurred in the patient (transference); the other occurred in the clinician (countertransference). These two phenomena are universal and can shape the nature of clinician–patient relationships (Goldberg, 2000). The transference often develops in the patient in relation to the clinician in ways that mimic an important relationship with a significant other (usually a primary caregiver, a parent, or even a lover) in the patient's past. Transference can be viewed as a repetition of an infantile object relationship that causes the patient to resist the treatment unless the resistance is countered appropriately by the clinician (Gabbard, 1994). Empathy plays an important role in the emergence of transference and in the development of the therapeutic alliance (Book, 1988). The importance of transference in the context of medical care, particularly in the primary care setting, has been discussed by Zinn (1990).

Because the patient unconsciously identifies the clinician with the former significant other, the patient is likely to behave *as if* the clinician is the significant other. The patient's need for understanding and reassurance, especially when experiencing illness and pain, triggers the unconscious tendency to view the clinician as an authoritative parental figure (Novack, 1987), thus increasing the likelihood of transference. The clinician is viewed in the patient's mind as the former significant other, which prompts the patient to reexperience the intense emotions associated with the relationship with the significant other in the past. According to Kohut (1959), this complex phenomenon, called transference in the psychoanalytic literature, plays an active role in the development of empathic engagement in the context of patient care. Awareness of the patient's inner world is possible not only through the senses (hearing, seeing, smelling, and touching) but also through understanding and analysis of the transference phenomenon. Empathic understanding can be enhanced if the clinician handles the phenomenon by an appropriate countertransference.

Countertransference

Transference is by no means confined to the patient. The clinician may, in response, develop mixed feelings toward the patient. The way a clinician handles the patient's transference is called countertransference. Lending oneself to becoming a wise figure to resolve the patient's past frustrations and conflicts is an example of an appropriate countertransference, which would lead to a positive patient outcome. In contrast, a clinician who projects his or her irrationalities and past unresolved conflicts onto the patient's transference relationship is an example of an inappropriate countertransference, which would lead to a negative patient outcome (Katz, 1984). According to Book (1988), countertranferential difficulties arise when the clinician uses empathy defensively to gratify his or her own psychological needs. According to Zinn (1990, p. 293), physicians bring their own "biases and emotional needs to the encounter, resulting in a dynamic interaction that ultimately shapes the outcome of the relationship." Clinicians' awareness of the transference phenomenon and their skill in handling it can empower them to make their interventions more effective even in ambulatory practice settings (Schmidt & Baker, 1986).

By handling the patient's transference properly, the clinician paves the way for an empathic engagement and becomes a secure base the patient can use to resolve past frustrations and explore options for a healthy personal and social life. Although the transference and countertransference phenomena are believed to occur in intense psychoanalytic relationships, their presence in medical consultations cannot be ruled out (Zinn, 1990).

Medical students and physicians tend to eschew probing for psychological factors during interviews with patients for fear of being unable to handle such factors properly (Smith, 1984). The presence of this fear was confirmed in a study with medical students, the great majority of whom expressed feelings of being unable to handle talking with patients about fears associated with cancer and death because they were afraid of harming the patients (Smith, 1984). Medical educators should pay more attention to teaching medical students and residents the psychodynamics of interpersonal encounters, including transference and countertransference, to improve their understanding of the peculiarities of clinical encounters and to enhance their capacity for empathic engagement with their patients.

Empathy-Enhancing Factors in Clinician–Patient Encounters

A number of factors contribute to the quality of relationship between clinician and patient. Some of the factors that are more relevant to the enhancement of empathy are discussed briefly in the following sections.

The Placebo Effect

White (1991) proposed that once an empathic clinician–patient relationship is formed, the clinician becomes a powerful placebo-like agent, an "X" factor in healing, that has a tangible positive influence on patient outcomes. It is further suggested that the placebo effect of the clinician–patient relationship is independent from any other placebo like intervention (Hróbjartsson & Gøtzsche, 2001).

The placebo effect, defined as an intervention that simulates medical treatment but is not believed to be a specific treatment for the target condition

(Brody, 1985), has a long history in medicine. The existence of the placebo effect is, in itself, a testimony to the notion that psychosocial factors have a tangible influence on the pathophysiology of disease (Spiro, 1986). The reported rate of response to placebos ranges from 15% to 58% (Turner et al., 1994). However, the notion that a placebo may be an effective treatment in one-third of cases remains the standard in clinical research (Hróbjartsson & Gøtzsche, 2001). (This rate was first suggested about half a century ago by Beecher, 1955.) Although no convincing evidence exists concerning the underlying mechanisms of the placebo effect, some authors have speculated that expectation, reduced anxiety, learning, and an endorphin-mediating effect may explain the placebo response (Turner et al., 1994). Research suggests that the placebo effect is more pronounced when patients comply with clinician's orders (Turner et al., 1994). Better compliance is a function of clinician–patient empathic engagement (Pumilia, 2002). Thus, through leading to better compliance, the empathic relationship can prompt a more positive placebo effect and a better patient outcome.

Recognition of Nonverbal Cues

In clinician–patient encounters, recognition of nonverbal cues and explicit acknowledgment of patients' feelings, concerns, and experiences are important to establish "rapport" (Matthews et al., 1993), which is the essential element of empathic relationships. Rapport also can be strengthened by physicians' ability to decode and encode nonverbal messages and convey their understanding of those messages to their patients (DiMatteo, 1979). Some nonverbal behaviors that are said to promote rapport include clinicians' efforts to match patients' postures, gestures, respiration rates, tempo and pitch of speech, and language patterns (Matthews et al., 1993). Also, tone of voice, gaze and aversion of gaze, posture, silence, laughter, teary eyes, facial expression, hand and body movements, trembling, touch, physical distance, leaning forward or backward, sighs, and other signs of distress or comfort are among important nonverbal cues in clinical encounters (Fretz, 1966; Wolfgang, 1979) (see Chapter 3 for a detailed discussion about nonverbal communication in a general context).

Physicians' ability to decode nonverbal cues is an important component in forming empathic relationships with their patients (DiMatteo, 1979). Using the Profile of Nonverbal Sensitivity Test (PONS Test) (Rosenthal, Hall, DiMatteo, Rogers, & Archer, 1979), DiMatteo and associates found that a patient's perception that the physician listened was predicted by the physician's ability to decode nonverbal cues, such as smiles, grimaces, finger tapping, and a high-pitched voice (DiMatteo, Taranta, Friedman, & Prince, 1980).

Other authors have pointed out that leaning forward during interpersonal interactions is perceived as an indication of a warm, intimate, attentive, and empathic relationship (Fretz, 1966; Harrigan & Rosenthal, 1983; Hasse & Tepper, 1972; Trout & Rosenfeld, 1980). Authors also have reported that postural congruency (positioning one's head, hands, and legs in a corresponding manner when interacting with another person) is an indication of nonverbal social rapport among friends, colleagues, and those engaged in conversation with a common goal (Buchheimer, 1963; Trout & Rosenfeld, 1980). Postural congruency may be a remnant of synchronized behavior between mother and child (Chapter 4), a reflection of the understanding and sharing that are important in empathic relationships.

Other components of nonverbal behavior can influence patients' perceptions of rapport during encounters with physicians. For example, the physician who nods his head (indicating agreement and approval), leans toward the patient (indicating attentiveness, accessibility, closeness, and empathic concern), and sits with his hands resting on his lap (indicating openness, confidence in his ability, and readiness to respond), rather than folding his arms across his chest, conveys a positive rapport that opens the gate to more empathic exchanges (Harrigan & Rosenthal, 1983). Arms and legs in the open position convey less defensiveness and a more positive attitude than closed arm and leg positions do (Mehrabian, 1969).

In addition, the degree of eye contact can indicate the nature of clinician–patient empathic engagement. For example, Mehrabian (1969) reported that a higher degree of eye contact is maintained when the interacting pair like, rather than dislike, one another. However, cultural and sex factors help to determine the desirable degree of eye contact in clinician–patient encounters. For example, Mehrabian (1969) indicated that in American culture, people tend to maintain more eye contact when they are dealing with high-status individuals. In some non-Western cultures described as collectivistic (as opposed to individualistic) (Triandis, 1995), direct eye contact between people of the opposite sex or of different status is avoided.

The face is recognized as a primary channel for affective communication (Ekman & Friesen, 1974). Changes in facial expression (e.g., expressions conveying pain) are often accompanied by parallel changes in autonomic arousal and subjective feelings (Vaughan & Lanzetta, 1981). Facial expressions and nonverbal cues often "leak" unconscious messages (DiMatteo et al., 1980). However, when assessing nonverbal cues and detecting deception, one may make more accurate judgments by observing the body rather than the face (Ekman & Friesen, 1974). In psychoanalytic interviews, the psychoanalyst sits behind the patient, who is laying on the couch, to prevent the patient from viewing the analyst's facial expressions and emotional reactions (Slipp, 2000). Hearing hidden messages beyond spoken words with "the third ear" and seeing nonverbal cues emitted often beyond conscious behavior with "the mind's eye" paves the road for empathic engagement in encounters between clinician and patient.

The "Third Ear" and the "Mind's Eye"

For a better understanding of interpersonal dynamics in clinical encounters, clinicians must learn to hear their patients not only with their anatomical ears but also with their "third ear" to get beyond the spoken words. In addition, to enhance their empathic understanding, clinicians must view their patients' inner worlds not only with their anatomical eyes but also with their "mind's eye." The rapport between clinician and patient will be stronger and the empathic understanding between them will become deeper if the clinician listens to the patient's narrative account of illness with the third ear and sees the personal, psychological, social, and cultural factors involved in the patient's interpersonal relationships with the mind's eye. The more that is said, the more that is heard, and the more that is understood, the deeper the relationship becomes (Jackson, 1992). The seeds of empathy are sowed by listening with the third ear and seeing with the mind's eye.

During the 19th century, seeing was more prominent than hearing in the realms of sickness and healing (Jackson, 1992). As a result, observation of nonverbal cues was given an important place in the diagnosis and treatment of illness. Waisman (1966) suggested that in clinical medicine, physicians needed to look at the hidden aspects of a patient's illness not only by observation (seeing with the mind's eye) but also by listening with their third ear.

In the therapeutic relationship, listening is a crucial method for acquiring information from the help seeker, for understanding the problem, and for bringing about the help seeker's healing (Jackson, 1992). This tradition is attributed to William Osler, who said: "Listen to the patient, he is telling you the diagnosis" (cited in Jackson, 1992, p. 1630). According to Samuel Coleridge (1802), to submerge ourselves in the thoughts of another being, we must have "the eye of a North American Indian" tracking the footsteps of the enemy upon the leaves that strew the forest, "the ear of a wild Arab" listening to the silent desert, and "the touch of a blind man" feeling the face of a darling child. In the context of patient care, these qualities translate into a clinician's ability to listen with the third ear, to see with the mind's eye, and to possess the capacity for empathy to understand the patient beyond spoken words and observable behavior.

Listening from the "outside" only with one's anatomical ears is insufficient in these encounters. According to Greenson (1960), clinicians must shift their attention to listening and feeling from the "inside." As Jackson (1992) pointed out, such listening can be initiated from an empathically attuned position. Research has demonstrated that teachers who attempt to listen to their students with a third ear by using an empathic response were better able to help them with academic and behavioral problems (Cleghorn, 1978).

Empathy, according to Schwaber (1981), is a "mode of analytic" listening. Similarly, Theodore Reik (1948) pointed out that a clinician must hear not only what the patient's words do say but what the words do not say as well. To achieve that goal, Reik emphasized that the clinician "must learn to listen with the third ear" (p. 144). By listening with the third ear, clinicians can catch what other people feel and think but do not say; therefore, they need to learn how one person's mind "speaks" to another person in silence. To form an empathic relationship with patients to provide them with optimal care, clinicians must tune in and listen with the third ear to understand what the patients intend to say beyond the spoken word (Good, 1972).

Listening with a third ear can be accomplished by becoming more vigilant during verbal communication with patients, and seeing with the mind's eye can be accomplished better by becoming more observant of nonverbal clues in clinician–patient encounters. Spoken language is more than a vehicle for the transfer of information; it can influence thoughts as well (Hunt & Agnoli, 1991). In a broader context, Lee Whorf (1956) said back in the mid-19th century that language can convey more than perspectives and feelings; it can shape the thoughts of a culture as well. Therefore, in the context of patient care, the voice that can be heard by the anatomical ear can have more powerful meaning when processed with the third ear. Charles Darwin (1965, p. 354) proposed that the "force of language is much aided by the expressive movements of face and body." Thus, important information about a person's cognitive and affective states can be communicated through nonverbal cues (Lanzetta & Kleck, 1970) that show a wider picture through the mind's eye. Empathic understanding can be enhanced by recognizing hidden and unspoken messages by decoding nonverbal cues with the mind's eye.

Cultural Factors

Culture, defined as "the set of attitudes, values, beliefs and behaviors shared by a group of people, communicated from one generation to the next" (Sternberg, 2004, p. 325) determines how people connect with one another. People in different cultures have strikingly different views of self and others (Markus & Kitayama, 1991) that can influence their help-seeking and help-giving behaviors. Sociocultural factors in clinical encounters, according to Weissman and colleagues (2005), can influence clinician–patient communication and clinical decision making. Cultural norms, racial or ethnic differences, religious beliefs, sex stereotyping, and other embodied sources of identity can influence empathic engagement in the context of patient care. Comas-Diaz and Jacobsen (1991) postulated that ethnocultural factors can not only influence the individual's presentations and interpretations in clinical encounters, they also can significantly affect the process and outcomes of patient care.

For a better understanding of interpersonal dynamics of care-seeking and caregiving behaviors, these behaviors must be examined in the cultural context, because culture is inextricably interlinked to any kind of behavior. For example, in a cross-cultural study of care-seeking attitudes, it was found that a Belgian sample expressed less care-oriented and more cure-oriented attitudes toward health care (DeValck et al., 2001). A recent study by Nelson and Baumgarte (2004) showed that unfamiliarity with cultural norms of others reduces empathic understanding mediated by a lack of perspective taking on the part of the observer. Thus, the clinician's familiarity with the patient's culture is another factor that must be considered when studying empathic engagement in patient care. Little empirical research has been conducted on this topic, however. Although similarities have been noted in Western and non-Western (e.g., Japanese) cultures with regard to physician–patient communication and patient satisfaction (Ishikawa, Takayama, Yamazaki, Skei, & Katsumata, 2002), it is crucial to recognize that clinician–patient encounters are determined by cultural factors that bring cognitive and affective content as well as therapeutic values, expectations, and goals to the relationship (Kleinman et al., 1978).

Despite the importance of cultural awareness in clinical encounters, a recently published study shows that only 8% of the medical schools in the United States and no medical school in Canada offer formal courses about cultural issues in patient care (Flores, Gee, & Kastner, 2000). In a recent study on cross-cultural medical education among a national sample of residents in different specialties in the United States, it was found that although 96% of the residents indicated that it was important to understand cultural issues when providing care, two-thirds reported that no evaluation was made with regard to their skills in the cross-cultural aspects of communication with patients (Weisman et al., 2005).

Cultural differences can influence the clinician–patient empathic engagement as well as the outcomes of patient care to a significant degree (Hall, Roter, & Katz, 1988; Hooper, Comstock, Goodwin, & Goodwin, 1982; Kleinman et al., 1978; Waxler-Morrison, Anderson, & Richardson, 1990). Cultural differences have been observed in physicians' behavior when revealing cancer diagnoses to patients (Holland, Geary, Marchini, & Tross, 1987). For example, in some Asian cultures, diagnosis of terminal illnesses is withheld from patients based on the assumption that disclosure may generate such fear that progression of the disease will accelerate. Evidence suggests that this assumption may not be entirely baseless because increased fear has been reported to be a major factor in "voodoo death" (Cannon, 1957). The power of suggestion often observed in research on hypnosis and imagery is a testimony to the belief that disclosing a serious illness to some patients may result in making their situation worse rather than better.

Hopelessness generated by revealing a fatal diagnosis can cause sudden death among some patients (Richter, 1957). Revealing the diagnosis of a terminal disease is viewed as cruel, inhumane, and unempathic in some cultures and as ethical and empathic in other cultures (Holland et al., 1987). An international survey of oncologists from 20 countries revealed that less than 40% of physicians in Africa, Hungary, Iran, Panama,

Portugal, and Spain would disclose a cancer diagnosis to patients, whereas more than 80% of physicians in Austria, Denmark, Finland, the Netherlands, New Zealand, Norway, Switzerland, and Sweden would reveal the diagnosis (Holland et al., 1987). Clinical realities are culturally constituted, and the nature of physician–patient relationships varies in different cultures and in different ethnic groups within a culture (Kleinman et al., 1978). Clearly, culture can exert an important influence on the nature and contents of clinician–patient communication. However, empathic understanding is always beneficial in clinical encounters regardless of cultural peculiarities.

Furthermore, despite the highly recommended advice that physicians must share their treatment decisions with patients to obtain the patients' input and compliance, such is not the case in the training and practice of physicians in all cultures. In a study by Ali, Khalil, and Yousef (1993) in which American and Egyptian cancer patients were compared, it was found that Egyptian patients preferred not to be involved in decision making; instead, family had an important role in making decisions. Disclosure of a serious diagnosis was socially unacceptable. Emotional support was considered to be the responsibility of the family, not of the health care provider (Ali et al., 1993). Many Moslem patients, for example, believe in the doctrine of predestination, fatalism, and stoicism. With this group of patients, empathic physician–patient relationships can be better formed when physicians covey to them that it is God's will that provided the opportunity for the patient–physician encounter.

In some Asian cultures, physicians are paternalistic figures who have absolute authority to dictate any treatment they deem necessary regardless of the patient's input. In those authoritarian cultures, the patient-centered approach to medical care is likely to covey the physician's lack of determination and competence! Therefore, because empathic concern has a different connotation in different cultures, clinicians' awareness of their patients' cultural peculiarities can enhance empathic understanding. For this reason, cultural issues must receive serious attention in undergraduate, graduate, and continuing medical education programs.

Personal Space

Everyone knows that most animals display territoriality by marking off certain areas as their own space. Human beings exhibit a similar tendency by establishing an invisible bubble around themselves called "personal space" (Hall, 1966; Sommer, 1969). The boundaries of that space determine the distance individuals need to preserve their privacy. Overcrowding that interferes with one's personal space (or territory) can lead to aggressive behavior (Calhoun, 1962). It is interesting to note that the boundaries of personal space are reduced to a minimum in intimate and empathic relationships (Hall, 1966).

Shamasundar (1999) postulated that interpersonal interactions represent an enmeshment of personal spaces in exchange for affective and cognitive information that results in empathic understanding. Sharing of personal spaces is the essence of an empathic relationship—the more overlap in personal spaces, the deeper the empathic understanding.

The nature of the relationship, sex, personality, and cultural factors determine the desirable amount of personal distance. People who are emotionally disturbed or have low self-esteem tend to maintain more personal space (Shamasundar, 1999). Furthermore, the desirable amount of personal space varies in different individuals and in different cultures. For example, in the United States, a maximum of 18 inches of personal space was observed in most intimate encounters (e.g., romantic relations), and a personal space ranging from 1 to 4 feet was considered a desirable distance between friends and acquaintances (Hall, 1966). People who like each other and form empathic relationships with one another tend to maintain less personal space between them when conversing than strangers do (Mehrabian, 1969).

Encroaching on a person's personal space can elicit negative attitudes if the relationship is not empathic (Mehrabian, 1969). For example, violation of an individual's personal space can lead to anxiety or irritability and, sometimes, to increased aggression and the breakdown of interpersonal communication. One study found that people sit closer when expecting approval and sit farther away when expecting disapproval (Rosenfeld, 1965). In the context of clinician–patient encounters, a desirable degree of personal space should be maintained to facilitate empathic interpersonal exchanges.

Boundaries

On the basis of Carl Rogers's description of empathic relationships in clinical encounters (Rogers, 1959), one can perceive another person's internal frame of reference "as if" one were the other person (see Chapter 1). If the "as if" condition is lost, a sense of profound emotional involvement (sympathy) in the clinician–patient relationship can develop, leading to potential risks (see Chapter 1), including the clinician's increased susceptibility to the patient's pain and suffering on the one hand and the patient's dependence on the clinician on the other hand.

In clinician–patient relationships, sharing of emotions always necessitates setting limits or boundaries regarding affective involvement. Although boundaries in clinician–patient encounters are often unspoken and unwritten, they are mutually understood (Gabbard & Nadelson, 1995). Boundaries imply the refraining from intense emotional and erotic involvements. Some boundaries are spelled out in codes of professional ethics. Clinicians violate boundaries when they purposefully exploit the patient's trust and dependency and respond unprofessionally to the patient's desires and expectations. Sexual relationships, dual relationships, receiving inappropriate gifts or services, bartering, unusual time and duration of visits, use of seductive and erotic language, excessive self-disclosure, and inappropriate physical contact are among frequently reported violations of boundaries (Gabbard & Nadelson, 1995). All the aforementioned violations can sabotage the development of an empathic clinician–patient relationship.

The extent of intimacy in clinician–patient relationships is defined by boundaries that prevent the exploitation of both parties (Farber et al., 1997). On the one hand, patients who seek help are vulnerable and tend to form an emotional attachment to the clinician, who is viewed as an omnipotent authority figure resembling a wise parent (e.g., through the transference mechanism). On the other hand, being human beings, too, and thus vulnerable, clinicians must be vigilant about not bonding with a patient as a result of a strong emotional involvement (e.g., an inability to deal with the patient's transference).

Because "to err is human," errors can be made in clinician–patient relationships (Kohn, Corrigan, & Donaldson, 2000). However, education and the guidelines of professional ethics can minimize the violation of boundaries during encounters with patients (Sage, 2002). Several factors contribute to the maintenance or violation of boundaries in clinician–patient relationships: age, sex, ethnicity, culture, attitudes, developmental and family background, personality, education, and the capacity for empathic understanding.

Transgression of boundaries can occur in all specialties, but the likelihood of transgression is greater in psychological and psychiatric consultations because of the transference arising from the intense emotions generated in such consultations (Gabbard, 1994). Transgressions involving sexual issues are often initiated by patients (Gartrell, Herman, Olarte, Feldstein, & Localio, 1986). The oldest skill in medicine, as Thomas (1985) pointed out, is the physician's laying hands on the patient. Therefore, touching during physical examinations has traditionally been regarded as the opening gate to the diagnosis and sometimes to therapeutic benefits. Touching is not only a reminiscent of maternal stroking that generates a feeling of security but also conveys affection and empathic support (Mayerson, 1976). However, the inappropriate use of touch is certainly a transgression of boundaries that diminishes trust and ruins the empathic relationship.

When medical students and physicians are insufficiently trained with regard to potential transgressions of interpersonal boundaries, medical education is often blamed (Gartrell et al., 1986); but the problem is that the "rules of engagement" concerning identification of boundary transgressions are vague and therefore not easy to teach. Needless to say, empathic engagement in clinician–patient relationships can help to avoid the transgression of boundaries.

Recapitulation

Empathic engagement in the context of patient care is a complex phenomenon driven by many factors operating in the dynamics of clinician–patient relationship. Factors that bind clinicians and their patients together include the need for human connection, particularly at the times of crisis; the need for survival; the clinician's position as an authority figure; role expectations in the patient-care environment; psychological dynamics of clinical encounters; and clinicians' ability to understand patients by listening with the third ear and seeing with the mind's eye. Empathic engagement in patient care can also be influenced by cultural factors, personal space, and boundaries. When two people are empathically connected, there are many factors beyond spoken words and observable behavior that provide the glue for binding them together.

9

Empathy as Related to Sex, Personal Qualities, Clinical Competence, and Career Choice

Man is essentially a bulb with many thousands of roots.

(George Christoph Lichtenberg, 1742–1799; cited in Strauss, 1968, p. 285)

Preamble

In this chapter, I describe the link between empathy, sex, personality, and selected psychosocial variables. Women are endowed with a greater capacity for empathy than men are because they begin demonstrating more sensitivity to social stimuli and emotional signals at an early age and because of their care-oriented qualities resulting from evolutionary history and social learning. Empathy correlates positively with prosocial and altruistic behaviors and with a number of desirable personal qualities, including sociability, social skills, likeability, flexibility, tolerance, emotional intelligence, moral judgment, sense of humor, and sensitivity. A long list of undesirable personal attributes, including aggressiveness, externalization, antisocial behaviors, hostility, depression, anxiety, introversion, conduct disorders, neurotic or psychotic disturbances, lying, stealing, physical abuse, and dogmatism correlate negatively with empathy. Also, satisfaction with the early relationship with the mother, selection of a career in medicine for humanistic reasons, and attention to psychosocial issues in medicine have been linked to empathy. Empirical data suggests that scores on empathy are associated with indicators of clinical competence and with career choice. Individuals who choose people-oriented specialties are more likely to obtain higher average scores on empathy than those interested in procedure- or technology-oriented specialties.

Introduction

Empathy, like any other personality attribute, varies among individuals with different constitutional, developmental, experiential, and educational backgrounds. This chapter reviews findings regarding differences in empathy between men and women and describes the link between empathy, personal qualities, academic attainment, and career choice.

Sex Differences

Differences in personal qualities between men and women have long been discussed, and the implications of those differences have been hotly debated. A recent meta-analytic study reported that similarities between the sexes are overwhelmingly more than the overinflated claims of sex differences (Hyde, 2005; Spelke, 2005). Because men and women are similar in many psychosocial variables, Hyde (2005), recently suggested that sex similarities rather than differences, should be tested in research hypotheses. Although most sex differences have been attributed to social learning and role adaptation, recent studies on brain imaging suggest that some differences may be "prewired"—that is, beyond social learning (Cahill, 2005; Singer et al., 2006). In an atmosphere of political correctness, there is a tendency to overlook sex differences for fear of adverse reactions from others and inappropriate social implications, but the fact remains that despite many similarities, variations observed between the sexes are real and are the essence of life. Empirical evidence consistently indicates that the sexes do differ significantly from one another with respect to specific attributes that are relevant to the capacity for empathy.

Sensitivity to Social Stimuli

Sex differences in responses to social stimuli can be observed in children at an early age. For example, female newborns are more responsive than male newborns are to auditory and social stimuli and are able to maintain eye contact for longer periods of time (Hittelman & Dickes, 1979; Osofsky & O'Connell, 1977). Female neonates also smile more and show less rapid buildup of arousal and excitement (Osofsky & O'Connell, 1977). A study of neonates (mean age, 36.7 hours) in which a human face and a mobile were presented simultaneously found that the females exhibited a stronger interest in the human face, whereas the males showed a greater interest in the mobile (Connellan, Baron-Cohen, Wheelwright, Batki, & Ahluwalia, 2000).

Female newborns also showed less irritability than male newborns did (Moss, 1967), and infant girls had less difficulty regulating emotions and displayed less irritation than infant boys did when confronted with their mother's expressionless face (the still-face experiment described in Chapter 4) (Weinberg et al., 1999). Obviously, these early differences cannot be attributed to socialization and adaptation to sex roles.

Perception of Emotions and Decoding of Emotional Signals

Empirical research suggests that from an early age, females seem to be more sensitive to emotional signals than males are. For example, female infants exhibit more reactive crying when another crying infant is present than male infants do (Sagi & Hoffman, 1976) (in Chapter 5, a reactive crying response was described as an indication of a primitive empathic response).

A significant difference has also been observed in favor of women regarding the transmission and detection of nonverbal emotional cues (Brown & Dunn, 1996; Buck, 1984; Buck, Savin, Miller, & Caul, 1972). Women's ability to understand emotional cues has been observed in a number of studies in both children and adults (Brown & Dunn, 1996; Davis, 1983, 1994; Eisenberg and Lennon, 1983, Eisenberg & Strayer, 1987a; Feshbach, 1982; Hogan, 1969; Hojat et al., 2001b, 2002b, 2002d; Jose, 1989; Litvack-Miller et al., 1997).

The ability to perceive the emotions of another person and to "send" and "receive" nonverbal signals through facial expressions and body language contributes significantly to empathic engagement. Women are more receptive to emotional signals than men are (Trivers, 1972) and are more perceptive about their meaning (Baron-Cohen, 2003; Bjorklund & Kipp, 1996; Buss & Schmitt, 1993). Despite the fact that women are generally better at perceiving other people's emotions and are less socially constrained about expressing their emotions, they are not always superior to men in the expression of certain emotions. For example, although women generally are better at expressing fear, sadness, love, and happiness, men are better at expressing anger and hatred (Wagner, Buck, & Winterbotham, 1993), characteristics that are not conducive to empathy. Women have been stereotyped as nurturant and interpersonal oriented (Eisenberg & Lennon, 1983), characteristics that have been identified as central components of female identity (Jack, 1993).

Women not only understand other people's facial expressions better than men do, they are also more facially expressive than men are (Buck, Miller, & Caul, 1974). In one experiment, female pairs were more skillful than male pairs at understanding nonverbal emotional cues (by observing on closed-circuit television the facial expressions of a person who was watching slides with varied emotional content) (Buck et al., 1972). Hall's review (1978) of 75 studies on sex differences in the ability to decode other people's emotional states confirmed women's superiority in decoding visual and auditory cues. Another study (Zuckerman, DePauls, & Rosenthal, 1981) found that women could even detect negative aspects of interpersonal behavior, such as deception, better than men could. Obviously, the ability to interpret nonverbal cues and another person's state of mind correctly is relevant to the capacity to form empathic relationships.

Interpersonal Style, Verbal Ability, Aggressive Behavior, and Caring Attitudes

Men and women have different interpersonal styles. Research has shown that men are more likely to interrupt when women are talking with each other, whereas women are less likely to interrupt when men are talking with each other (McMillan, Clifton, McGrath, & Gale, 1977). In addition, men speak more assertively than women do during verbal communication (Kramer, 1974). Taylor and colleagues (2000) reported that men and women often exhibit different biobehavioral responses to stressful events that reflect differences in their neuroendocrine and physiological systems. The authors suggested that men generally tend to react to stress with the "fight-or-flight" response, whereas women's response tends to be characterized as "tend-and-befriend," a pattern involving nurturant activities developed during human evolutionary history to protect the self and offspring. Taylor and colleagues suggested that the underlying biobehavioral mechanism responsible for this "tend-and-befriend" pattern might be set in motion by the attachment system described in Chapter 4 and by hormones, such as oxytocin in conjunction with other female reproductive hormones, and the activities of endogenous opioid peptides. Obviously, these differences in interpersonal styles and biobehavioral responses can influence the formation of empathic relationships.

In interpersonal interactions, smiling is the best single predictor of warmth (Bayes, 1972) and an indicator of prosocial behavior and positive affect. Appropriate use of smiling serves as a positive signal in interpersonal communication. A meta-analytic study of sex differences with regard to smiling found that women and adolescent girls were significantly more likely to smile than men and adolescent boys were (LaFrance, Hecht, & Levy Paluck, 2003).

Women's superiority on tests of verbal ability has been documented in many empirical studies (e.g., see Maccoby and Jacklin, 1974). Girls often begin talking at an earlier age than boys do, and they maintain their superior verbal ability thereafter (Rutter et al., 2005). In addition to verbal skills, women surpass men in sociability. For example, Hall (1985) reported that women make more eye contact during interpersonal interactions than age-matched men do.

Women also tend to understand the social context of certain matters better than men do (Willingham & Cole, 1997). For example, female college students identified with story characters to a greater degree than the male students did. The researcher found that such identification correlated positively with scores on the Empathic Concern subscale of Davis's Interpersonal Reactivity Index (IRI) (Jose, 1989).

Women's typical characteristic of expressing their emotions (e.g., externalizing) and men's typical characteristic of concealing their emotions (e.g., internalizing) prompts the two sexes to reveal their emotions differently (Buck et al., 1972). Femininity has been found to correlate with empathy. An empirical study reported that the men and women who received higher femininity scores on the Gender Role Orientation Inventory (Bem, 1974) also had significantly higher empathy scores on the IRI (Karniol, Gabay, Ochion, & Harari, 1998).

Although some sex differences in interpersonal styles and verbal skills can be attributed to socialization and learned sex roles (Eagly, 1995), evidence suggests that these differences may be hard-wired, partially biological in origin (Baron-Cohen, 2003), and deeply rooted in the human evolutionary history (Buss, 2003). In a recent study by Singer and colleagues (2006) using functional magnetic resonance imaging, it was noticed that while both men and women exhibited empathy-related activation in areas that register pain (fronto-insular and anterior cingulated cortices), the empathy-related brain activities were significantly reduced in men when observing a cheater in pain.

Some authors have argued that the difference in levels of prenatal testosterone in male and female fetuses supports the notion that the hormone has an important role in forming sex-specific interpersonal styles and verbal ability (Baron-Cohen, 2003; Connellan et al., 2000). For example, a study in which an inverse relationship was found between levels of fetal testosterone and size of the vocabulary in children at 18 and 24 months of age supported the importance of fetal testosterone levels in verbal ability in men and women (Lutchmaya, Baron-Cohen, & Raggatt, 2002).

Verbal aggression and aggressive behavior reflect a negative affect, which interferes with the formation of empathic relationships. Women are generally less likely than men to exhibit aggressive behavior (for a meta-analytic study, see Eagly & Steffen, 1986). Sex differences in the expression of aggression may be attributable not only to hormonal differences but also to social learning and stereotypical sex roles that lead men to become tougher, more assertive, and more behaviorally aggressive than women. However, it is important to note that social learning explains only part of the picture because research indicates that aggression is more pronounced in male than in female children (Hyde, 1984).

Women express aggression in different ways than men do and toward different targets. For example, women tend to be verbally, rather than physically, aggressive and to direct their aggression toward other women, not men (Eagly & Steffen, 1986). Feelings of guilt about aggressive behavior often prohibit women from expressing aggression, and research has shown that they experience more guilt and anxiety about their aggression than men do (Frodi & Macauley, 1977).

Control of aggression is a self-regulatory behavior that promotes empathic relationships. By using the "still-face" procedure described in Chapter 4, investigators found that male infants had greater difficulty than female infants did in maintaining emotional regulation (Weinberg et al., 1999).

Thus, women seem to have more control over regulation of their emotions, which leads to better interpersonal interactions.

Social stereotypes often portray men who help others as heroic and chivalrous (e.g., those who risk their own life to save others from harm) and portray women as nurturant and caring (Eagly & Crowley, 1986). A meta-analytic review of the literature revealed that, in general, men were more likely than women to give help and women were more inclined to receive help (Eagly & Crowley, 1986). However, women historically have been more inclined than men to place the needs of others, especially those of their children, above their own (Chodorow, 1978) and are more oriented toward caring (Gilligan, 1982). Charles Darwin also noticed this quality. In his seminal book, *The Descent of Man*, Darwin (1981) indicated that women exhibit greater tenderness in social relationships than men do, and because of their maternal instincts, their tenderness toward their infants is likely to extend toward others.

According to Reverby (1987) and Trivers (1972), women's caring attitude toward their offspring, which can be generalized to other humans, has evolutionary roots. Women's caring attitude toward their children often takes precedence over other important matters. For example, caring attitudes toward offspring can often interfere with a woman's career advancement in ways that have nothing to do with the barrier known as the "glass ceiling" effect. Male and female faculty members of academic medical centers who did not have children showed equivalent career accomplishments, but female faculty members who had children progressed more slowly in their careers because of their involvement in child raising (Carr, Ash, & Friedman, 1998). This phenomenon is an indication of the intrinsic motivation that prompts women toward caring and contributes to sex differences in empathy.

Empathy as a Function of Sex Differences

Consistent with the characterizations of women described in this chapter so far, empirical studies have reported that women often outscore men on measures of empathy (Davis, 1983; Eisenberg et al., 1983; Hoffman, 1977; Hogan, 1969; Jose, 1989; Karniol et al., 1998). Block (1976) reported that the results of most of the studies she examined favored women with regard to empathy. However, Eisenberg and Lennon (1983) reported a significant sex difference in empathy favoring women when the measures of empathy were self-report inventories but noted no sex difference when the measures of empathy were either physiological or unobtrusive observations of behavior. These findings indicate that women may have an image of themselves as empathic that is reflected in their self-report measures of empathy.

Studies with adults indicate that women are more skillful than men are at initiating empathic relationships. They typically exhibit behaviors described as "communal" (e.g., social sensitivity, caring, friendliness), whereas men tend to manifest behaviors described as "agentic" (e.g., controlling, independent, dominant) (Eagly, 1995). Also, Rokeach (1973) found that women place more emphasis on the emotional aspects of their interactions than do men, who place more emphasis on the rational aspects. Consistent with Rokeach's findings, a study of undergraduate students found that women differed significantly from men on emotional empathy (akin to sympathy) but not on perspective taking (Riggio, Tucker, & Coffaro, 1989). Other authors have reported that women tend to adopt care-oriented moral reasoning, whereas men tend to have a more justice-oriented moral perspective (Gilligan, 1982; Sochting, Skoe, & Marcia, 1994). In a study of nursing and medical students, the differences in judicial and moral considerations regarding patient care appeared to be explained by sex, rather than by differences in professional roles (Peter & Gallop, 1994). When the students were faced with a hypothetical clinical dilemma, female students, regardless of academic major, were more care-oriented than their male counterparts were.

Sex differences in empathy have been observed among various professionals. For example, in a study of nurses, social workers, and teachers, women obtained significantly higher empathy scores than men did on Mehrabian and Epstein's Emotional Empathy Scale (Williams, 1989). In another study with students in the first and final years of a medical school in Poland (Kliszcz, Hebanowski, & Rembowski, 1998), women scored higher than men on both the Emotional Empathy Scale and the IRI. A survey of physicians showed that the female physicians rated themselves as more empathic than their male counterparts rated themselves (Barnsley, Williams, Cockerill, & Tanner, 1999). Similarly, female residents in internal medicine (Day, Norcini, Shea, & Benson, 1989) and family medicine (Abbott, 1983) outscored their male counterparts on a measure of humanism.

In our studies, we consistently observed that female medical students obtained higher scores on the JSPE than male students did (Hojat et al., 2001b, 2002a). We also observed that female physicians not only had higher average scores on the JSPE than male physicians did but had higher scores on each individual item of the scale as well (Hojat et al., 2002b). The differences favoring female physicians were particularly pronounced on items that measured the "perspective taking" factor. Inconsistent with our findings, however, Kupfer and colleagues (1978) found no sex differences in the scores of medical students at the University of Pittsburgh School of Medicine on an abbreviated version of Hogan's Empathy Scale. In a study of positive role models in medicine, however, female physicians scored higher than their male counterparts did on measures of personality facets that were conceptually relevant to empathy, such as openness to new experiences, aesthetics, and feelings (Magee & Hojat, 1998).

Despite their advantage in interpersonal style and empathic capability, women seem to be more vulnerable than men are when working under stressful conditions. This differential vulnerability to stress prompts women to appraise stressful events as being more devastating than men do (Barnett, Biener, & Baruch, 1987). In our study with medical students, we found that women were more sensitive than men were to stressful life events and consequently appraised stressful events as more disturbing (Hojat, Glaser, Xu, Veloski, & Christian, 1999; Hojat, Gonnella, Erdmann, & Vogel, 2003). These results indicate that although female physicians have an advantage when it comes to establishing empathic engagement with their patients, vulnerability to professional stress puts them at a disadvantage. It should also be noted that although empathy enhances patient outcomes (see Chapter 10) and is valued by both physicians and patients, research shows that empathy is not associated with promotion (Carmel & Glick, 1996), and this may affect women more than men. In one large-scale study involving 5,314 medical students, we found that female medical students at the beginning of their medical education expected, on the average, 23% less financial gain from the practice of medicine regardless of their planned specialties than their male counterparts did (Hojat et al., 2000b). These findings are consistent with the notion that women are more likely than men to choose medicine for altruistic reasons (Gross, 1992) than for financial gain (Stamps & Boley Cruz, 1994).

Sex Differences in the Practice of Medicine

It seems reasonable to speculate that sex differences concerning empathy could influence male and female physicians' style of practice and provision of patient care, and some empirical studies have confirmed this speculation (Bertakis, Helms, Callahan, Azari, & Robbins, 1995; Bylund & Makoul, 2002; Fruen, Rothman, & Steiner, 1974; Henderson & Weisman, 2001; Maheux, Duford, Beland, Jacques, & Levesque, 1990; Weisman & Teitlebaum, 1985).

Female physicians were more likely than male physicians to engage patients in positive talk, discuss psychological and social issues in health and illness with them, use more positive statements, engage in more verbal exchanges with patients, and spend a longer time with them (Cooper-Patrick, Gallo, & Gonzales, 1999; Hall, Irish, Roter, Ehrlic, & Miller, 1994; Meeuwesen, Schaap, & Van der Staak, 1991; Roter & Hall, 1997; Roter, Hall, & Aoki, 2002; Roter, Lipkin, & Korsgaard, 1991). On the average, female physicians spent 3 or 4 more minutes with their patients than their male counterparts did, engaged in more humorous conversations with their patients, and shared more decision-making responsibility with them (Charon, Greene, & Adelman, 1994). Female physicians also are more prevention-oriented than their male counterparts are (Bertakis et al., 1995; Frank & Harvey, 1996; Maheux et al., 1990). Furthermore, they provide more screening and more preventive counseling about sensitive topics, particularly with female patients (Henderson & Weisman, 2001). These sex differences in practice style, according to Bylund and Makoul (2002), can the result of the female physicians' tendency to communicate at a higher degree of empathy with their patients than their male counterparts do.

Charon and her colleagues (1994, p. 216) observed that female physicians acted as if they were alert to their patients' emotional and daily life concerns—concerns that otherwise "tend to be muted in medical interactions." Their observation agreed with the idea posed by others that women, more than men, can bring empathy to the healing relationship (Bickel, 1994; Bylund & Makoul, 2002). Charon et al. also found that patients reacted to male and female physicians differently. Patients of both sexes reported that female physicians were more willing to discuss medical topics and probe about personal habits, such as smoking, alcohol, drug use, sex, and sleep, and psychological issues, such as family, work, finances, and emotional problems.

In a study of patients' satisfaction, both male and female patients gave more favorable ratings to the care they received from female residents than from male residents (Linn, Cope, & Leake, 1984). However, Howell, Gardiner, and Concato (2002) found that although a greater number of patients preferred female over male obstetricians, their satisfaction with medical care was unrelated to a physician's sex. With regard to medical malpractice claims, the fact that female physicians have a better record than male physicians do is attributed more to better physician–patient relationships than to taking less risky patients (Sloan, Mergenhagen, Burfield, Bovjerg, & Hassan, 1989). In the area of clinical competency, our study showed that directors of residency training programs rated female residents higher than their male counterparts on the "socioeconomic aspect of patient care" at the end of the first year of postgraduate medical education (Hojat et al., 1994). These findings suggest that female and male health care providers have different practice styles resulting from their differences in interpersonal style reflected in their empathic engagement with patients.

Psychosocial Correlates of Empathy

Prosocial Versus Aggressive Behaviors

Prosocial behavior has been defined as a person's voluntary act that can benefit another person (Eisenberg & Miller, 1987). The notion that empathy is a determining factor in altruism and prosocial behavior has been widely discussed and accepted (Aronfreed, 1970; Batson & Coke, 1981; Eisenberg & Miller, 1987; Hoffman, 1981; Staub, 1978).

Prosocial behavior can be initiated by an egoistic motivation (e.g., the expectation of a reward, an attempt to avoid aversive stimuli or punishment, or an attempt to reduce distress by helping others) or by an altruistic motivation (e.g., the act of helping to reduce other people's distress, even if the act is harmful to oneself, without expecting any reward). One study found that people who were more empathic behaved more altruistically: that is, they were willing to help others, even when their own welfare was jeopardized (Krebs, 1975). In a later study, teachers' ratings indicated that children's empathy was associated with their helpful behavior (Litvack-Miller et al., 1997).

Some authors have argued that empathy-induced helping behavior can be the result of merging self with others. In certain circumstances, feelings of oneness emerge so that human beings experience others as "we," rather than as "they" (Hornstein, 1978). In these circumstances, we may be psychologically indistinguishable from the others and will understand their experiences better. And when this feeling of oneness emerges, the two shall become one, and, as reported by Lerner and Mindl, "If the empathic tie is dominant, it would be natural for us to engage in acts which we or others might label as self-sacrifice or martyrdom" (Lerner & Meindl, 1981, p. 227). In summarizing their research findings, Batson and colleagues (1997b, p. 508) reported that "empathy evokes concern for the other, distinct from oneself, that is beyond self-interest."

Prosocial behavior initiated by altruism has been studied in relation to empathy (Eisenberg & Miller, 1987). However, in an earlier meta-analytic review of 11 studies, most of which involved children, the investigators found no consistent link between empathy and prosocial behavior (Underwood & Moore, 1982). This unexpected result can be explained by the finding that the evaluation of empathy in children could be confounded by such factors as validity issues regarding measurements of empathy and the evaluators' sex (Chapter 5). In addition, Eisenberg and Miller (1987) proposed that the association between empathy and prosocial behavior is weaker among children than among adults because emotional or cognitive responses and prosocial behavior become more integrated with age. In a later meta-analytic study of a larger number of research articles involving adults in which more recent empirical studies and doctoral dissertations were reviewed, Eisenberg (1983) reported a significant link between empathy and prosocial behavior.

Individuals with high scores on Mehrabian and Epstein's Emotional Empathy Scale were more likely to demonstrate helping behavior than were individuals with low scores (Barett et al., 1980; Rushton, Chrisjohn, & Fekker, 1981). In a review of studies on empathy and individual differences, scores on the Emotional Empathy Scale were not only significantly correlated with altruistic behavior but also with greater physiological arousability (greater skin conductance and increased heart rate), more emotionality (a greater tendency to weep), spending more time with and displaying more affection to children, higher moral judgment, more volunteerism, and less aggressive behavior (Mehrabian et al., 1988).

College students who scored higher on empathy were more eager than low-scoring students to help neurologically handicapped children who could benefit from a volunteer's efforts (Barnett, Feighney, & Esper, 1983). College students who were members of help-oriented groups, such as those helping the underprivileged, scored higher on the Emotional Empathy Scale than did students who were members of self-interest organizations, such as the biology honors fraternity (Van Orum, Foley, Burns, DeWolfe, & Kennedy, 1981). In a study with prison inmates, the investigators observed that the inmates who volunteered to help disadvantaged individuals in the prison scored higher on Hogan's Empathy Scale than nonvolunteers did (Gendreau, Burke, & Grant, 1980).

Personal Qualities

A number of empirical studies have addressed the relationships between empathy, personality, and psychosocial measures. In an earlier empirical study (Kerr & Speroff, 1954), significant correlations were reported between students' scores on a measure of empathy (developed by the study authors) and scores of popularity and likeability measured by a sociometric method developed by Moreno (1934). Also, empathy scores in that study were correlated with the smiles observed at a commencement exercise and with feelings for others. Kerr and Speroff (1954) reported a positive link between empathy scores and automobile salesmen's sales records and their merit rankings. However, a later study by Lamont and Lundstrom (1977) found that the performance of successful industrial salesmen was negatively correlated with scores on Hogan's Empathy Scale but was positively related to a measure of endurance.

In the early 1970s, Hogan and colleagues conducted several studies comparing scores on Hogan's Empathy Scale with scores obtained on other measures of personal qualities. Hogan and Mankin (1970) reported a significant correlation between scores on the Empathy Scale and those on a measure of likeability. Two years later, Hogan and Dickstein (1972) found a significant correlation between empathy and mature moral judgment. A year later, Greif and Hogan (1973) reported a significant link between college students' scores on the Empathy Scale and a personality factor called "person-orientation" they derived from the California Personality Inventory.

Medical students' scores on Hogan's Empathy Scale were positively and significantly correlated with measures of intellectual efficiency, flexibility, tolerance, good impression, and extraversion and were significantly but negatively correlated with depression, anxiety, and introversion (Hogan, 1969). The following adjectives had the highest positive correlations with scores on Hogan's Empathy Scale: pleasant, charming, friendly, dreamy, cheerful, sociable, sentimental, imaginative, discreet, and tactful. In contrast, the following adjectives correlated most highly but negatively with scores on Hogan's Empathy Scale: cruel, cold, quarrelsome, hostile, bitter, unemotional, unkind, hard-hearted, argumentative, and opinionated (Hogan, 1969). Hogan's findings paint a picture of an empathic person as one who is emotionally stable and socially mature—that is, a person who possesses the major attributes described more than two decades later as emotional intelligence (Goleman, 1995; Salovey & Mayer, 1990). Investigators reported that scores on a measure of emotional intelligence were positively correlated with empathic perspective taking (Schutte et al., 2001).

Moral judgment and helping behavior were significantly correlated with scores on Mehrabian and Epstein's Emotional Empathy Scale (Eisenberg-Berg & Mussen, 1978). Students who scored higher on a modified version of the Emotional Empathy Scale were more assertive, less narcissistic, more sensitive, less self-focused, and more concerned about a healthy life-style (Kalliopuska, 1992a). It also was reported that people living in the countryside obtained a higher average score on the Emotional Empathy Scale than did those living in towns (Kalliopuska, 1994). Significant and positive correlations have been observed between scores on the IRI and measures of hypnotic susceptibility and self-absorption (Wickramasekera & Szylk, 2003). Among nurses, effective leadership has been linked to scores on the IRI (Mansen, 1993).

A meta-analytic study conducted in the late 1980s found that empathy was negatively related to aggressive, antisocial, and externalizing behaviors, such as conduct disorders, lying, and stealing as well as to physical abuse (Miller & Eisenberg, 1988). Physically and emotionally abusive parents scored significantly lower than a comparison group of foster parents on the Perspective Taking, Empathic Concern, and Personal Distress subscales of the Davis's IRI (Wiehe, 2003). When Hogan's Empathy Scale was administered to incarcerated child molesters, their scores showed deficits in empathy (Marshall & Maric, 1996). The findings in these studies reveal that individuals who are deficient in empathy naturally possess less capacity to understand and respond to the needs of others, including their own children.

Negative relationships were reported between scores on Hogan's Empathy Scale; measures of anxiety, phobia, obsession, and depression (Kupfer et al., 1978); and indicators of neurotic and psychotic disturbances (Hekmat, Khajavi, & Mehryar, 1974, 1975). Scores on Mehrabian and Epstein's Emotional Empathy Scale were inversely related to a measure of psychopathic personality (Sandoval, Hancock, Poythress, Edens, & Lilienfeld, 2000). In addition, negative correlations were reported between scores on Hogan's Empathy Scale and measures of state and trait anxiety (Deardroff, Kendall, Finch, & Sitartz, 1977). Scores on the Emotional Empathy Scale were negatively correlated with a measure of narcissism among undergraduate students (Watson, Grisham, Trotter, & Biderman, 1984) and among young baseball players in Finland (Kalliopuska, 1992b).

Symptoms of depression and dogmatism among medical students were negatively correlated with scores on Hogan's Empathy Scale (Streit-Forest, 1982). In a study of medical students at the Louisiana State University Medical Center, perceptions of changes in empathy during medical school (measured by a single item) were strongly associated with students' perceptions of changes in their sensitivity, helpfulness, and concern for patients (Wolf, Balson, Faucett, & Randall, 1989).

In an attempt to validate Hogan's Empathy Scale for medical students at Monash University in Australia, researchers found a significant correlation between the students' scores on Hogan's scale and the ratings of peers concerning the students' social skills, sense of humor, and awareness of the impression they made on others (Hornblow et al., 1977). Furthermore, medical students in that study obtained higher average empathy scores than did psychiatric patients diagnosed with a personality disorder.

Streit-Forest (1982) studied first-year medical students at the University of Montreal and found that students with a more positive attitude toward the physician–patient relationship and students who chose medicine for humanistic reasons scored highest on Hogan's Empathy Scale. The author also noted that the students who were more likely to watch television in their leisure time scored lower on empathy than did classmates who were more likely to spend their leisure time on a hobby.

In a study with medical students in Canada (Streit, 1980), significant and positive correlations were observed between scores on Hogan's Empathy Scale and scores on the following subtests of the Attitudes Toward Psychosocial Issues in Medicine (Parlow & Rothman, 1974): Doctor–Patient Relations (recognition of the importance of interpersonal clinician–patient relationships in effective patient care), Social Factors (recognition of the importance of social factors as determinants of health and illness), General Liberalism (open-mindedness about social issues outside of medicine), Preventive Medicine (recognition of medicine's role in maintaining health), and Government Role (endorsement of government's involvement in regulating health care costs).

In a study with medical students, scores on the Empathic Concern and Perspective Taking subscales of the IRI were correlated with a measure of femininity that included such qualities as gentleness, warmth, helpfulness, kindness, understanding emotions, devotion to others, and awareness of other people's feelings (Zeldow & Daugherty, 1987). In another study with medical students, empathy was correlated with a measure of androgyny (Yarnold, Martin, & Soltysik, 1993).

Age and professional experiences also have been correlated with empathy in a few studies. For example, younger nurses with a moderate amount of professional experiences expressed more empathy toward elderly patients than older nurses did (Pennington & Pierce, 1985). Similarly, younger, less experienced physicians showed more empathic concern for their patients than did older, more experienced physicians (Hall & Dornan, 1988). These findings raise concerns about a possible decline in empathy as a result of older age or more professional experience that need to be studied in the future.

In a study with nurses, social workers, and teachers (Williams, 1989), the respondents' scores on the Emotional Empathy Scale were significantly and positively correlated with both emotional exhaustion and personal accomplishment. The investigator suggested that high emotional empathy—as opposed to cognitive empathy (Chapter 1)—may predispose helping professionals to emotional exhaustion that must be mediated by personal accomplishment to avoid depersonalization and burnout (Williams, 1989).

By imagining how other people feel when watching someone whose hand was strapped in a machine, Stotland (1969) demonstrated that perspective-taking was a major mechanism that generated empathy. In a later study, Stotland (1978) reported that scores on the Fantasy–Empathy Scale (Chapter 5) were correlated with altruism, more palmar sweat, and more vasoconstriction while study participants were observing others in pain. Stotland attributed this finding to the tendency of more empathic individuals to understand and feel another person's experiences.

Hogan (1969) reported that young delinquents and prison inmates scored approximately one standard deviation lower on the Empathy Scale than college students did. Hogan (1976) also reported that inmates scored lower on the empathy scale than Air Force officers did. Furthermore, incarcerated delinquents scored lower on the Empathy Scale than nondelinquent undergraduate students did (Kurtines & Hogan, 1972). Individuals with low scores on the scale were more likely to be deficient in morality. A group of repeat offenders scored lower on Hogan's Empathy Scale than did first-time offenders and research participants from the general public (Deardroff, Finch, Kendall, Liran, & Indrisano, 1975). Also, men with high scores on the Emotional Empathy Scale were influenced to a significantly lesser degree by a female potential coworker's physical attractiveness than were men with low scores (Crouse & Mehrabian, 1977).

Mehrabian and colleagues (1988) found that empathy measured with the Emotional Empathy Scale was associated with emotional arousability. The investigators explained their findings by suggesting that arousability indicates the degree to which a person's emotions are influenced by events. Similarly, emotional empathy indicated an individual's tendency to be affected by other people's emotional experiences. Therefore, it followed that scores on emotional empathy (that was viewed as analogous to sympathy in Chapter 1) would be positively linked to arousability.

In our study of 422 first-year medical students (Hojat et al., 2005b), we found that higher scores on the JSPE were associated with higher scores on sociability and lower scores on aggression–hostility on the short version of the Zuckerman–Kuhlman Personality Questionnaire (ZKPQ) (Zuckerman, 2002). Similar findings were reported by Beven, O'Brien-Malone, and Hall (2004), who found a positive correlation between empathy measured by the Perspective Taking subscale of the IRI and a measure of socialization but found a negative correlation with a measure of impulsivity in a sample of violent offenders.

Furthermore, our study of medical students (Hojat et al., 2005b) showed that higher scores on the JSPE were associated with higher levels of self-reported satisfaction with the early relationship with the mother, but not with the father. These results were consistent with our earlier findings (Hojat, 1998) that medical students' perceptions of satisfaction with the early relationship with their mother were predictors of higher self-esteem; better peer relationships; less loneliness, depression, and anxiety; and more resilience when faced with stressful life events. We did not find such associations regarding students' perceptions of their early relationship with their father.

In a study of physicians in postgraduate training, we found a significant link between the physicians' perceptions of their early relationship with their mother and their clinical competence in relation to their interpersonal skills and attitudes assessed by the directors of the training programs (Hojat, Glaser, & Veloski, 1996). Again, this link was not observed in relation to the physicians' perceptions of their early relationship with their father. These findings provide support for the developmental aspect of empathy discussed in Chapter 4—that the quality of the relationship with a primary caregiver (usually the mother) early in life can be a precursor of empathy in adulthood.

Academic Attainment and Clinical Competence

Few attempts have been made to examine relationships between measures of empathy and indicators of academic attainment. In one early study, scores on a test of empathy developed by the investigators proved to be independent of intelligence, reading level, mechanical comprehension, spatial relations, and aptitudes in chemistry and mathematics (Kerr & Speroff, 1954). A later study showed a lack of correlation between empathy and academic performance (Hogan & Weiss, 1974).

In the late 1970s, a study of five classes of medical students at the University of Pittsburgh School of Medicine found that scores on a brief version of Hogan's Empathy Scale and scores on the Medical College Admission Test (MCAT) were positively correlated in one class, negatively correlated in another class, and not correlated at all in the three remaining classes (Kupfer et al., 1978).

At Wake Forest University's Bowman Gray School of Medicine, medical students' scores on Hogan's Empathy Scale were not correlated with either their scores on Parts 1 and 2 of the National Board of Medical Examiners medical licensing examinations or with their grades on preclinical and clinical examinations (Diseker & Michielutte, 1981). Furthermore, all correlations between the students' scores on Hogan's Empathy Scale and the Verbal, Quantitative, Science Problems, and General Information subtests of the MCAT were negative and negligible. Two later studies involved assessments of medical students by standardized patients. In one study, Colliver, Willis, Robbs, Cohen, and Swartz (1998) reported that the patients' assessments of empathy among fourth-year medical students were associated with indicators of better clinical performance. In another study, Coutts and Rogers (2000) found low correlations between medical students' scores on a measure of humanism in medicine and assessments of their academic performance in medical school. Among these low correlations, the highest one ($r = 0.31$) was obtained between the standardized patients' assessment of the students' history-taking skills and the students' "humanism" scores.

In our own study of 371 third-year medical students (Hojat et al., 2002a), we found that the students' scores on the JSPE were not significantly correlated with their performance on objective (e.g., multiple choice) tests, such as examinations on sciences basic to medicine in the first 2 years of medical school; the MCAT's Biological Sciences, Physical Sciences, and Verbal Reasoning subtests; and Steps 1 and 2 of the United States Medical Licensing Examination. However, we observed a statistically significant link between the students' JSPE scores and the faculty's global ratings of students' clinical competence in third-year core clerkships in family medicine, internal medicine, obstetrics and gynecology, pediatrics, psychiatry, and surgery. These results agreed with those of Colliver et al. (1998). Our findings were expected because the students' understanding of patients' feelings and experiences measured by the JSPE could be reflected in their interpersonal communication with patients, a factor usually considered when assessing students' clinical competence. However, because such personal qualities cannot be measured with objective tests of medical or clinical knowledge, we did not expect to find a significant link between students' empathy scores and measures of knowledge attainment.

Choice of a Career

A student's choice of a career and interest in a particular specialty can be influenced by a number of variables, including constitutional factors, aptitudes, personality, developmental and educational experiences, skills, social trends, role models, cultural factors, and market forces (Bland, Meurer, & Maldonado, 1995; Christodoulou, Lykousras, Mountaokalakis, Voulgari, & Stefanis, 1995; Kassebaum & Szenas, 1994; Powell, Boakes, & Slater, 1988; Reed, Jernstedt, & Reber, 2001; Richard, Nakamoto, & Lockwood, 2001; Sierles, Vergare, Hojat, & Gonnella, 2004; Weissman, Haynes, Killan, & Robinowitz, 1994). Some empirical studies have reported a link between empathy and career interest. For example, Hogan (1969) reported that college students majoring in psychology, education, and medicine obtained the highest scores on his Empathy Scale, whereas engineering and architecture students and military officers obtained the lowest scores. Rovezzi-Carroll and Fitz (1984) found that students majoring in physical therapy scored high on Hogan's Empathy Scale and were more people-oriented and that those majoring in medical technology were more task-oriented.

Studies With Medical Students.

Medical students in Israel scored higher on a Hebrew version of Mehrabian and Epstein's Emotional Empathy Scale than did college students majoring in psychology, social work, economics, physics, and chemistry (Elizur & Rosenheim, 1982). However, the investigators found that the medical students unexpectedly scored lower than the other students did in their attention to psychosocial areas related to health and illness. They interpreted this unexpected finding as an indication that medical schools overemphasize achievement in the sciences and fail to devote adequate attention to the development of psychosocial skills. In a Canadian study, medical students who had high scores on Hogan's Empathy Scale had chosen medicine for humanistic reasons, whereas the students who had low scores had chosen medicine for scientific reasons (Streit-Forest, 1982).

A study at Baylor College of Medicine found that medical students interested in family medicine, general internal medicine, and pediatrics obtained the highest mean scores on humanistic attributes (measured by ratings given by standardized patients during the clerkship's Objective Structured Clinical Examinations), whereas students interested in anesthesiology, pathology, radiology, emergency medicine, and physical medicine and rehabilitation obtained the lowest mean rating scores (Coutts-van Dijk, Bray, Moore, & Rogers, 1997). Using the Physician Belief Scale (Ashworth et al., 1984), a measure of psychosocial orientation in patient care, the researchers observed a similar pattern of results. A study with medical students at the University of Washington School of Medicine found that interaction with patients was among the major factors that prompted students to choose primary care as their specialty (Burack, Irby, Carline, Ambruzy, Ellsbury, & Stritter, 1997).

Although Harsch (1989) observed no relationship between medical students' scores on Hogan's Empathy Scale and the specialties they were interested in, a later study with medical students contradicted that report. The researchers who conducted the later study reported that after sex was controlled for in the statistical analyses, the students who expressed interest in pursuing "core" specialties, such as family medicine or pediatrics, scored significantly higher on the Emotional Empathy Scale than did students who were interested in pursuing "noncore" specialties, such as radiology or pathology (Newton et al., 2000).

In her doctoral dissertation, Bailey (2001) reported that medical students who planned to pursue a career in specialties requiring extensive and prolonged encounters with patients received significantly higher average scores on the IRI than did their counterparts who planned to pursue procedure-oriented specialties.

Studies With Physicians.

Truax, Altmann, and Millis (1974) compared the scores of general practitioners, other medical professionals (e.g., nurses), and nonmedical professionals (e.g., clergymen, lawyers) on the Accurate Empathy subscale of Truax and Carkhoff's Relationship Questionnaire (Chapter 5) and on measures of warmth and genuineness. They reported that the general practitioners received the highest scores. These results are consistent with the findings of another study that ongoing interpersonal relationships with patients and their families and interprofessional collaboration with colleagues in other specialties were among the features ascribed to primary care physicians (Hennen, 1975). In a 1983 study comparing physicians in family medicine, internal medicine, and surgery, the family physicians obtained the highest mean score on a humanism scale, the surgeons obtained the lowest mean score, and the mean score of the internists fell in between (Abbott, 1983).

In a survey of 327 physicians representing five graduating classes in the School of Medicine at the University of Missouri-Kansas City, views of a group of primary care physicians were compared with those of a group of non-primary care physicians (Arnold, Calkins, & Willoughby, 1997). The results showed that the primary care physicians assigned significantly higher ratings to such professional qualities as a pleasant personality, the ability to relate to people, and the ability to empathize. Among personal values, the primary care physicians also gave a higher rating to empathy and a lower rating to competition than the other group did.

In our study involving 704 physicians, we noticed that psychiatrists obtained the highest mean score on the JSPE, followed by physicians in internal medicine, pediatrics, emergency medicine, and family medicine (Hojat et al., 2002e). The lowest mean scores were obtained by anesthesiologists, orthopedic surgeons, neurosurgeons, and radiologists. When sex was controlled for, the differences in empathy scores among physicians specializing in psychiatry, internal medicine, pediatrics, emergency medicine, and family medicine did not reach the conventional level of statistical significance ($p < .05$). However, the psychiatrists' mean score differed significantly from the mean scores of anesthesiologists, orthopedic surgeons, neurosurgeons, radiologists, cardiovascular surgeons, and obstetricians and gynecologists. A higher mean score by psychiatrists was expected because of their specific interpersonal training and findings that showed they scored high on a measure of tolerance for ambiguity (Geller, Tambor, Chase, & Holtzman, 1993), which facilitates empathic engagement with patients.

In two other studies, we compared two groups of physicians (Hojat et al., 2001a, 2002c). Group 1 included 462 physicians in "people-oriented" specialties, such as family medicine, general internal medicine, pediatrics, emergency medicine, obstetrics and gynecology, and psychiatry. Group 2 included 242 physicians in "technology- or procedure-oriented" practices, such as anesthesiology, radiology, pathology, surgery, and surgical subspecialties. The physicians in Group 1 outscored their counterparts in Group 2 not only on the total JSPE scores, but on all 20 items of the JSPE as well (Hojat et al., 2002c). However, the differences were statistically significant for only 11 of the 20 items. The results of the two studies remained unchanged when the effect of sex was controlled for.

Interestingly, the pattern of malpractice claims against physicians in different specialties has proved to be consistent with research findings on empathy among physicians practicing in different specialties. For example, in a large-scale study involving 12,829 physicians, the following specialists experienced the highest rates of malpractice claims: neurosurgeons, orthopedic surgeons, obstetricians and gynecologists, general surgeons, and anesthesiologists. The lowest rates occurred among specialists in psychiatry, pediatrics, and internal medicine (Taragin et al., 1994). The specialists who experienced low rates of malpractice claims in that study scored highest on empathy in our study (Hojat et al., 2002d).

Clinical Importance of the Differences

Differences in empathy among physicians in different specialties or between male and female physicians do not necessarily indicate a deficiency in empathy in the low-scoring groups. It is important to emphasize this point for two reasons.

First, according to the information available so far, almost all the statistically significant differences in empathy among medical students and physicians of each sex and in different specialties appear to be clinically unimportant. With the exception of our own studies, none of the studies discussed in this chapter so far have reported the effect-size estimate, an important statistical index that reveals whether the relationships or differences obtained are of practical importance and are clinically meaningful (Cohen, 1987; Hojat & Xu, 2004). In our studies, most estimates of the effect size were small, and only a few fell in the moderate range, indicating that the differences were not large enough to raise serious concerns about empathy scores that fall outside the normal range (Hojat et al., 2002c, 2002e).

Second, the duties involved in the procedure- and technology-oriented specialties obviously are primarily procedural and therefore may not demand the degree of empathic understanding necessary in the people-oriented specialties. For example, understanding patients' experiences and emotions is more crucial in primary care settings than it is in radiology or pathology departments.

An important question is whether differences in empathy scores among physicians in different specialties are a result of a different emphasis in interpersonal skills training of residents in psychiatry, family medicine, and internal medicine versus procedure-oriented specialties or are a function of personal qualities formed before students enter medical school. For example, in some medical school clerkships and residency programs, such as family medicine, internal medicine, pediatrics, and psychiatry, more emphasis is placed on training in interpersonal skills and physician–patient relationships. Therefore, a stronger empathic orientation could be expected to develop among individuals subjected to such training.

To address the issue of whether the differences in empathy among students interested in different specialties can be detected when students enter medical school (empathy attributed to personal qualities) or after they have been subjected to medical training (empathy attributed to medical education), we administered the JSPE to 422 students on orientation day, before they were exposed to the medical school curriculum (Hojat et al., 2005b). We also asked the new students about the medical specialty they planned to pursue after graduating from medical school. Because some students may have lacked a clear plan regarding a choice of specialty, we presented them with the following four scenarios and asked them to choose the one they were most interested in at that moment.

1. *Procedure-oriented specialties*: Performing specialized diagnostic procedures or basic applied laboratory research and major contact with colleagues, not patients. Primarily hospital-based (e.g., radiology, pathology).

2. *Technology-oriented specialties*: Performing highly skilled and specialized therapeutic techniques or procedures; serving as an expert consultant. Primarily hospital-based, with some office activities (e.g., orthopedic surgery, neurosurgery, ophthalmology). Patients are often referred by a primary care physician.

3. *Non-primary care specialties*: Providing episodic or long-term care of a specific and limited number of medical problems and a mix of ambulatory and hospital-based practice (e.g., cardiology, gastroenterology, dermatology, emergency medicine, psychiatry, obstetrics, and gynecology).

4. *Primary care specialties*: Providing first-encounter appraisal of health or illness and preventive education and intervention and episodic and long-term comprehensive care of a wide variety of medical conditions and primarily office-based (e.g., family medicine, general internal medicine, general pediatrics).

Our results indicated that students who were interested in primary care (Scenario 4) as a career obtained the highest mean score on the JSPE, followed by students interested in nonprimary care (Scenario 3), a technology-oriented specialty (Scenario 2), and finally a procedure-oriented specialty (Scenario 1) (Hojat et al., 2005b). Inferential statistical analyses indicated that the mean scores of students who were interested in the primary care specialties were significantly higher than the mean score of students who were interested in technology- or procedure-oriented specialties.

These results suggest that medical students often come to medical school with a preconceived idea about a career specialty that is consistent with their already developed personal attributes. However, the findings cannot eliminate the possibility that educational experiences or the interaction of personal qualities and educational experiences can also influence the choice of medical specialty. We are currently conducting a prospective 5-year longitudinal study to examine changes in empathy and interest in particular specialties from the beginning of medical school to completion of the first year of residency and to examine if change of interest in specialty in medical school is associated with changes in empathy scores.

Recapitulation

Empathy, like many other personal attributes, is associated with an individual's sex and a number of psychosocial variables. A large number of desirable personal qualities are positively related to measures of empathy. Conversely, a number of undesirable personal attributes are negatively linked to measures of empathy. Because of their capacity to engage empathically with the patients, individuals with high empathy scores demonstrate greater clinical competence and are more interested in people-oriented than technology- or procedure-oriented specialties.

Patient Outcomes

10

The secret of the care of the patient is in caring for the patient.

—(Francis W. Peabody, 1927/1984, p. 818)

The failure to empathize is the basis of most of the unhappy doctor–patient relationships.

—(Harry A. Wilmer, 1968, p. 248)

Preamble

The theoretical link between empathy and positive patient outcomes is based on three assumptions: When empathic engagement is formed, (a) the constraints of relationship will vanish, leading to a more accurate diagnosis, (b) the clinician becomes a trusting attachment figure and serves as a secure base from which to explore the unknowns of illness and the uncertainty of the future, and (c) the patient perceives the clinician as a helping member of a social support system with all the beneficial health effects of human connection. This chapter presents research findings on clinician–patient relationships in general and on empathic engagement in patient care in particular, in support of the following positive clinical outcomes: patients' greater satisfaction with their health care providers, better compliance with their physician's advice and a firmer commitment to the treatment plan, and a reduced likelihood of malpractice litigation. Further empirical confirmation is needed to support a direct link between measures of empathy and some objective indicators of patient outcomes.

Introduction

In this chapter, I briefly discuss the link between empathy and patient outcomes and present some theoretical framework and empirical evidence in support of that link. Presumably, any factor that contributes to enhancement of the clinician–patient relationship, including empathy, should in theory, have a beneficial effect on patient outcomes (Mercer & Reynolds, 2002). The expectation that an empathic clinician–patient relationship will result in positive patient outcomes is theoretically sound. Practically speaking, however, more empirical data are needed to support this expectation.

A Theoretical Framework

The theoretical link between empathic clinician–patient engagement and positive patient outcomes is based on three assumptions. First, from a *medical perspective*, it is assumed that when an empathic relationship is formed between a clinician and a patient, the constraints against disclosure will be lifted, the truth will emerge, and the result will be reflected in a more precise medical history and thus more accurate diagnostic information. Abundant evidence is available in support of this proposition, some of which was reported in Chapter 8.

Second, from a *psychological perspective*, in an empathic relationship, the patient perceives a clinician as a trustworthy attachment figure, an omnipotent authority similar to a protective wise parent. Therefore, the clinician becomes a secure base from which the patient can explore the unknowns of the illness, disclose real concerns without fear, and thus experience genuine human connection free of anxieties and concerns. Evidence supporting this assumption also is plentiful, some of which was presented in Chapter 4.

Third, from a *sociological perspective*, the patient views an empathic clinician as a helpful member of a social support system and therefore can benefit from all the positive effects of that system on his or her physical, mental, and social well-being. Ample evidence is available to support this claim as well, some of which was reported in Chapter 2.

On the basis of the three assumptions just described, an empathic clinician–patient relationship must lead to positive patient outcomes. However, despite the abundance of reports in the medical, psychological, and sociological literature about these three assumptions, empirical evidence supporting the direct link between empathy and measurable patient outcomes in medical and surgical care is difficult to find. As I indicated in Chapters 1 and 6, the dearth of empirical evidence in support of a direct link between empathy and patient outcomes is the result of two factors. First, the conceptual ambiguity regarding empathy in clinician–patient relationships has been an obstacle to the development of an operational definition of empathy in patient care. Second, until recently, the lack of a psychometrically sound measure of empathy designed specifically for use in the context of patient care has been an impediment to empirical investigation of empathy and its outcomes in the context of medical and surgical care. However, because empathy is the backbone of clinician–patient relationships, we can safely assume that the majority of research findings about the effects of physician–patient relationships on patient outcomes could be applicable to empathic engagement in patient care as well.

The Clinician–Patient Relationship and Patient Outcomes

A large volume of research has accumulated in support of the notion that the quality of the clinician–patient relationship can facilitate the process of patient care and thus have a positive influence on patient outcomes (Butow, Maclean, Dunn, Tattersall, & Boyer, 1997; Neuwirth, 1997; Roter et al., 1998; Sanson-Fisher & Maguire, 1980; Staudenmayer & Lefkowitz, 1981; Stewart, 1996). The relevance of such research findings to the theme of empathy in patient care is evident if one assumes that empathic engagement is a core ingredient of successful clinician–patient relationships.

The medical literature contains abundant evidence in support of the notion that the quality of physician–patient relationships has a tangible effect on clinical outcomes. For example, a review of 21 published studies revealed that 16 (76%) of the articles reported a positive, statistically significant relationship between effective physician–patient communication and health outcomes (Stewart, 1996). Among the elements of effective communication were physicians' empathic engagement, supportive role, and concern about patients' feelings and experiences (Stewart, 1996).

The following sections present some empirical evidence from the medical literature in support of the notion that high-quality physician–patient relationships positively influence patients' satisfaction and compliance and reduce the likelihood of malpractice litigation.

Patient Satisfaction

Patient satisfaction is a widely recognized outcome measure in health care research (Hall et al., 1988). The relationship between patients' satisfaction with their health care providers and their recall of and compliance with the providers' medical advice suggests that satisfaction is an important determinant of the outcome of health care (Hall & Dornan, 1988).

Patients' overall satisfaction with their health care providers is often moderately high (in the 70s or 80s on a 100-point scale) (Hall & Dornan, 1988). Interpersonal exchanges between physician and patient have often proved to be significant predictors of patients' satisfaction (Butow et al., 1997). For example, a meta-analytic study found that such factors as nonverbal cues (e.g., touch, forward lean, closer distance, eye contact, nods, gestures), social–emotional conversation (about nonmedical issues), positive talk, and length of encounter contributed to the patients' satisfaction with health care providers (Hall et al., 1988). Other determinants of patients' satisfaction were patients' participation in the therapeutic process (Speedling & Rose, 1985), commitment to the therapeutic relationship (i.e., willingness to return to the physician for care), the length of time the physicians spent with their patients, and the physicians' willingness to listen and to be accessible when needed (DiMatteo, Prince, & Taranta, 1979).

Moreover, physicians' ability to communicate their concern, warmth, and interest to their patients also leads to patients' satisfaction (Speedling & Rose, 1985). Physicians' general sensitivity to patients' emotions and their ability to express feelings were associated with patients' satisfaction (DiMatteo et al., 1980). All the qualities of physicians just described are among the ingredients of empathic engagement between physician and patient.

One explanation for the positive link between physicians' empathy and patient outcomes is that empathic engagement can help patients formulate their health problems more clearly, thus leading to more accurate diagnoses, more acceptable solutions to their health problems, and thus better compliance with treatment regimen (Stiles, Putman, Wolfe, & James, 1979). For example, patients infected with the human immunodeficiency virus (HIV) indicated that the quality of interpersonal relationships with medical staff was an important factor in their satisfaction with clinical outcomes (Stein, Fleisman, Mor, & Dresser, 1993). In another study, patients' perceptions of their physicians' interpersonal and communication skills contributed more to their satisfaction with clinical outcomes than physicians' knowledge did (Clearly & McNeil, 1988).

Investigators who conducted a study with residents in internal medicine and their patients noticed that patients' satisfaction was related more to interpersonal relationships reflected in physicians' courtesy and giving of information than to physicians' nonverbal behavior, such as eye contact and body posture (Comstock, Hooper, Goodwin, & Goodwin, 1982).

Reports that patients are generally more satisfied with an empathic health provider (Beckman & Frankel, 1984; Bertakis, Roter, & Putman, 1991; Francis & Morris, 1969; Korsch, Gozzi, & Francis, 1968b; Zachariae et al., 2003) and comply more with physicians who understand them better (Blackwell, 1973; Davis, 1968; Hall et al., 1988; Squier, 1990; Stewart, 1996) provide one explanation for positive clinical outcomes of empathy in patient care. Patients generally view physicians' conduct as a key determinant of their satisfaction with medical care (Moss, 1967). The finding that the physicians' understanding of their patients' perspective is related to the patients' perceptions of being helped (Eisenthal, Emery, Lazare, & Udin, 1979) provides additional support for the link between empathic understanding and patient outcomes. In a factor analytic study, 52% of the variance in patent's ratings of their satisfaction with medical care was accounted for by the physician's level of interpersonal warmth and respect (Kenny, 1995). In a study with diabetic patients, dieticians' empathic understanding was predictive of the patients' satisfaction and the success of consultations (Goodchild, Skinner, & Parkin, 2005). To summarize, the practice style reflected in a clinician's empathic concern for patients can lead to more satisfaction on the patients' part.

Adherence and Compliance

Adherence to and compliance with treatment regimens are additional, widely used indicators of clinical outcomes (Hall et al., 1988; Kim, Kaplowitz, & Johnston, 2004; Ong, DeHaes, Hoos, & Lammies, 1995; Roter et al., 1998; Sackett & Haynes, 1976; Stewart, 1996). Although the terms adherence and compliance are often used interchangeably in the literature, their meaning is not identical. For example, compliance reflects a biomedical paradigm of disease that reinforces passivity in patients (Roter et al., 1998) and refers to the patient's acceptance of the clinician's orders or advice without participating in the decision-making process (Kelman, 1958). When the patient follows the clinician's instructions as a participant in the process, however, adherence is the more appropriate term. Adherence implies a more active patient–clinician collaboration involving patient's choice in planning the treatment (Eisenthal et al., 1979; Roter et al., 1998; Squier, 1990).

An abundance of evidence suggests that empathy in physician–patient relationships not only contributes to patients' satisfaction with their health care providers and adherence to the providers' advice but also leads to adequate disclosure of problems, all of which can have a significant impact on patient outcomes (Beckman & Frankel, 1984; Butow et al., 1997; Falvo & Tippy, 1988; Sanson-Fisher & Maguire, 1980). Physicians' understanding of their patients was found to be significantly correlated with adhering to treatment and feeling better on the part of their patients (Eisenthal et al., 1979). In a pediatric health care setting, investigators reported that mothers of sick children adhered more closely to the care provider's advice when they perceived that the provider attempted to understand their concerns (Francis & Morris, 1969; Korsch, Gozzi, & Francis, 1968a). In a similar study, physicians' empathic understanding, reflected in their expression of positive affect, increased adherence to the physicians' advice among mothers after emergency visits to a children's hospital (Freemon, Negrete, Davis, & Korsch, 1971).

Patients' adherence to treatment reportedly varied from 25% to 94%, depending on several factors, including interactions between physician and patient (Eisenthal et al., 1979). Despite the important benefits patients derived from following their physician's advice, two studies reported that a significant number of patients (30%–60%) failed to follow that advice (Kaplan & Simon, 1990; Luscher & Vetter, 1990). This can be attributed to a lack of empathic engagement. Physicians' empathic skills and interpersonal style have been cited as crucial factors determining whether patients adhere to treatment regimens (DiMatteo et al., 1993). Indicators of a physician's empathy, such as sensitivity, decoding skills, tone of voice, and nonverbal communication, were related to patients' compliance with scheduled appointments (DiMatteo, Hays, & Prince, 1986). Furthermore, in situations where the physician failed to demonstrate empathic engagement, the patient easily forgot their advice and was likely to miss follow-up appointments (Falvo & Tippy, 1988). In addition, physicians who expressed willingness to answer patients' questions without being concerned about the time had a positive influence on patients' adherence to treatment (DiMatteo et al., 1993). These studies suggest that an interpersonal style that reflects a physician's empathic understanding of patients can enhance patients' adherence to treatment.

Malpractice Claims

Research indicates that a problematic physician–patient relationship can increase the likelihood that a patient will initiate a legal action against the physician. A physician's style of communication, in particular, is an important factor in a plaintiff's decision to take such an action (Beckman, Markakis, Suchman, & Frankel, 1994; Hickson, Clayton, Githens, & Sloan, 1992; Levinson, Roter, Mullooly, Dull, & Frankel, 1997; Meyers, 1987; Shapiro, Simpson, & Lawrence, 1989). Empirical evidence suggests that a positive physician–patient relationship reduces not only the actual malpractice claims but also patients' intention to take such action, regardless of the severity of the adverse medical outcomes (Moore, Adler, & Robertson, 2000). In a survey conducted in the mid-1980s, malpractice attorneys indicated that more than 80% of malpractice suits were based on unsatisfactory physician–patient relationships (Avery, 1985).

One study found that physicians who exhibited empathic concern for their patients were better diagnosticians and provided better treatments (Barsky, 1981), and another study reported that better diagnosis and treatment reduced the risk of malpractice litigation (Levinson et al., 1997). Conversely, poor communication skills on the physicians' part, which led to inadequate empathic engagement with patients, proved to be the most important factor prompting patients to file a lawsuit against a physician (Beckman et al., 1994).

In a study examining rates of malpractice claims for different medical specialties, Taragin and colleagues (1994) controlled for confounding factors (e.g., physicians' age, training, and certification status and the severity of the diseases they treated) and concluded that the variation in claim rates could not be explained by differences in the physicians' academic achievements. Consistent with these findings, researchers in another study found no relationship between malpractice claims against obstetricians and the technical quality of physician's care (Entman et al., 1994).

Among mothers of infants who had been permanently injured or had died, dissatisfaction with the obstetrician's interpersonal style (e.g., not listening, not talking openly, and not discussing long-term outcomes) was a major factor in determining whether the obstetrician was sued (Hickson et al., 1992). Compared with obstetricians who had been sued, those who had never been sued were viewed as concerned, accessible, and willing to talk (Hickson et al., 1994). Other studies have shown that the physician's communication skills and empathic concern are the factors that reduce the risk of malpractice litigation (Beckman et al., 1994; Levinson et al., 1997).

A review of allegation transcripts revealed that physicians' failure to understand the perspectives of their patients or their patients' families, a clear indication of a lack of empathic engagement, was among the important factors that contributed to patients' decision to sue (Beckman et al., 1994; Levinson et al., 1997).

Physicians' Empathy and Patient Outcomes

Although some studies show a link between empathic engagement and patient outcomes in the context of medical and surgical treatments (Luborsky, Chandler, Auerbach, Cohen, & Bacharach, 1971; Nightingale et al., 1991), empirical evidence in support of empathic engagement and patient outcomes has been reported more often in the context of psychotherapy (Free et al., 1985; Gladstein, 1977; Kurtz & Grummon, 1972). For example, premature termination of therapy has been reported among clients who gave their therapists low ratings on a measure of empathy (Burns & Nolen-Hoeksema, 1992). Some reviews of the literature have linked the therapist's empathy, warmth, and genuineness to positive changes in clients (Patterson, 1984). Other reviews have reported positive patient outcomes resulting from empathic engagement between patients and nurses (Bennett, 1995). However, fewer studies have shown a direct empirical link between empathy and the outcomes of medical and surgical treatments (Stewart, 1996).

Research on psychotherapeutic outcomes, for example, has reported a high level of empathic clinician–patient engagement as the most important factor in the reduction of symptoms (Rogers, Gendlin, Kiesler, & Truax, 1967). Also, therapists' scores on the Accurate Empathy Scale of Truax and Carkhuff's Relationship Questionnaire (see Chapter 5) were significantly higher in successful than in unsuccessful therapy cases. Bacharach (1976) reported that a therapist's empathy was consistently correlated with other qualities such as regard, genuineness, concreteness, and self-disclosure that are associated with treatment outcomes. Some studies have provided evidence supporting the causal role of empathy in psychotherapeutic outcomes (Burns & Nolen-Hocksema, 1992; Greenberg et al., 2001). Nonetheless, there are other studies that have not confirmed a direct link between therapists' empathy and positive patient outcomes (Bohart et al., 2002; Luborsky et al., 1971; Meltzoff & Kornreich, 1970). The conceptualization and measurement issues described in Chapter 1 could be the reasons for a lack of correlations reported between empathy and patient outcomes in these studies.

A meta-analytic review found that the typical effect size in studies on empathy and patient outcomes is in the 0.20s (Bohart et al., 2002). According to the operational definitions of effect sizes (Cohen, 1987; Hojat et al., 2004), an effect size of this magnitude is trivial. However, the magnitude of effect size for the relationship between empathy and patient outcomes varies, depending on the conceptualization of empathy (e.g., cognitive or emotional empathy) and the instruments designed to measure it, the format of the assessment (e.g., self-rated or observer-, peer-, or client-rated), the type of therapy (e.g., group, cognitive, psychoanalytical, or behavioral therapy), the therapist's experience, the patient's receptivity, and so on (Bohart et al., 2002).

Empathic engagement, determined by standardized patients' assessments, was significantly correlated with patients' level of comfort and feelings of being important in a study with 1,048 fourth-year medical students (Colliver et al., 1998). In that study, the students whose empathic engagement was evaluated as insufficient (judged to be empathic by less than three of the seven standardized patients) also received lower ratings concerning their skills in history taking and physical examinations (Colliver et al., 1998).

Staudenmayer and Lefkowitz (1981) found that physicians' empathic concern (determined by peers' ratings of their sensitivity) was related to the length of hospitalization and concerns about medications: Highly sensitive physicians were more concerned about the side effects of medications and kept their patients (with asthma and other pulmonary problems) in the hospital for longer periods. MacPherson, Mercer, Scullion, and Thomas (2003) reported that the perceptions of acupuncture patients concerning their care providers' empathy was significantly associated with patients' enablement, which in turn was highly correlated with self-reported patient outcomes.

Levinson (1994) reported that patients' satisfaction and adherence to treatment were directly associated with their physicians' empathic skills, whereas patients' dissatisfaction and malpractice claims were associated with their physicians' lack of those skills. In another study, physicians regarded empathic behavior as the most important quality for being a "good physician" in improving patient outcomes; however, the physicians themselves listed empathic behavior as the least important factor for being promoted in the hospital setting! (Carmel & Glick, 1996).

An experiment conducted in the General Medicine Clinic at Cook County Hospital in Chicago showed that physicians' empathic, as opposed to sympathetic, responses to patients can lead to different measurable influences on their practice behavior and on patient outcomes (Nightingale et al., 1991). The sample in that experiment consisted of 96 residents and fellows whose preference for responding empathically or sympathetically to patients was determined by the following scenario:

> Your next patient enters the office, sits down, and says: "Doctor, my husband/wife died and I feel terrible!" The English language gives you two basic ways to respond to the patient: (A) "I understand how you feel" or words to that effect, or (B) "I feel sorry for you" or words to that effect. Which do you use?

The A option was considered to be an empathic response, and the B option was considered to be a sympathetic response. The physicians who chose the empathic response (60% of the sample) ordered fewer laboratory tests, performed cardiopulmonary resuscitation for a shorter period of time before declaring their efforts unsuccessful, and showed less preference for intubating a hypothetical patient with end-stage lung disease. The investigators concluded that physician's empathic or sympathetic responses could lead to significant differences in their style of practice and the use of resources. In another study it was reported that empathy can reduce the cost of medical care (Yarnold, Greenberg, & Nightingale, 1991.)

In a recent study on the effect of physicians' empathy on patients' satisfaction and compliance with treatment (Kim et al., 2004), a set of questionnaires was administered to 550 outpatients at a university hospital in South Korea. The results indicated that patients' perceptions of physicians' empathy, measured by a modified version of the Barrett-Lennard's Relationship Inventory, could have a significant influence on the patients' satisfaction and compliance. The researchers concluded that enhancement of physicians' empathic communication skills is among the best approaches to improving patient satisfaction and compliance with treatment. In another study, expressions of empathy and support contributed to patients' satisfaction with their physicians (Thompson, Hearn, & Collins, 1992).

Dubnicki (1977) reported that psychotherapists' high scores on Hogan's Empathy Scale were predictive of more accurate prognoses. Kendall and Wilcox (1980) found that when therapists formed an empathic relationship with hyperactive, uncontrolled children, the children's behavior improved. Physicians' empathy, determined by positive interactions between pediatricians and the mothers of sick children, improved the mothers' satisfaction with the children's care and reduced their concern about the illness (Wasserman, Inui, Barriatua, Carter, & Lippincott, 1984). Another study found that physicians' empathy, responsiveness, and reliability were significant determinants of patients' satisfaction with their health care (Bowers, Swan, & Koehler, 1994).

The majority of studies on the link between physicians' empathy and patient outcomes relied on physicians' self-reports. However, patients' own perceptions of their therapist's empathy, rather than the therapist's self-report, could be a better predictor of clinical outcomes (Free et al., 1985; Kurtz & Grummon, 1972).

Recapitulation

One can speculate that physicians' positive interpersonal conduct, as an indicator of empathic engagement, is associated with positive patient outcomes, including more accurate diagnoses, better adherence by patients to treatment regimens, patients' greater satisfaction with their physician's care, and less likelihood of malpractice litigation. Abundant research supports this speculation. Although studies that confirm a correlation between physician–patient empathic engagement and patient outcomes in medical care are convincing, more empirical evidence is needed to verify a direct link between measures of empathy in the context of patient care and objective indicators of patient outcomes.

11 Enhancement of Empathy

You couldn't love something you didn't understand.

—(Forrest Carter, 1976, p. 38)

Preamble

Although empathy is viewed as an important element of professionalism in medicine, a few obstacles to the development and implementation of empathy exist in medical education and practice. For example, students tend to become cynical during their medical education, a paradigm shift is taking place in the health care system, and the system has become overly reliant on biotechnology. Thus, attention to the enhancement of empathy in medical education and the practice of health care not only is timely and important but also is a mandate that must be acted on by educators in the health professions. Research often shows that empathy is an attribute that is amenable to change as a result of educational experiences. Approaches used to enhance empathy include interpersonal skills training, exercises in perspective taking, role playing, role models, imagining, and exposure to educational activities that resemble patients' experiences in encounters with health care providers and hospital staff. In addition, the Balint approach to improving physician–patient interpersonal relationships has also been used to improve physicians' empathy. The study of literature and the arts and the improvement of narrative skills are specifically recommended as ways of enhancing empathy through a better understanding of human emotions, pain, and suffering. Empirical research is needed to confirm the effectiveness of programs designed to enhance empathy and to support their long-term effects.

Introduction

This chapter begins with a discussion of professionalism in medicine and describes some factors that hamper the development of empathy among students and practitioners in the health professions. Then I present some of the approaches that psychologists and researchers in health education have used to enhance empathy.

Professionalism in Medicine

Professionalism in medicine is defined as an array of personal qualities beyond the requisite medical knowledge and procedural skills that health care professionals must possess to deliver high-quality health care to their patients that leads to positive clinical outcomes (Veloski & Hojat, 2006). Medical educators currently are encouraged to make every effort to foster professionalism in medicine by offering programs at the undergraduate, graduate, and continuing education levels.

Although no consensus exists regarding the number and nature of personal qualities required for professionalism in medicine, compassionate care and empathy have frequently been mentioned as its key components (Arnold, 2002; Barondess, 2003; Linn et al., 1987). In his book *Humanism and the Physician*, Edmund Pellegrino (1979) described the empathic way of helping patients as an important aspect of the physician's humanistic attributes. Senior residents at Laval and Calgary universities in Canada listed empathy, respect, and competence as the three most important elements of professionalism in medicine (Brownell & Cote, 2001).

Cultivating humanistic values, including empathy, is among the important goals of education in the health care professions. The Medical Schools Objectives Project of the Association of American Medical Colleges, (2004) includes enrichment of empathy among the educational objectives of medical schools, emphasizing that the schools should strive to produce altruistic physicians who provide compassionate care to patients and demonstrate empathy by conveying their understanding of the patients' perspective. In a position paper, the American Board of Internal Medicine, (1983) recommended that humanistic attributes, including empathy, should be instilled in and assessed among residents as an essential part of their medical training.

Despite the consensus regarding the healing potential of empathic encounters in patient care, insufficient attention has been given to enhancement of the capacity for empathy in the design of medical education curriculum. As a result, the concept of empathy in patient care, according to Novack (1987), seems to be fading away in modern medical education, with the exception of a few lonely souls who attempt to treat empathy with respect, as if it were an endangered species on the verge of extinction. The current system of medical education does not seem to be seriously concerned about physicians' losing their healing touch, treating it instead "as if it were a relic of an unscientific past" (Novack, 1987, p. 346).

The lack of attention to empathy in patient care is partially the result of overreliance on computer-based diagnostic and therapeutic technology and partially the result of changes in the health care system, with its ripple effect on medical education and practice. In the biotechnologically advanced atmosphere of patient care, what computers spit out seems to receive more attention from some practitioners, who trust the machines more than their skills in detecting clinical signs of disease or their patients' narrative accounts of illness.

Although the pathophysiology of disease may be detected by examining computer output and electronic images, an accurate diagnosis of illness is possible only by listening to the patient and conducting physical examinations in clinical encounters (Spiro, 1986). Today, the public pleads desperately for physicians who are more communicative and empathic in their encounters with patients (Fishbein, 1999). Despite the current emphasis on the development of professionalism, enhancement of empathy in the education of health care professionals has not yet received systematic and sufficient attention. According to Girgis and Sanson-Fisher (1995), although most physicians are well equipped to provide high-quality technical services, they are often ill equipped to provide empathic care.

Obstacles to Empathy in Patient Care

Some of the factors that impede the development and implementation of empathy in education and practice in the health professions are described in the following sections.

Cynicism

Medical students often embark on becoming physicians with idealism and enthusiasm for curing disease and preventing infirmity. Despite the intention of medical school faculty to nurture these qualities, it is ironic that some have noticed a decline in humanitarianism, enthusiasm, and idealism among students during medical training (Kay, 1990; Maheux & Beland, 1989; Sheehan, Sheehan, White, Leibowitz, & Baldwin, 1990; Silver & Glicken, 1990; Wolf et al., 1989; Zeldow & Daugherty, 1987).

The effects of medical education on personal qualities were addressed empirically more than four decades ago, with some disturbing results (Becker & Geer, 1958; Eron, 1958). One longitudinal study conducted in the 1950s (Eron, 1958) found that medical students became more cynical and less humanitarian as they progressed through medical school, whereas this pattern was not observed among law students! In that study, a typical question used to measure cynicism was, "If you don't look out for yourself, nobody else will," and a typical question for measuring humanism was, "When I hear about the suffering of a particular individual or group, I want very much to help."

A similar concern about medical students' progression toward cynicism during medical school was raised in the early 1980s (Silver, 1982). Another study found that as many as three-fourths of medical students became more cynical about academic life and the medical profession as they progressed through medical schools (Sheehan et al., 1990). This metamorphosis in the character of medical students was likened to the "battered child syndrome" and was attributed to inappropriate treatment of students by the medical schools (Rosenberg & Silver, 1984; Silver & Glicken, 1990). The terms "dehumanization" (Edwards & Zimet, 1976) and "traumatic de-idealization" (Kay, 1990) also were used to describe the cynical transformation occurring during medical education.

Several additional studies conducted in the 1980s reported other disturbing findings. A study at the University of Texas Health Science Center in San Antonio found that medical students underwent a significant hedonistic change in personality between the freshman and junior years of medical school: They became less inhibited and more self-indulgent (Burnstein et al., 1980). In a longitudinal study conducted at the same medical center, a decline in students' scores on the "need to understand" scale of a personality inventory also raised concern about the negative influence of medical education on students' personalities (Whittemore, Burstein, Loucks, & Schoenfeld, 1985). Students in the senior year at the Louisiana State University School of Medicine reported that the top two changes in attitude during medical school were more cynicism (76%) and more concern about making money (60%) (Wolf et al., 1989).

The alarm bells became even louder in 2002, when a nationwide study found that 61% of residents in American residency training programs believed that they had become more cynical during their medical education (Collier, MaCue, Markus, & Smith, 2002). Cynicism was more prominent among female residents than it was among male residents (63% versus 56%, respectively). Interestingly, however, residents with children reported less cynicism and more humanistic feelings during their medical education (Sanson-Fisher & Maguire, 1980).

In an atmosphere of declining humanism, the emphasis some modern medical educators place on "detached concern" and "affective distance" for the purpose of increasing objectivity in clinical decision making is accelerating the dramatic metamorphosis occurring in medical education and patient care (Coulehan & Williams, 2001; Evans et al., 1993; Farber et al., 1997). Although well intended, the advice of those educators can be misinterpreted, thus adding to the factors contributing to the ultimate diminishment of empathy's importance in medical education and practice (Ludmerer, 1999; Starr, 1982). Among other factors fueling increased cynicism in medical education are lack of role models (Diseker & Michielutte, 1981; Kramer, Ber, & Moore, 1987) and lack of dedicated educational programs for nourishment of humanistic qualities in patient encounters.

Paradigmatic Shift in the Health Care System

As Gonnella, Hojat, Erdmann, and Veloski (1993a, 1993b) suggested, in addition to factors related to physicians and patients, the environment of health care delivery exerts a significant influence on patient outcomes. Recent developments in the organization, financing, and delivery of health care, notably in the expansion of managed care and the restriction of physicians' autonomy, pose challenges that contribute to physicians' discontent with the practice of medicine and a lack of opportunity for empathic engagement in clinical encounters (Burdi & Baker, 1999; Magee & Hojat, 2001).

Anecdotal reports suggest that financial incentives and insurance regulations in the current environment of health care have forced a number of physicians to trade off their patients' interest. The golden principle that the patient's best interest must be the primary consideration of patient care may lose its priority in such a market-driven health care environment. According to a survey of physicians, the significant decline in the time physicians spent with patients and their inability to control the length of patients' hospital stays and their own work schedules exacerbated their dissatisfaction with the current atmosphere of the health care environment (Burdi & Baker, 1999). When Burdi and Baker (1999) compared a sample of physicians surveyed in 1991 with another, cohort-matched sample of physicians surveyed in 1996, they found that the number of physicians who said they would have chosen medicine if they had been college students declined by 10% during the 5-year period. This decline reflects the evolving changes in the health care system leading to physician dissatisfaction.

In a survey of 2,608 physicians conducted in 2004, 58% of them said their enthusiasm for medicine had declined in the past few years, and 87% said their morale had declined because of changes in the health care system (Zuger, 2004). The discontent of physicians is an inevitable outcome of the restrictions on their autonomy and use of resources imposed by the health care system and the health insurance industry (Hojat et al., 2000c; Kassirer, 1998; Magee & Hojat, 2001). Physicians' discontent with the practice of medicine, especially among those who have been "wounded" by malpractice allegations, matters because it influences the interpersonal quality of care and empathic engagement in clinical encounters. An analysis of how physicians are depicted in the movies showed that their portrayal as positive figures has declined in recent years. In current films, they are often depicted as greedy, egoistic, uncaring, and unethical (Flores, 2002).

The "time" factor is another impediment caused by the growing emphasis on cost containment that has contributed to shortening the time spent in clinical encounters, thus hindering the formation of empathic relationships. The medical profession, once the most respected of all the professions (Thomas, 1985), is now under siege, and physicians are frequently blamed, often mistakenly, for the problems created by nonphysician managers of health insurance organizations. These structural and functional shifts in the health care delivery system can hamper the potential benefits of forming empathic clinician–patient relationships. The ripple effect of changes in the American health care system also has had a profound effect on medical students (Hojat et al., 1999b) and nurses (Steinbrook, 2002).

Research shows that physicians' discontent leads to patients' noncompliance with treatment (DiMatteo et al., 1993) and dissatisfaction with their health care providers (Hass et al., 2000; Linn, Yager, Cope, & Leake, 1985). Such discontent among physicians can be reflected in pessimism manifested in their communication with patients. Furthermore, research suggests that pessimism is significantly associated with mortality among physicians as well as their patients (Hollowell & De Ville, 2003).

As a result of the paradigmatic shift described earlier, the health care delivery system has been transformed into a profit-driven enterprise, with less emphasis on clinician–patient interactions and more emphasis on financial efficiency (Merlyn, 1998). Diminished prestige, loss of autonomy, and deep personal dissatisfaction are among the outcomes of paradigmatic shifts in health care systems. Research shows a widespread "professional malaise" among physicians, who are caught between the desire to provide high-quality care to their patients on the one hand and the need to satisfy the insurers and regulators on the other hand (Zuger, 2004).

According to psychoanalytic theories, this type of approach-avoidance psychic conflict (e.g., a desire to help patients and avoid conflicts with insurers at the same time) can lead to frustration and neurotic-type distress that threaten physicians' physical, mental, and social well-being. Poor clinical management and substandard medical care resulting from a system that restricts physicians' autonomy in dealing with patients inevitably lead to hostile reactions by the public, often directed toward physicians, who themselves are victims of the system's crippling effects.

Added to this paradigmatic shift in the health care delivery system is the dramatic rise in the number of malpractice suits. The inevitable result is greater discontent with medicine among practitioners and even greater dissatisfaction with health care services among patients (Mello et al., 2004). In an atmosphere in which the physician–patient relationship resembles an encounter between consumer and retailer, little room obviously is left for compassion and empathy.

The primary concern of powerful players in the health care system—notably, nonphysicians employed by government agencies and the health insurance industry—is cost containment. The new arrangements created by this shift of emphasis have intruded in the clinical autonomy of physicians, led to the inability of physicians to preserve their altruistic image, and eroded the public's trust and support (Schlesinger, 2002). In a hostile atmosphere where physician–patient encounters are based on fear of allegations of malpractice, rather than on trust, the physician–patient relationship is likely to be shaken at best and violated or broken at worst (Thom, Hall, & Pawlson, 2004). As a result of all the changes occurring in the health care system, the adverse effects on the clinician–patient relationship are more threatening to the outcomes of care than ever before (Simpson et al., 1991). Needless to say, an empathic relationship is highly unlikely to form in an atmosphere in which physicians view each patient as a potential adversary for malpractice litigation (Mello et al., 2004).

In 2002, the American Board of Internal Medicine, the American College of Physicians, the American Society for Internal Medicine, and the European Federation of Internal Medicine jointly published a report titled *Medical Professionalism in the New Millennium: A Physician Charter* (Sox, 2002). The report not only confirmed the existence of the problems described here but also underscored their severity by concluding that the "changes in the health care delivery systems in countries throughout the industrial world threaten the values of professionalism" (p. 234). These trends in medicine, with their ripple effect on medical education, have resulted in brief consultations, the goal of which is to identify one physical problem as the "chief complaint" (Shorter, 1986), thus shifting the attention from the patient as a person to a disease as a case. One hopes that the recent attention to professionalism in medical education and practice will bring empathic engagement between physician and patient to the forefront of health care once again.

Overreliance on Biotechnology

The new millennium offers either the best or the worst clinical care, depending on whether one views the "glass" as half full or half empty. The glass is half full, given the fact the biotechnological developments can certainly help to prevent many diseases worldwide at a rapid pace, to make more accurate diagnoses much earlier than before, and to treat patients more aggressively. The glass is half empty, however, given the fact that computerized medicine is gradually replacing "the laying on of hands," trivializing the importance of face-to-face encounters between physician and patient and reducing opportunities to form empathic physician–patient engagement as a result. Even telephone calls to family physicians (who used to make home visits in the good old days) are answered by automatic messages instructing desperate patients to call back during office hours or go to the emergency room for help. Obviously, these trends are not conducive to empathy in patient care.

During visits to a physician's office, patients are sometimes required to undergo a series of laboratory tests, unnecessarily in some cases (Divinagarcia, Harkin, Bonk, & Schluger, 1998; Sandler, 1980), and wait until the physician receives the results and makes a diagnosis, overlooking the clinical signs and symptoms that have been used successfully by physicians for hundreds of years. In this era of biotechnology, many physicians tend to view the results of laboratory tests and computerized diagnostic procedures as the holy script—despite the well-known errors associated with the sensitivity and specificity of the tests—rather than pay more attention to the patients' clinical signs and illness narrative. Thus, patients are treated as objects of technical services (Coulehan & Williams, 2001), rather than as subjects for human services. This style of dealing with patients defies Peabody's stated purpose of patient care: "The treatment of a disease may be entirely impersonal; the care of a patient must be completely personal" (Peabody, 1984, p. 814). In a survey of patients who either changed their physicians or were thinking of changing their physicians, the following comment made by a patient deserves serious attention in medical education: "Students should be taught to use technology as a backup and not as the primary factor of the examination of the patient" (Cousins, 1985, p. 1423).

The strain in the physician–patient relationship caused by the shift from the patient's trust in the physician's healing touch to the physician's trust in computerized diagnostic procedures has led to the public's perception that physicians have become too "detached" to be concerned about their patients (Mangione et al., 2002). As a result, the medical profession is increasingly faced with the criticism that physicians are losing their human touch (Johnston, 1992). Indeed, a number of studies have supported this view by confirming that medical students, residents, and practicing physicians have become more cynical and less compassionate during medical training and practice (Feudtner et al., 1994; Kay, 1990; Lu, 1995; Maheux & Beland, 1989; Self, Schrader, Baldwin, & Wolinsky, 1993; Sheehan et al., 1990; Silver & Glicken, 1990; Wolf et al., 1989; Zeldow & Daugherty, 1987).

The above-mentioned issues are only some of the challenges facing medical education and practice today. However, despite all the bad news, the good news is that it is possible to enhance empathy through dedicated educational programs and through demonstrations of its beneficial effects on patient outcomes.

The Amenability of Empathy to Change

A number of studies have shown that during the course of medical education, a person's capacity for empathy can undergo positive, negative, or no change. Although the inconsistent research findings are troublesome and may reflect issues involving conceptualization, measurement, and methodology, the fact that some studies have noted a change in empathy, either positive or negative, indicates that this attribute is amenable to change—welcome news for medical educators.

The State-Versus-Trait Debate

The idea of enhancing empathy during education for the health professions depends heavily on the belief that the capacity for empathy is amenable to change. Thus, it is important to address this issue at the outset because, if empathy proved to be a stable personality trait that cannot be easily changed, discussion of educational programs designed to enhance empathy would be pointless.

Psychologists have long been concerned about the possibility of changing people's motivations, attitudes, values, personality, and behavior. It is generally believed that some human attributes are more resistant to change than others. In the behavioral and social sciences, personal qualities, such as excitability, that are highly stable and difficult to change, are often called *traits*, whereas relatively unstable personality attributes, such as moods, that are easy to change are called *states* (Cole, Martin, & Steiger, 2005). The findings of longitudinal research concerning the stability of the so-called traits are inconsistent. For example, some findings suggest that traits can change over time (Roberts & DelVecchio, 2000), and other findings indicate that traits continue to show stability over a period of 15 years (Caspi & Silva, 1995).

The notion that empathy has an evolutionary root (Chapter 3) suggests that under normal circumstances, normal individuals are naturally programmed to demonstrate empathy. The extent to which the potential for empathy can be actualized or enhanced in a particular person will depend on the interaction of several factors, including the person's constitutional makeup, early life experiences, motivation, and a facilitating environment as well as exposure to specific educational programs. Therefore, empathy, in my view, is neither a highly stable personality trait nor a state that can be changed without effort. In a sense, empathy resembles the notion of attachment that is rooted in evolutionary, genetic, developmental, experiential, situational, and educational ground, and its deficit can be improved by therapeutic approaches.

Changes in Empathy During Professional Education

Positive Change

Some studies that offered a targeted educational program reported an improvement in empathy. For example, residents who participated in a comprehensive interpersonal skills training course demonstrated greater use of empathy when dealing with patients (e.g., they asked more open-ended questions and provided emotion-related responses) (Kause, Robbins, Heidrich, Abrassi, & Anderson, 1980).

A study of Israeli medical students found that a clerkship in psychiatry improved their scores on Mehrabian and Epstein's Emotional Empathy Scale and that the students retained the effect of the program for at least 6 months (Elizur & Rosenheim, 1982). In another study, the investigators noticed that medical students and physicians who participated in an interpersonal skills workshop demonstrated improved empathic behavior, as determined by their increasing use of supportive behaviors, such as listening, responding empathically, and calming the patients (Kramer, Ber, & Moores, 1989).

At the University of Missouri School of Medicine in Kansas City, empathy training offered to students in the early years of medical school resulted in increased scores on Carkhuff's Empathic Understanding in Interpersonal Processes Scale (Feighny, Arnold, Monaco, Munro, & Earl, 1998). However, the students' scores on Davis's Interpersonal Reactivity Index (IRI) did not increase, probably because of its lower sensitivity in the clinical context. Finally, over the years, training in communication skills provided in various formats (lectures, workshops, and audio- or videotapes) has proved to be useful in improving empathy-related skills (Evans et al., 1993; Fine & Therrien, 1977; Kramer et al., 1989; Sanson-Fisher & Poole, 1978; Winefield & Chur-Hansen, 2000). Stepien and Baernstein (2006) reviewed articles on empathy education programs in medical schools and found that many of the articles reported an improvement of empathy. However, these authors suggested that research on enhancement of empathy in medical education poses challenges because of the lack of consensus about the conceptualization and definition of empathy, the lack of adequate research designs and control groups, and variation among the instruments used to measure empathy.

Negative Change

Another group of studies showed a decline in empathy among medical students and residents during the course of their medical education in the absence of a targeted educational program. For example, after a period of clinical experience, medical students at the Bowman Gray School of Medicine in North Carolina showed a slight decrease in scores on Hogan's Empathy Scale (Diseker & Michielutte, 1981). Another study reported that a sample of medical students developed a hedonistic personality pattern during medical school that contributed to the decline in empathy (Whittemore et al., 1985).

In a study of changes in empathy, humanism, and professionalism during medical education at a major academic center, Marcus (1999) analyzed approximately 400 dreams reported by healthy medical students and house staff and traced the development of empathy and humanistic attitudes in different years of medical education. Marcus reported that identification with cold and uncaring role models; increasing reliance on the technological aspects of treatment, rather than on the humanistic side of patient care; and development of a sense of elitism or of belonging to a privileged group were among the factors that became noticeable among students in the third year of medical school, as inferred from dream analyses.

At the University of Pennsylvania Hospital, Bellini, Baime, and Shea (2002) administered the IRI to first-year residents in internal medicine and reported a decline in the residents' scores on the Perspective Taking and Empathic Concern subscales of the IRI. Conversely, the residents' scores increased on the IRI Personal Distress subscale—a result that was not conducive to empathic patient care. A follow-up study 3 years later showed that the decline in scores on the Empathic Concern subscale remained throughout the 3 years of the residency program (Bellini & Shea, 2005).

In a study of residents in internal medicine in three different years of residency at Thomas Jefferson University Hospital, we noticed a progressive decline in scores on the Jefferson Scale of Physician Empathy (JSPE) as the residents progressed from one level of training to the next (Mangione et al., 2002). Although systematic, the observed decline did not reach the conventional level of statistical significance ($p < .05$). In a subsequent study, we administered the JSPE to 125 third-year medical students at the beginning and end of the academic year and observed a statistically significant decline in the students' average scores by the end of the year (Hojat et al., 2004). Sherman and Cramer (2005) also observed a significant decline in dentistry students' scores on the JSPE as the students progressed through dental school.

Research results indicating that empathy declines during education for the health care professions is deeply troubling and should not be viewed as a trivial matter. To restore respect to the medical profession, the most humanistic profession in existence, the factors that contribute to the decline of empathy and other humanistic values must be investigated seriously. A medical education system that produces physicians who are unable to apply the science of medicine in conjunction with the art of healing represents an unfinished business. The physician who has learned the science but has no sense of the art of healing is, in the words of Saadi, the 12th-century Persian poet, like "a man who ploughs, but sows no seed."

No Change

There is yet a third group of studies that shows no change in empathy during medical education. For example, a course in behavioral science offered to medical students did not change the students' orientation toward viewing the patient as a person (Markham, 1979). In another study with medical students, researchers at the Bowman Gray School of Medicine exposed the students to a one-semester course in human communication and observed no change in the students' scores on Hogan's Empathy Scale (Diseker & Michielutte, 1981).

In the late 1980s, researchers reported that they observed no significant changes in medical students' empathy and other personal qualities measured with the Empathic Concern and Perspective Taking subscales of the IRI

(Zeldow & Daugherty, 1987). A study in which the IRI was administered to nursing students during their third year of nursing education found no change in the students' empathy during the 9-month training period (Becker & Sands, 1988).

The majority of findings reported in the previous section indicate that empathy is amenable to either positive or negative change during professional education. Even the negative findings can be viewed optimistically because if empathy can decline in the absence of appropriate educational programs, it has the potential to increase if appropriate educational remedies are provided. The possibility of teaching empathy (Spiro, 1992) and other human virtues (Shelton, 1999) during medical training has already been discussed. However, do we all agree that educators in the health professions must assume responsibility for improving the students' personal attributes, such as empathy, in addition to imparting knowledge to them and developing their clinical and procedural skills? Although this question may generate some debate concerning the applications of behavioral modification with students and practitioners in the health professions, my own answer is an affirmative one because of my belief that medicine is a public service profession and therefore must produce professionals who can better serve the public. Consequently, in addition to opportunities to acquire up-to-date knowledge and develop clinical and procedural skills, their training should provide them with opportunities to develop personal qualities that lead to positive patient outcomes (Knight, 1981; Shelton, 1999).

As the research findings just described attest, assuming that students in the health professions will automatically develop empathic understanding and other humanistic qualities during their professional education obviously is unrealistic (Hornblow, Kidson, & Ironside, 1988). Therefore, because not everyone develops the capacity for empathy by default, enhancement of empathy among health care professionals will require targeted educational programs, appropriate experiences, and exposure to humanistic role models.

Approaches to the Enhancement of Empathy

Several approaches have been used to enhance empathy, most of them by social psychologists and some by medical and nursing educators. I will briefly describe some of them, focusing primarily on the methods used by medical educators. Among the many approaches to improving empathy are parental training (Gladding, 1978; Therrien, 1979), skills-development workshops (Black & Phillips, 1982; Hatcher et al., 1994; Kremer & Dietzen, 1991; Pecukonis, 1990), perspective-taking exercises (Coke et al., 1978), role taking and role playing (Kalisch, 1971; Moser, 1984), communication or interpersonal skills training (Kause et al., 1980; Yedidia et al., 2003), films and videos (Gladstein & Feldstein, 1983; Simmons, Robie, Kendrick, Schumacher, & Roberge, 1992; Werner & Schneider, 1974), role modeling

(Dalton, Sunblad, & Hylbert, 1976; Gulanick & Schmeck, 1977; Shapiro, 2002), or a combination of these and other approaches (Beddoe & Murphy, 2004; Benbassat & Baumal, 2004; Erera, 1997; Kipper & Ben-Ely, 1979).

Although didactic teaching methods are effective for improving beginners' empathic communication skills (Gladstein et al., 1987), more advanced techniques, such as role playing, simulation, and audiovisual methods, are useful for advanced training in empathy. In the following sections, I briefly describe some of the approaches used to enhance empathy in the fields of social and counseling psychology and then discuss some of the methods used among students and practitioners in the health care professions.

Social and Counseling Psychology

In early laboratory experiments, social psychologists used the classical conditioning paradigm to demonstrate that empathic responses could be elicited. For example, two studies indicated that watching others who appeared to be receiving electric shocks followed by a warning signal could cause observers to form empathic reactions to the warning signal (Berger, 1962; DiLollo & Berger, 1965). The observers terminated the electric shocks more quickly when they believed they were able to help (Weiss, Boyer, Lombardo, & Stich, 1973). These studies suggest that the empathic response can be elicited by classical and operant conditioning.

An empathy enhancement program called Parent Effectiveness Training, which included lectures, tape recordings, role playing, and role modeling, also was implemented for parents who wished to improve their parent–child communication (Therrien, 1979). The results showed that parents who participated in the program were able to function at a higher level of empathy, as measured by the Accurate Empathy Scale of Truax and Carkhuff's Relationship Questionnaire. The improvement was maintained over a period of 4 months.

In a series of studies on the use of imagination, Stotland and colleagues demonstrated that when an observer was instructed to "stand in another person's shoes" by simply imagining the pain experienced by a person whose hand was strapped to a machine generating painful heat, the observer exhibited a more intense empathic response than did other observers who passively watched the distressed person's actions and appearance (Stotland, 1969; Stotland et al., 1978). This finding suggests that a cognitive process of taking the role of the other person or imagining the other person's experience (i.e., standing in the other person's shoes) can elicit empathic responses reflected in the role taker's behavior, heartbeat, and skin conductance.

Imagination also is used as a method of inducing an empathic response. Two kinds of imagination are used. One kind is imagining another person in a specific situation (e.g., a person whose parents have been killed in an automobile accident). The question is what the other person might feel and experience. The other kind is imagining oneself experiencing another person's concerns, feelings, and experiences as vividly as possible. Empathic behavior determined by physiological responses or self-reports can be generated by such imaginings.

Because prejudice against specific groups leads to psychological distance, some psychologists have attempted to reduce prejudice and improve prosocial behavior by enhancing empathy. If an important ingredient of empathy is the ability to understand other people's pain and suffering, such an understanding can reduce prejudice and bridge the gap between people. Efforts to understand others will diminish hatred toward them, and helping behavior presumably would follow when empathic understanding is formed (Batson, 1991; Batson & Coke, 1981; Davis, 1994).

One approach to understanding others is to read about them—their values, culture, pain, and suffering. Most programs designed to increase cultural sensitivity focus on the simple principle that understanding different cultures reduces prejudice and increases the sense of common identity. When people were asked to read stories about a particular group of sufferers, such as patients with AIDS, homeless people, or prisoners on death row, they developed more positive attitudes toward these groups (Batson et al., 1997a).

Those who read vignettes about racial discrimination and were instructed to empathize with the victims (by standing in the other person's shoes) improved their attitudes toward the victims (Stephan & Finlay, 1999). When college students participated in a "dialogue group" to discuss diversity, race, and ethnic issues, the researchers observed both short- and long-term improvements in the students' empathic understanding of minority groups (Gurin, Peng, Lopez, & Nagda, 1999; Lopez, Gurin, & Nagda, 1998). Such dialogues concerning people's similarities and differences can create a sense of a common identity that reduces prejudice and increases helping behavior. Research also has demonstrated that people who participate in multicultural educational programs, read relevant materials, watch videos, and engage in conversation with people from other racial, ethnic, and cultural groups increase their insight and their empathic understanding of the views held by those groups (Banks, 1997).

More than a quarter century ago, Bridgman (1981) suggested that prosocial behavior could be measured by cognitive developmental processes through role taking. In a study based on this suggestion, children from different groups who took the role of a person from another group in specially designed educational programs worked cooperatively together and improved their empathic understanding of each other (Bridgman, 1981). These findings have implications for education in the health professions with regard not only to improving practitioners' understanding of patients and other staff members from diverse sociocultural backgrounds and experiences but to promoting collaboration and teamwork as well. Our studies have shown that when medical students and nurses work together, the students' understanding of the importance of nursing services to patient care increases and their attitudes about collaborative relationships improve significantly (Hojat et al., 1997; Hojat & Herman, 1985).

Krebs (1975) and Stotland and colleagues (Stotland, 1969; Stotland et al., 1978) indicated that taking another person's perspective can lead to increased intensity of the motivation to help and, consequently, to an empathic response. Batson and associates reported that empathic behavior could be developed in a two-stage model of training (Batson, Coke, & Pych, 1983; Coke et al., 1978). In Stage 1, adopting the perspective of another person, such as a patient, increased empathic concern. The motivation to help was elicited in Stage 2 as a result of adopting another person's perspective.

Crabb, Moracco, and Bender (1983) developed a training program for lay helpers (church volunteers) based on the microcounseling interviewing technique (Ivey, 1971) and the skilled-helper training method (Egan, 1975) and offered the program to a large group of church volunteers. After administering Carkhuff's Empathic Understanding in Interpersonal Processes Scale to the participants, the authors reported that a large-group format for teaching the skills of empathy can be effective (Crabb et al., 1983).

In another study, undergraduates were taught active listening skills (e.g., identifying expressions of emotion and communicating this understanding verbally) either through training tapes (the self-directed method) or through highly intensive programs presented by teachers (Kremer & Dietzen, 1991). Although both approaches improved the students' empathy skills, the investigators concluded that empathy skills could be taught effectively in a large-group format without intensive programs and with direct contact with a teacher as a necessary component.

Another important finding was that an observer's empathic responses could be demonstrated better when the person observed was involved in a distressing, not pleasant situation (Stotland et al., 1978). In other words, human beings tend to empathize with people who need help to reduce their pain, and suffering, rather than empathize (rejoice) with people who want to share their joy and ecstasy. This finding is relevant to physician–patient encounters, where there is always a patient in pain and in need of help and a clinician in a position to offer help. Such is the condition in which an empathic relationship is waiting to form.

The Health Professions

Since the 1970s, a number of researchers have argued that empathy is far too important to be taught only to health professionals (Ivey, 1971, 1974). Egan (1975) and Therrien (1979) recommended that everyone should receive empathy training to improve human relationships in general and to face crises of life more effectively. Others have suggested that the capacity for empathy can serve as a foundation for building interpersonal relationships that have a buffering effect against stress and can be an essential step in conflict resolution (Kremer & Dietzen, 1991).

Researchers in the health professions have attempted to enhance empathy by offering educational programs. Most of the programs address the broader goal of improving students' interpersonal skills that implicitly mean enhancement of the capacity for empathy. It is assumed that the capacity for empathy is an essential prerequisite to demonstrate empathic behavior (Book, 1991). The following studies are examples of the training programs designed to enhance empathy among students and practitioners in the health professions.

Helping Professions

In a study at the University of Haifa, social work students participated in an empathy training program developed and implemented for helping professionals (Erera, 1997). Designed to enhance participants' cognitive sensitivity, the program consisted of four activities: (a) recording students' interviews with clients, (b) reviewing the interviews for the purpose of developing hypotheses or speculating about statements clients made during the interviews, (c) developing hypotheses about the students' statements, and (d) verifying the hypotheses or speculations by analyzing possible reasons for the statements students made during exchanges with clients. For example, "What did the client try to convey by using a specific statement?" or "What did the student infer from the client's statement?" A statistically significant improvement in scores on Mehrabian and Epstein's Emotional Empathy Scale was observed among the students who participated in the program.

Sensitivity to nonverbal cues is an important skill in establishing an empathic clinician–patient relationship. When a group of mental health professionals was exposed to a 90-min program designed to increase their ability to interpret nonverbal cues, the results demonstrated that such skills could be learned (DiMatteo, 1979; Rosenthal et al., 1979). The brief presentation included information about the importance of nonverbal communication in clinical settings, demonstrations of how one can understand nonverbal expressions of affect by noting changes in tone of voice, and practice in judging emotions by observing facial expressions, bodily movements, and postures. The participants had no difficulty learning the apparent meaning of certain nonverbal cues. For example, folded arms were likely to indicate defensiveness, coldness, rejection, or inaccessibility, whereas moderately open arms were likely to convey acceptance and warmth (DiMatteo, 1979).

Nursing

In an early study designed to improve empathy among nursing students, the students underwent didactic training that involved role playing, and exposure to a role model (Kalisch, 1971). Although the investigator noticed an increase in the students' self-reported empathy on Barrett-Lennard's Relationship Inventory, no increase occurred in patients' ratings of the nurses' empathy.

LaMonica, Carew, Winder, Haase, and Blanchard (1976) developed an empathy training program for hospital nursing staff based on Carkhuff's human relationship model (1969). During the brief program, nurses learned to interpret patients' nonverbal behaviors and expressions of anger, engaged in empathic role playing, and practiced responding empathically. Despite a significant increase in the nurses' empathy scores, the authors reported that the majority of participants needed more training.

Layton (1979) attempted to enhance nursing students' empathy by conducting an experiment based on Bandura's observational social learning theory (1977). The students observed interviews with simulated patients that consisted of three components: (a) a modeling component demonstrating the interviewers' empathy (positive modeling) or lack of empathy (negative modeling), (b) a labeling component in which segments of the modeling component were played back, followed by a narrative explaining the presence or absence of empathy depicted on the videotapes, and (c) a rehearsing component, during which the videotapes were stopped briefly after each verbal and emotional expression made by a patient. During each pause, the students were asked to construct their own responses to the patient's expressions. When the experiment ended, Layton found that the junior-year students' scores on Carkhuff's Empathic Understanding in Interpersonal Processes Scale had improved, whereas the scores of the senior students had not. Layton speculated that one explanation for the disparate results was that the modeling approach may have been more effective for less advanced students.

As a result of extensive work in nursing education and research in the 1960s and 1970s, Orlando (1961, 1972) developed a model of therapeutic encounters proposing that when nurses interacted with patients, they should validate their perceptions to ensure that they had an accurate understanding of the patients' experiences. More than two decades later, Olson and Hanchett (1997) adopted Orlando's model as a suitable method of studying empathy and patient outcomes and hypothesized that if nurses understood their patients' needs accurately and shared that understanding with patients, who in turn confirmed its accuracy, patient outcomes would improve. Accordingly, Olson and Hanchett initiated a study involving 70 staff nurses and 70 patients to test the hypothesis that nurses' empathy would reduce patients' distress and overlap with the patients' perceptions of the nurses' empathy, as measured by the Empathic Understanding subscale of Barrett-Lennard's Relationship Inventory. At the end of the study, the authors reported a moderate but statistically significant relationship between the nurses' self-reported empathy and the patients' perceptions of the nurses empathy: i.e., the hypothesis was confirmed.

In a recent study, Beddoe and Murphy (2004) exposed nursing students to an 8-week "mindfulness-based stress reduction" program to explore the program's effects on stress and empathy. At the end of the 8 weeks, the authors reported favorable changes in the students' scores on the Personal Distress and Fantasy subscales of the IRI.

Medical Education and Practice

Werner and Schneider (1974) used a variation of a technique called "Interpersonal Process Recall" to enhance medical students' interviewing skills and awareness of patients' affective messages. The students were videotaped as they interacted with simulated patients with certain health problems; the videotapes were then played back so the students could view their interactions with patients and receive critical analyses from instructors and other students about their interactions. Positive results were noted.

Later, Sanson-Fisher and Poole (1978) subjected medical students in Australia to eight videotaped training sessions in empathy. After the training, the students' scores on the Accurate Empathy subscale of Truax and Carkhuff's Relationship Questionnaire increased significantly compared with the scores of a control group of students who did not participate in the program.

In a study conducted at the University of Missouri-Kansas City School of Medicine, medical students participated in a three-stage multidimensional training program on empathy (Feighny et al., 1998). In Stage 1, the students developed a clinical presentation of an illness, such as diabetes, from a patient's perspective (cognitive empathy). In Stage 2, the students tried to experience the situation as if they were patients (emotional empathy). In Stage 3, the students were provided with corrective feedback about their communication skills (behavioral empathy). The investigators noted that the students' scores improved significantly on Carkhuff's Empathic Understanding in Interpersonal Processes Scale but did not change significantly on the IRI. The investigators attributed the discrepancy to the IRI's lack of sensitivity in the context of patient care. In her doctoral dissertation at Iowa University, Stebbins (2005) reported that exposure to interactive interpersonal communication enhanced empathy (measured by the JSPE) among second-year osteopathy students.

Winefield and Chur-Hansen (2000) reported that 81% of medical students who participated in two brief sessions on effective communication with patients felt better prepared to engage in empathic interviews. Concerning the positive effect of empathy training, Anthony and Wain (1971) found that medical corpsmen who were exposed to 10 hours of empathy training functioned at a significantly higher level of empathy than a control group did. Yedidia and colleagues (2003) reported that practicing communication skills and engaging medical students in self-reflection on their performance improved students' overall communication competence as well as their skills in relationship building in patient care.

Some investigators have suggested that faculty in undergraduate and graduate medical education can serve as role models or mentors to improve the students' capacity for empathy (Campus-Outcalt, Senf, Watkins, & Bastacky, 1995; Ficklin, Browne, Powell, & Carter, 1988; Skeff & Mutha, 1998; Wright, 1996). Despite the fact that exposure to role models is an important factor in the enhancement of empathy, the results of a mailed survey of medical students at four different medical schools in Canada (Maheux, Beaudoin, Berkson, Des Marchais, & Jean, 2000) raised a question about students' exposure to appropriate role models: 25% of the second-year students and 40% of the seniors said they did not agree that their medical school faculty behaved as humanistic physicians and teachers. A study of medical students in South Africa (Mclean, 2004) found that as the students progressed through medical school, they selected more faculty members as role models. However, the role models they selected most often were their own parents, and notably their mothers, who were described as caring, sympathetic, and self-sacrificing mentors. These findings are consistent with the notion I described in Chapter 4: that mothers are the key figure in the development of a child's capacity for empathy.

At the University of Arkansas for Medical Sciences, first-year medical students participated in a Patient Navigator Project in which each student "shadowed" a patient (with the patient's permission) during visits to a surgical oncologist and observed the patient throughout treatment (Henry-Tillman, Deloney, Savidge, Graham, & Klimberg, 2002). Seventy percent of the students said they experienced empathy while participating in the program.

At the University of California-Los Angeles Medical School, healthy second-year medical students who had completed their training in the basic sciences and had no previous history of hospitalization participated in a program designed to examine whether the experience of being hospitalized would increase their empathy for hospitalized patients (Wilkes, Milgrom, & Hoffman, 2002). The students were admitted to the hospital under an assumed name and reported that the experience was useful because it enhanced their understanding of patients' problems. Interestingly, the students gave the nursing staff more favorable ratings concerning encounters with hospital staff as "new patients" than they gave to physicians! Because of the effect of hospitalization on physician's understanding of patients, Ingelfinger (1980) suggested that hospitalization experiences during the adolescent or adult years should be used as a criterion for admission to medical schools to increase the number of empathic physicians!

At the University of Minnesota Medical School, Pacala, Boult, Bland, and O'Brien (1995) used an educational program to enhance students' empathy toward elderly patients. The program was a modified version of the "aging game," originally developed to enhance students' empathy toward geriatric patients and to stimulate their interest in caring for such patients (McVey, Davis, & Cohen, 1989). The program included role playing and simulation exercises, followed by having students assume the roles and identities of elderly people aged 65–85 years. The students wore earplugs to simulate hearing loss, heavy socks to simulate pedal edema, and popcorn kernels in their shoes to simulate the discomfort of arthritis. A facilitator, playing the role of a care provider, conveyed increasingly negative attitudes toward elderly people at some stations (testing sites) and responded empathically at other stations. Using a measure of empathy they developed consisting of two statements—"I believe I can truly empathize with older patients" and "I believe I understand what it feels like to have problems associated with aging"—Pacala and colleagues observed a significant improvement in the students' empathy scores when the program ended.

Platt and Keller (1994) developed a program to enhance empathic communication among physicians facing difficult encounters with patients who expressed strong negative emotions (e.g., anger, fear, sadness) and were unwilling to assume responsibility for their own health. During the program, the participants attempted to increase their awareness of a patient's emotional clues by trying to understand the emotion, naming the emotion for the patient to insure they had identified the emotion correctly, acknowledging and justifying the patient's emotion, and affirming the patient's behavior and offering help. The authors concluded that empathic communication is a teachable and learnable skill.

One way to teach empathy to health professionals is to constantly remind them to view things from the patient's perspective and ask themselves "What would it be like if I were in the patient's shoes?" (Surrey & Bergman, 1994, p. 129). Other skills that can enhance empathic relationships include eliciting and discussing feelings and experiences, paraphrasing to convey understanding of the patient's concerns, showing that the health care provider shares the patient's concerns, using silence appropriately during conversations to allow for additional thoughts and insights, listening with the third ear to indicate that one understands the meaning of the patient's experiences beyond the spoken words, viewing events with the mind's eye to understand the patient's experiences more completely, and paying attention to nonverbal cues to gain insight into the patient's sensitivities, feelings, and affective reactions.

In a randomized clinical trial conducted at the Johns Hopkins University School of Hygiene and Public Health, 69 physicians were assigned to one of three groups: two experimental groups and one control group (Roter et al., 1995). Physicians in the experimental groups received 8 hours of training designed to increase their communication skills and reduce their patients' emotional distress. However, the patients in one group were actual patients and those in the other group were simulated patients. During the training, the physicians asked patients about their concerns and expectations, reassured them, and acknowledged their psychosocial problems. The results showed that the empathic skills of the physicians who participated in either training course improved significantly without increasing the time spent with individual patients.

Suchman and colleagues (1997) examined transcripts and videotapes of physician–patient encounters and observed that, rather than expressing their emotions, feelings, and inner experiences verbally, patients provided nonverbal clues that physicians tended to let pass. Thus, after asking patients to elaborate, physicians needed to respond with accurate and explicit acknowledgments so that patients realized they were heard and understood. As a result of their observations, Suchman and colleagues proposed a comprehensive model to improve empathic communication in medical settings consisting of the following three steps: (a) detecting patients' clues and recognizing their emotions, (b) probing and encouraging patients to elaborate on their emotions, and (c) acknowledging patients' concerns so they felt their concerns had been heard.

On their first day in the Emergency Medicine Department at the University of Florida Health Sciences Center, 25 residents participated in a study in which they were instructed to register as patients (the nurses were not aware of the experiment) (Seaberg, Godwin, & Perry, 1999, 2000). Although the study was brief, ending when the examining physician entered the examination room, the results suggested that this brief experience enhanced the residents' empathy, as indicated by their reports that the experiment improved their attitude toward patients in the emergency room.

Another approach to enhancing empathy among physicians was originally introduced by Michael Balint (1957) of the Tavistock Institute in London. Balint designed a program to counteract a problem that Houston (1938) had described nearly two decades earlier. Because medical trainees spent virtually their entire training in the laboratory and the hospital ward, they had few opportunities to develop skills for dealing with the interpersonal aspects of patient care. Balint's program provided physicians with opportunities to compensate for deficits in interpersonal communication and awareness of psychosocial aspects of illness by having them meet in small groups of 10 to discuss cases they felt were difficult, particularly in relation to the physician–patient relationship. The 1- or 2-hour meetings were held every 1 to 3 weeks for 1 to 3 years. The group format was unstructured, open, and supportive, and the primary focuses were on behavioral, cognitive, and emotional issues related to communication between physician and patient. The discussions were often coordinated and led by a psychologist or psychoanalyst. The twofold purpose of the program was to impress on group members the importance of physician–patient interactions and to illustrate the differences between patient-oriented versus disease-oriented approaches in physician–patient communication.

In the last decade or so, Balint's program has been receiving attention in some residency programs in the United States, particularly in family medicine (Brock & Salinsky, 1993; Cataldo, Peeden, Geesey, & Dickerson, 2005) because educational programs in this specialty place emphasis on psychosocial aspects of illness (Gaufberg et al., 2001). Although the Balint training program seems to be potentially useful for enhancing empathy among physicians, convincing empirical evidence to support the program's effectiveness is currently lacking. In their recent study, Cataldo and colleagues (2005) compared residents in family medicine who participated in a Balint training program with counterparts who had not been exposed to such a program. Residents who completed the Balint training expressed more satisfaction with their choice of family medicine as their career. However, their scores on the JSPE were not significantly different from the scores of residents who did not participate in the training, probably because of insufficient exposure to training.

The Study of Literature and the Arts

In his book *A History of Medicine*, Castiglioni (1941) quoted Hippocrates as saying, "Where there is a love for man, there is also a love for the arts." The statement indicates that there is a bridge connecting the human heart and the arts together.

Numerous authors have proposed that in addition to reading the medical literature, medical students and physicians should read literature unrelated to medicine because it would expose them to a rich source of knowledge and insights about the emotions, pain, and suffering, and perspectives of other human beings and would improve their capacity for forming empathic connections (Acuna, 2000; Charon et al., 1995; Herman, 2000; Jones, 1987; McLellan & Hudson Jones, 1996; Montgomery Hunter et al., 1995; Peschel, 1980; Szalita, 1976) (for an annotated bibliography of works in medical and nonmedical literature, see Montgomery Hunter et al., 1995). In support of the impact of physicians' familiarity with the literature and arts on patient outcomes, Mandell and Spiro (1987, p. 458) suggested that "the humanities will not improve the technical care of our patients, but they may help to civilize that care."

Borrowing from Jungian concepts, Knapp (1984) suggested that by studying classical literature, the reader can develop insight into the "collective unconscious" of the human mind and better understand the archetypal images in myths, legends, literature, and the arts. The simulated worlds offered by famous novels, short stories, poems, plays, paintings, sculptures, music, and films enable us to learn how emotions are expressed in human relationships (Oatley, 2004). Thus, the study of literature and the arts can provide students and practitioners in the health professions with values and experiences in areas of concern in clinical practice, such as aging, death, disability, and dying (Montgomery Hunter et al., 1995). The study of literature and the arts also can aid the development of otherwise hard-to-teach clinical competencies, such as accurate observation, interpretation, imagination, ethical issues, and moral reflection (Montgomery Hunter et al., 1995).

In addition, studying literature and reading poetry not only facilitates clinicians' understanding of other people's feelings and expressions of their inner world but also can be used as an ancillary tool through which both clinician and patient can find different meanings in and ways of expressing emotion, pain, and suffering (Lerner, 1978, 2001). Furthermore, literature and the arts provide clinicians with the ability to use metaphor in encounters with patients that can help them to enhance mutual clinician–patient understanding (Blanton, 1960; Lerner, 1978).

Charon and colleagues (1995) indicated that in addition to increasing one's understanding of human suffering and ability to use metaphor, studying literature and the arts can help health professionals to "contextualize" and "particularize" the ethical issues in patient care. Other authors have indicated that health professionals can gain new insights into the moral and ethical issues posed by their profession through the lens of literature, poetry, and the arts (Calman, Downie, Duthie, & Sweeney, 1988; Charon et al., 1995; Coles, 1989; Flagler, 1997; Marshall & O'Keefe, 1994; Radley, 1992). The quandaries and decision-making processes of characters in literary narratives are useful for teaching ethical guidelines to students and practitioners in the health professions (Coles, 1989). The thoughts, feelings, sensations, and intuitions influenced by immersing oneself in literature can serve as a powerful impetus toward understanding the human mind (Schneiderman, 2002).

Reading literature can result in higher mental processes leading to greater imagination and better interpretive skills that reinforce empathic understanding (Calman et al., 1988; Charon et al., 1995; Clouser, 1990; Downie, 1991; Radley, 1992; Starcevic & Piontek, 1997; Younger, 1990). Literature can enrich students' moral education, increase their tolerance for uncertainty, and give them a rich grounding for empathic understanding of their patients. Lancaster, Hart, and Gardner (2002) offered a 1-month course in which medical students read works, such as Tolstoy's *The Death of Ivan Ilych*, that improved their narrative skills. When the course ended, the students assigned their highest rating to the enhancement of empathy as a result of their participation in the course. Although it is assumed that engagement with literature can deepen medical students' understanding of illness experiences, increase their capacity for self-reflection, and enhance their capacity for empathy, resistance among medical students to a course on literary inquiry has been observed (Wear & Aultman, 2005). Denying the relevance of studying literature to medicine, discounting the value of literary inquiry to patient care, and distancing the arts from science are among the reasons for medical students' resistance to studying literature and improving their narrative skills (Wear & Aultman, 2005). Students' motivation can be improved by convincing them of the link between literary inquiry and medicine.

In addition to the study of literature, theatrical performances (e.g., simulated, standardized, and virtual patients) have been used as educational tools in medical education. For example, performances by real patients or by professional actors portraying patients have been used to enhance empathy among medical students and practitioners in the health professions. Shapiro and Hunt (2003) presented medical students at the University of California-Irvine College of Medicine with performances by two patients. One patient chronicled his experiences with AIDS through narrative and song. The other patient, a survivor of ovarian cancer, described her experiences on hearing the diagnosis, undergoing treatment, and coping with the psychological effects of the ordeal and the spiritual journey on which she embarked while dealing with the illness. After the presentations, the students reported that watching the presentations increased their empathic understanding of patients with AIDS or ovarian cancer. The performing arts also have been used to increase medical students' understanding of patients' grief (Stokes, 1980) and of death and dying (Holleman, 2000).

In addition to providing educational messages, dramatic and tragic theatrical performances can generate insights in the observer that arise from climactic intellectual, emotional, or spiritual enlightenment (Golden, 1992). In his theory of catharsis, Aristotle explained that observing the hero's tragic experiences can generate a calming effect (a catharsis) that serves to separate the observer from the hero's suffering while understanding the hero's pain. A healthy society needs the performing arts, and students and practitioners in the health care professions need them for the same reason, because they learn about the experiences of others and can experience catharsis by being drawn into their patients' tragic stories while remaining separate from patients (Trautmann Banks, 2002). In other words, empathy can arise from the cathartic effects of these stories.

Another explanation for the beneficial effects of the performing arts on empathy is the involvement of the human mirror neuron system. As I described in Chapter 3, when a person observes another person performing an act, the mirror neuron system is activated and contributes to empathic understanding. It also is well known, particularly from studies involving hypnosis and imagery, that imagination can produce real physiological effects (Wester & Smith, 1984). These neurological and physiological activities may explain how studying literature, reading poetry, and watching theatrical or cinematic performances can induce neurophysiological effects leading to a greater empathic understanding. Of course, empirical verification of this explanation awaits further research. Despite the importance of humanities in enhancing empathy, only a third of all the medical schools in the United States had incorporated literature into their curriculum as of the mid-1990s (Charon et al., 1995; Jones, 1997; Montgomery Hunter et al., 1995). Other medical schools should be encouraged to follow their lead.

Narrative Skills

It is said that human beings are storytelling animals (Hurwitz, 2000), that the universe is made of stories (Feldman & Kornfield, 1991), and that physicians are immersed in patients' stories (Steiner, 2005). Humans are described by Dawes (1999, p. 29) as "the primates whose cognitive capacity shuts down in the absence of a story." It is suggested that the human brain is evolved to process stories better than any other forms of input (Newman, 2003). Narrative, defined by Smith (1981, p. 228) as "someone telling someone else that something happened," is the royal road to a patient's world. It is physicians' attentive listening to their patients' narratives of illness (narrative skills), rather than "clinical interrogation," (Kleinman, 1995) that opens a window of opportunity to empathic engagement. In clinician–patient encounters, listening to the patient's stories of illness with the third ear while taking the history of the patient's current illness is described as a "narrative communication" that, when skillfully performed, not only has diagnostic value but has therapeutic benefit as well (Adler, 1997). The narrative account of the patient's illness is the beginning of the healing process as well as a pathway to a correct diagnosis (Adler & Mammett, 1973). Patients often carefully monitor the clinician's attentiveness to their illness narrative, detect the signs of the clinician's empathic receptiveness, and feel better when the clinician appears to be in tune with the narrative themes (Brody, 1997). In his article "Power of Stories over Statistics," Newman (2003) suggests that narrative skills enable physicians to make empathic connections with their patients.

Clinicians are often witnesses to their patients' pain and suffering: They listen to the patients' stories, and they prepare short narratives of the patients' experiences after taking their history and interviewing them. The clinicians' task, according to Kleinman (1988, p. 50), is "to witness a life story, to validate its interpretation, and to affirm its value." Because the feelings and experiences of others are captured in patients' narratives, their narratives can convey how they view their illness (Bruner, 1990). Evidence suggests that participating in programs on reflective writing can improve clinicians' empathic understanding (DasGupta & Charon, 2004; Lancaster et al., 2002; Shapiro & Hunt, 2003). According to Steiner (2005), clinical stories can be used to inform, to share, to inspire, to educate, and to persuade, with implications not only in forming empathic engagement but also in health research (to find a common theme) and in health policy (to formulate compassionate policies).

Clinicians' narrative skills gained by engaging with stories in the literature is pivotal when thinking about case histories in ethics (Charon & Montello, 2002). Rita Charon (2001b) has written extensively about narrative medicine and physicians' narrative competence in recognizing and interpreting the predicaments of their patients. She believes that a bridge exists between narrative skills and capacity for empathy (Charon, 1993) and that the effective practice of medicine requires narrative competence that includes the ability to understand, absorb, interpret, and act based on the stories and plights of patients (Charon, 2000, 2001a).

Narrative competence in medicine can be acquired by reading, writing, studying the arts and recognizing that all human beings are vulnerable to illness and death (Charon, 1993). According to DasGupta and Charon (2004), the ability to elicit, interpret, and translate patients' narrative accounts of their illness is the key to empathic communication. Reflective writing and narrative competence offer opportunities for empathic and nourishing medical care (Charon, 2001a). In a study involving 11 second-year medical students, 9 reported that reflective writing (e.g., writing about a personal illness or another person's illness) could enhance their understanding of patients and improve their ability to care for patients (DasGupta & Charon, 2004).

Narrative competence is beneficial not only for the clinicians who write the patients' stories of illness to make accurate diagnoses and select appropriate treatments but for the patients as well. For example, patients with mild or moderately severe asthma or rheumatoid arthritis who wrote about their stressful experiences achieved a significantly better clinical outcome (Smyth, Stone, Hurewitz, & Kaell, 1999).

Branch, Pels, and Hafler (1998) suggested that small-group discussions about medical students' narrative reports of critical incidents during encounters with patients can enhance the students' understanding of the clinician–patient relationship. In summary, the aforementioned studies indicate that studying literature and the arts, theatrical performances, and narrative skills can enhance empathic understanding in human encounters.

Effectiveness of the Programs

Although some studies cited in this chapter indicate that empathy can be enhanced, some clues suggest that the improvement cannot be retained without practice or reinforcement (Engler, Saltzman, Walker, & Wolf, 1981; Kause et al., 1980). Thus, the popular saying "Use it or lose it" may be applicable to empathy enhanced as a result of an educational program.

Furthermore, it is also important to bear in mind that when assessing any educational program designed to enhance empathy, it is desirable to examine not only the short-term but, more important, the long-term effects of the program. Although some studies have indicated that educational training programs designed to enhance empathy may have a relatively long-term effect (Kramer et al., 1989; Poole & Sanson-Fisher, 1980), the long-lasting effect of empathy training programs awaits more empirical scrutiny.

At a conceptual level, it makes sense to believe that studying literature and the arts and developing narrative skills cultivates empathy. However, according to Skelton, MacLeod, and Thomas (2000), the problem is the lack of empirical evidence to verify the truth of the belief. With regard to this challenge, McManus (1995) suggested that investigators who attempt to conduct empirical assessments of the humanities' contribution to medical outcomes must bite the bullet of definition and measurement. However, it is my hope that the conceptualization and definition of empathy in the context of patient care (Chapter 6) and the development of the JSPE (Chapter 7) can relieve us of the need to bite the bullet.

Recapitulation

Although the current emphasis on professionalism in medicine places a high value on enhancement of empathy in patient care, most students in the existing medical education programs do not routinely acquire the skills needed to demonstrate empathy. However, research shows that empathy can be enhanced effectively by dedicated educational programs. Counteracting current trends in medical education and practice that are not conducive to empathic engagement in patient care requires a mandate for the development and implementation of targeted educational programs at all levels of training in all academic medical centers. Only then will the public be better served and will all health professionals regain the respect they rightly deserve.

12

Parting Thoughts: A Paradigm of Empathy and Future Directions

Everything in the system is dependent on the previous state of the system.

—(Robert Lilienfeld, 1978, p. 14)

By becoming more and more aware of our roles in patient–doctor relationship—i.e., of our side-effects as drugs—our therapeutic efficiency will grow apace.

—(Michael Balint, 1957, p. 688)

Preamble

In this final chapter, empathy is viewed from a broader and more comprehensive perspective of systems theory. In a systemic paradigm of empathy in patient care, the contributions of major subsets of the system (e.g., clinician-related, nonclinician related, social learning, and education) and their related elements to clinical encounters, that lead to functional or dysfunctional system outcomes is discussed. An agenda for future research includes the following areas: (1) an examination of additional components of empathy; (2) the investigation of other correlates of empathy; (3) consideration of empathy as a criterion for admissions, selection, and employment; (4) the study of empathy as a predictor of career choice and professional success; (5) the development and evaluation of approaches for the enhancement of empathy in professional education; (6) consideration of patients' and peers' perspectives in outcomes of empathy research; and (7) an examination of neuroanatomical aspects and neurophysiological indicators of empathy. It is recommended that implementation of remedies for enhancement of empathy is a mandate that must be acted upon.

Introduction

Empathy is an attribute that is distributed unevenly in the population. Human beings are not created equal with regard to their capacity for empathy. It is a gift bestowed in abundance on some and in only meager amounts on others. It is an endowment that can grow like a tree if the condition are right. We embarked on a journey in this book to find out why people differ with respect to their capacity to form empathic connections.

Now that we have come so far, approaching the destination of our journey, I would like to reflect on what I have said so far. We embarked on this journey without a definition of the terrain we hoped to discover. Starting with the confusion reflected in research on the conceptualization and measurement of empathy, we attempted to achieve a better vision by resolving the confusion. We visited empathy's historical roots, developmental trajectories, psychosocial connections, and other related factors along the terrain. In passing along these paths, we learned about the antecedents, development, measurement, and consequences of empathic engagement in the context of patient care. Many additional issues remain to be studied, however.

An undefined concept can never be measured, and a well-defined concept is half-measured! On the basis of the premise that research findings are vulnerable to serious challenge when the definition of the phenomenon under study is unclear, I offered a definition of empathy in the context of patient care (Chapter 6) primarily as a cognitive, as opposed to an emotional, attribute. Although I do not expect this conceptual characterization to remain unchallenged, let us hope that it can help, to some extent, to resolve the longstanding and unsettled debate regarding the conceptualization and definition of empathy that has always haunted empathy research.

The concept of empathy as having both affective and cognitive components, adopted uncritically from psychology by educators in the health professions, fits poorly with clinical reality in physician–patient encounters (Morse et al., 1992). The golden principle of patient care, "Above all, do not harm" (*primum non nocere*), rules out intense emotional engagement between clinician and patient that may jeopardize the outcomes of patient care. In studying empathy in psychology in the context of prosocial behavior, emotions can often facilitate, rather than jeopardize, the positive outcomes. However, as I described in Chapters 1 and 6, in medical and surgical treatment, emotions must be curbed to maintain objectivity. Thus, to achieve positive patient outcomes, empathy in the context of patient care should be guided primarily by cognition, rather than emotion. Without such a distinction, we will be wrestling forever with the challenge of how to separate empathy and sympathy (Chapter 1). With that in mind, we also need to recognize that clinicians cannot remain completely emotionless when dealing with their patients. As part of human nature, emotions always play a role in any kind of human relationship. The challenging issue that remains to be debated is the extent to which emotions would be beneficial and to determine the point from which emotions become detrimental to patient outcomes.

A complex concept, such as empathy, cannot be the subject of scientific research in the absence of an instrument that produces quantifiable results. An instrument intended to measure empathy in patient care cannot pass the litmus test of face and content validity unless its contents are not only consistent with the definition of the subject under study but also relevant to the context of patient care. In addition, psychometric evidence must provide convincing support for the validity and reliability of the instrument. Let us hope that the Jefferson Scale of Physician Empathy (JSPE), the instrument discussed in Chapter 7, can help us resolve the measurement issues that have caused the confusion and uncertainty and have impeded empirical scrutiny of empathy in medical education and patient-care research.

Complex human attributes are not isolated entities; they always function in relation to other factors. As we learned in previous chapters, empathy is a multifaceted attribute that is deeply rooted in human evolution; it has genetic traces and a long history of development from conception to grave. Furthermore, as was discussed earlier, environmental, cultural, experiential, and educational factors contribute, independently and interactively, to the makeup of the attribute called empathy, and empathic engagement, or the lack of it, in the context of patient care will lead to virtually opposite outcomes.

Despite its deep evolutionary roots and genetic basis, the capacity for empathy is amenable to change to some extent when the conditions are right. Therefore, as the discussion in Chapter 11 illustrated, targeted educational programs, appropriate experiences, and environmental facilitators can enhance the capacity of health care providers for empathic engagement to a considerable degree.

Viewed from a broader perspective, a complex concept, such as empathy in patient care, requires a comprehensive model to depict its important elements, their interactions, and their outcomes. For that purpose, we can turn to systems theory to present a heuristic paradigm of empathy in the context of patient care.

A Systemic Paradigm of Empathy in Patient Care

The developmental trajectories and outcomes of a complex concept, such as empathy in patient care, can be viewed from the vista of systems theory. According to Pollak (1976), a systemic approach is the professional way of dealing with complexity. A system is defined as a set of interrelated subsets, each with an array of elements, no subset of which is unrelated to any other subset, and each element within a subset is related directly or indirectly to every other element in the system (Ackoff & Emery, 1981). A system will be functional only when all its subsets and all the elements within and between subsets function properly; otherwise, the system will be dysfunctional. A functional system has a purpose. The systemic purpose of empathy in patient care is to enhance mutual understanding between clinician and patient so that the goal of positive patient outcomes can be achieved.

More than 40 years ago, Gordon Allport (1960) suggested that human personality must be treated as an open system that should be viewed with

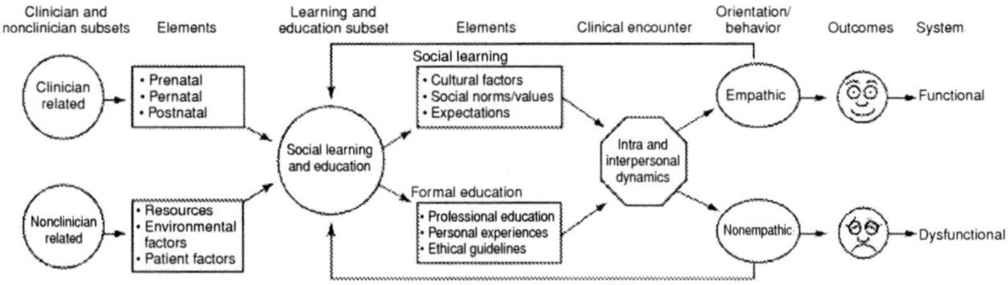

Figure 12.1 A systemic paradigm of empathy in the context of patient care.

an open mind. Active systems are often considered to be open systems because they are dynamic and therefore capable of responding and adapting to changes in the environment (Siegel, 1999). The combined functions of the elements within each subset of the system and the interrelationships among subsets prompt the system to generate a totality, a *gestalt*, in which the whole is greater than the sum of its parts. To achieve a better understanding of the antecedents, development, measurement, and outcomes of empathy in patient care, it seems desirable to view the concept, its major subsets, and the elements within each subset as an open system.

A complete understanding of any system requires an understanding of the subsets within the system and the nature of their interacting elements. For example, as Bateson (1971) indicated, if the family is viewed as a complex system, then an effective intervention in the context of family therapy requires a complete understanding of all subsets and elements of the system, including the roles, responsibilities, interactions, and functions of all family members within the family structure.

In the context of patient care as described in Chapter 8, the act of seeking help brings to the surface a need for connectedness that generates the energy to set the system of empathic engagement in motion. A clinician–patient encounter represents an open system in need of equilibrium brought about by the energy discharged in interpersonal connection. Achieving positive patient outcomes would indicate that the system is functional (i.e., a state of equilibrium), whereas negative patient outcomes would indicate that the system is dysfunctional (i.e., a state of disequilibrium). Empathic engagement in the clinician–patient relationship is the first step in maintaining systemic equilibrium. Figure 12.1 depicts a systemic paradigm of empathy in the context of patient care. It illustrates the major subsets of the system and the major elements within each subset that ultimately determine the functional or dysfunctional outcome of the system.

Major Subsets of the System

Let us elaborate briefly on the paradigm depicted in Fig. 12.1. Assuming that empathy in patient care resembles an open and purposeful system (i.e., a system that is amenable to change for the purpose of positive patient outcomes), the system would be set in motion by two interacting subsets: a clinician-related subset and a nonclinician-related subset (depicted on the left side of the figure as the entry to the model). Social learning and education are other subsets in the system.

The Clinician-Related Subset

This subset consists mainly of elements related to the clinician's personal qualities, which are offshoots of evolutionary, genetic, and constitutional factors (prenatal elements); events during childbirth (perinatal elements) that can contribute to later physical, mental, and social development; and such factors as early rearing environment, quality of attachment experiences with the primary caregiver, and family environment (postnatal elements). These elements, described in Chapters 3 and 4, are considered to be the bedrock on which a person's capacity for empathy is built.

The Nonclinician-Related Subset

According to Kurt Lewin (1936), manifestations of behavior are a function of personal qualities, environmental demands, and situational factors. In a paradigm of physicians' performance, Gonnella et al. (1993b) proposed that in addition to clinician's knowledge, clinical-procedural skills, and personal qualities, other factors that are not related to the physician and often are not under the physician's control contribute to patient outcomes. Hence, the term "nonclinician-related subset." The elements of this subset have often been ignored in evaluations of outcomes of medical education, appraisal of physicians' performance, and the assessments of patient outcomes. These elements include the availability of (a) human resources, such as technical and professional assistance and teamwork; (b) technical resources, such as diagnostic and treatment facilities, surgical equipment, and availability of laboratory tests; (c) environmental facilitators, such as physical facilities and facilitating rules and regulations; and (d) patient factors, such as personality, cultural values, attitudes, and life-style; willingness to seek timely help; and adherence to preventive guidelines and treatment regimens.

The Social Learning and Educational Subsets

The social learning subset consists mainly of elements related to cultural and social norms and values (e.g., ascribed social roles and modes of social behavior) and expectations (e.g., belief in a supernatural power, in the health care system, in health care providers, and in optimistic or pessimistic expectation of outcomes).

The education subset consists of an array of elements related to formal education and training experiences, such as professional education (e.g., undergraduate, graduate, and continuing education), personal educational experiences (e.g., influence of role models, observations, and clinical experiences), and professional ethics of conduct (e.g., ethical guidelines of professional organizations, such as the American Medical Association and the American Psychological Association, etc.). Targeted educational programs and educational experiences designed to enhance the capacity for empathy (see Chapter 11) also are among the elements of this subset.

The Clinical Encounter

Armed or disarmed with the elements of the aforementioned subsets, a clinician encounters a patient who is in a state of disequilibrium and is reaching out to someone for help. The system of empathic engagement begins to form. The intrapersonal and interpersonal dynamics described in Chapter 8 are triggered into operation during exchanges between the clinician and the patient. To form a functional system, the clinician should be armed with the skills needed to understand the patient's concerns and be motivated (an intrapersonal factor) to communicate this understanding to the patient (an interpersonal factor). As depicted in Figure 12.1, all elements of clinician-related, nonclinician-related, social learning, and education subsets come together in clinical encounters that can lead to either empathic or nonempathic clinician–patient engagements that, in turn, ultimately determine patient outcomes that will be positive in a functional system or negative in a dysfunctional system.

Outcomes

The interaction between intrapersonal and interpersonal dynamics described in Chapter 8 brings about cognitive processes that can lead to an orientation or a behavior. When the orientation or behavior is empathic, the likelihood of a positive patient outcome will increase. In this case, the system has achieved its purpose, and we can conclude that the system is functional. However, if the intrapersonal and interpersonal dynamics resting on the clinician-related, nonclinician-related, social learning, and formal educational subsets lead to a nonempathic orientation or behavior, the likelihood of a positive patient outcome will be drastically reduced. In this case, the system has failed to achieve its purpose, and we can conclude that the system is dysfunctional.

However, I must emphasize that because other unpredicted elements may intervene, the pathway to empathic engagement between clinician and patient is more complicated than the model depicted in Figure 12.1. Nonetheless, I hope that the systemic view of empathy just described can serve as a heuristic paradigm illustrating the major components that set the system in motion and show the complexity of the antecedents, development, measurement, and outcomes of empathy in the context of patient care.

An Agenda for Future Research

Training humane clinicians has long been a concern of education in the health professions. Because of the general societal changes that are taking place, particularly in the industrialized world, and directly or indirectly are weakening the power of important social support systems (see Chapter 2) and because of the changes that are evolving in the health care system and leading toward detached care (see Chapter 11), research on factors that contribute to the understanding and enhancement of empathy in patient care is now more important and timely than ever before.

Research on empathy in patient care deserves serious attention, not only because of its importance in training humane clinicians, but also because of its implications for the selection and education of clinicians. Empirical research on empathy in patient care is still in its infancy; therefore, much more research is needed to enhance our understanding of the antecedents, development, measurement, and outcomes of empathy in patient care. The questions discussed later present only a few of the areas that need to be included in the future research on empathy in patient care.

1 What Additional Constructs Are Involved in Empathy?

According to the findings determined by our factor analyses (Hojat et al., 2002e), empathy in patient care is a multidimensional concept involving at least three factors: "perspective taking," "compassionate care," and "standing in the patient's shoes." Similar factors that emerged in a recent factor-analytic study in which the JSPE was administered to dental students (Sherman & Cramer, 2005) and in another study with a large sample of medical students in Mexico (Alcorta-Garza, Gonzalez-Guerrero, Tavitas-Herrera, Rodrigues-Lara, & Hojat, 2005) have added to our confidence concerning the stability of the factors underlying empathy in different groups of health professionals. However, we need more evidence to support the factor structure of empathy in groups of students and practitioners in the different health professions (e.g., nursing, dietetics, psychology, social work).

It is important to bear in mind that the factors extracted in factor analytic studies obviously are a function of the number and contents of the items included in the measuring instruments. Therefore, the three underlying factors of empathy identified by the JSPE reflect the contents and intercorrelations of the 20 items included in the scale. Adding a sufficient number of items to address other factors, such as sociability, trust, and ethics, could result in a scale with a different underlying factor structure. More important, whether the current factor structure of the JSPE saturates the scale to the point where additional factors cannot account for more than a negligible amount of the variance or whether additional factors would contribute significantly to the scale's incremental validity (i.e., increase its criterion-related and predictive validity) need to be addressed in future research.

2 What Additional Variables Are Associated With Empathy?

As I described in Chapter 9, research has shown that empathy is linked to a number of demographic and psychosocial variables, indicators of clinical competence, and career interest. Evidence also suggests that empathic engagement in patient care is associated with physicians' diagnostic accuracy and patients' adherence to treatment, increased satisfaction with their health care providers, and a reduced tendency to file malpractice claims (Chapter 10). Also, as was described in Chapters 4 and 8 and depicted in Fig. 12.1, family environment, early attachment relationships, human and material resources, and environmental, social, and cultural factors contribute to the development and manifestation of empathy in patient-care situations.

It is important to study empirically and, ideally in prospective longitudinal studies, the relative contribution of early experiences, the quality of early and late attachment relationships, and social, cultural, educational, and other factors that can predict empathy scores. This line of research would have important implications for the development of programs to retain and enhance the capacity for empathy.

Empathy also was found to predict ratings of clinical competence among medical students and physicians (Chapter 9). However, further research is needed to address other measures of performance that are significantly correlated with empathy scores and patient outcomes. It is desirable to use prospective studies to examine the relationship between empathy scores and different measures of performance (e.g., disciplinary action against health care providers) at different levels of professional education.

Furthermore, the findings on sex differences in empathy scores call for more empirical research to discern whether the differences are more likely to be related to "intrinsic" sex characteristics or to "extrinsic" sex-role socialization. Such research is needed because determining the proportion of the variance in empathy scores that is accounted for by intrinsic or extrinsic factors in the analyses of sex differences is an important issue. The answer would potentially have different implications in relation to the selection and education of health professionals.

Further investigations also are needed on the unique contribution of empathy to accurate diagnoses, improved compliance, better patient satisfaction, reduced malpractice claims (Chapter 10), and other tangible clinical outcomes regarding control of chronic diseases, such as essential hypertension and diabetes mellitus. These outcomes are important to be studied, not only because of their impact on mortality and morbidity, but also because of the economic impact on the patients, their families, and the society at large. The extent of the impact of empathic engagement in clinical encounters needs to be empirically investigated.

It also is highly desirable, although complicated, to examine the relative contribution of the following factors to the capacity for empathy, as reflected in empathy scores: genetic factors; quality of early attachment relationships; early life experiences (e.g., parental divorce, death in the family, maternal employment, day care experiences); later personal life experiences (e.g., peer relationships, marital relationships, role models); environmental and social factors (e.g., sociopolitical conditions, cultural norms, ascribed roles); cultural and cross-cultural factors, particularly among immigrants; formal education; and the interactions among these and other factors.

Gonnella and colleagues (Gonnella & Hojat, 2001; Gonnella et al., 1993a, 1993b) proposed that to achieve optimal patient outcomes, a physician must perform three roles—clinician, educator, and resource manager. Thus, determining the extent to which each of these roles is affected by a physician's empathy is important. Furthermore, it would be interesting to investigate the relative contribution of different factors of empathy (e.g., perspective taking, compassionate care, and standing in the patient's shoes) to the three roles of a physician.

3 Should Applicants' Empathy Be Considered in Admissions to Medical Schools and Residencies?

Medical Schools

Almost all North American medical schools place great emphasis on applicants' undergraduate grade-point averages and scores on the Medical College Admission Test (MCAT) for screening of the applicants. Although grade-point averages and MCAT scores are relatively good predictors of a student's academic performance in the first 2 years of medical school (the basic sciences component of medical education), they have poor predictive validity regarding a student's performance in the third and fourth years (the clinical sciences component of medical education) (Glaser, Hojat, Veloski, Blacklow, & Goepp, 2004; Hojat, Veloski, & Zeleznik, 1985; Hojat et al., 2000a).

Kupfer and colleagues (1978) reported that considering personal qualities, including empathy, when deciding which applicants should be admitted to medical school would lead to excellence in the practice of medicine. Streit-Forest (1982) recommended that once a significant relationship has been established between personal qualities and indicators of academic and professional success, the personal qualities of applicants to medical school should be included among the criteria for admission. In longitudinal studies of medical students, my colleagues and I have shown that measures of personal qualities (e.g., sociability, satisfactory interpersonal relationships, and self-esteem) and measures of academic aptitude (e.g., grade-point averages, and MCAT scores) can equally predict performance measures in the first 2 years of medical school. However, the measures of personal qualities could predict ratings of clinical performance in the third year of medical school more accurately than grade-point averages or MCAT scores (Hojat et al., 1993, 1996; Hojat, Vogel, Zeleznik, & Borenstein, 1988). In other words, incremental validity can be improved significantly by including indicators of interpersonal skills and measures of personal qualities in multiple regression models (Hojat et al., 1988, 1993; Zeleznik et al., 1988).

In a recent study, Stern, Frohna, and Gruppen (2005) reported that none of the data on academic performance that are often used for admissions to medical schools could predict medical students' professional behavior. However, in that study, medical students' unprofessional behavior observed by faculty, clerkship directors, and fellow students could be predicted by students' failure to complete required course evaluations and to report immunization compliance. These findings support the notion that indicators of personal qualities can predict professional behavior beyond measures of academic attainment. Essential humanistic qualities, such as empathy, elude the measures of undergraduate academic achievement that are commonly used when selecting applicants for admission to medical schools. Although one purpose of letters of recommendation is to describe personal qualities of the applicant, too often these letters fail to add anything beyond a summary of a student's academic performance (Zeleznik, Hojat, & Veloski, 1983).

Undergraduate academic institutions do not routinely provide information about medical school applicants' interpersonal skills and other personal qualities relevant to the capacity for empathy. However, an examination of undergraduate elective courses or baccalaureate majors can provide hints about applicants' interests in humanities and literature that are linked to the capacity for empathy (Chapter 11). More information about applicants' interpersonal skills or capacity for empathy can be probed during admissions interviews once interviewers are trained to detect these qualities. The issue of whether undergraduate elective courses or majors could predict capacity for empathy also needs to be empirically addressed. In addition, the issue of whether training those who interview medical school applicants can lead to the selection of more empathic students needs to be studied.

Residency Programs

Graduate medical education programs often consider indicators of academic attainment in medical school and scores on medical licensing examinations, such as Steps 1 and 2 of the United States Medical Licensing Examinations, as important determinants in the selection of residents. A residency candidate's personal qualities are often either overlooked or ignored completely.

Although the purpose of interviewing candidates for residency programs is to assess their humanistic qualities, attitudes, motivation, and other personal qualities, guidelines for assessing such qualities are often vague or nonexistent. Interviews are often not structured to assess those human qualities, or the interviewers are not specifically trained to detect them. Information on humanistic qualities of candidates is often available from evaluations of students' behavior in clinical clerkships. Letters of evaluation that medical school deans write for graduates not only should summarize the students' academic attainment but also should include assessments of graduates' humanistic qualities when dealing with patients.

Long ago, Jamison and Johnson (1975) suggested that the public would be better served if volunteers for public services were selected on the basis of their empathy scores. Because medicine is a public service profession and the professional behavior of physicians includes compassionate care and empathy, should empathy be a criterion for selection of medical students and residents, or even for employment of physicians? This question deserves serious research attention. If research provides convincing empirical evidence that incorporating empathy into the criteria for selecting applicants to medical schools and residency programs can lead to the advancement of professionalism in medicine, we should set aside our hesitation and include important personal qualities, such as empathy, when selecting our future health care work force. One positive result could be that health care professionals might regain the respect that has been vanishing along with the changes taking place in the health care system (see Chapter 11). Meanwhile, we need to study the long-term consequences of using empathy as a criterion for selecting applicants to medical schools and residency programs.

4 Does Empathy Predict Career Choice and Professional Success?

Findings on differences in empathy among physicians in various specialties (Chapter 9) call for further research. The question of whether health professionals choose different specialties because of differences in their capacity for empathy prior to their professional education or because of effects of their professional education needs further investigation. The answer to the question will have implications for selection of students and trainees, career counseling, and curriculum development in academic health centers. If empathy predicts career choice and interest in particular specialties, any attempt to select empathic candidates or to enhance empathy could potentially influence the distribution of physicians in the different specialties.

5 How Can Empathy Be Enhanced During Professional Education?

The finding that in the absence of dedicated educational programs, empathy among medical students and residents tends to decline as their education progresses (Chapter 11) raises serious concerns. Consequently, prospective research is needed to investigate whether empathy scores decline *systematically* or *randomly* during the course of medical education. It also is important to determine what factors would contribute to the systematic decline of or systematic increase in empathy in different individuals at different levels of health education. In addition, it is important to determine which factors may be detrimental and which factors may be beneficial to all individuals. If the detrimental and beneficial factors do not affect all individuals equally, determining what individual characteristics or experiences account for the variation in effects would be an important research goal.

Finally, more research is needed to identify the best methods or the best combinations of approaches for enhancing empathy among students and practitioners (e.g., development of interpersonal skills, exposure to hospitalization experiences, role playing, exposure to role models, specifically targeted video or audio materials, workshops on perspective taking, theatrical approaches, study of literature and the arts, or improvement of narrative skills). Furthermore, both formative and summative evaluations are needed to confirm that programs developed to enhance empathy have achieved their stated goals and that both the short- and long-term effects of such programs have been carefully evaluated.

6 Do Patients' Perspectives and Peers' Evaluations Contribute to Empathic Outcomes?

Optimal and nonoptimal clinician–patient relationships cannot be studied if we fail to understand patients' perspectives regarding the empathy of their health care providers. In Chapter 10, I pointed out that a large majority of the medical malpractice claims filed are the result of patients' negative view of the relationship with their health care providers. Thus, it is important to study patient outcomes with respect not only to clinicians' self-reported empathy but also to patients' perceptions of their caregivers' empathy and to peers' evaluations of clinicians' empathy.

Furthermore, it is important to examine health care providers' specific behaviors, such as punctuality, sense of humor, nonverbal behavior, and verbal expressions, that patients regard as significant determinants of an empathic engagement. The patients' perspectives are particularly important because one key concept in the definition of empathy was clinicians' ability to communicate their understanding to their patients (Chapter 6). Thus, future research should focus on the relationship among three sets of variables: (a) physicians' self-reported empathy, (b) patient's perceptions of physicians' empathy, and (c) peers' evaluations of physicians' empathy. To enhance our understanding of factors that determine final outcomes of rendering care, the relative contribution of these variables to patient outcomes must be investigated.

7 What Are the Neurophysiological Indicators of Empathy?

The recent discovery of mirror neurons that are activated in the brain when a person sees another person performing a goal-directed act or hears another person who is in distress (Carr et al., 2003; Kohler et al., 2002) opens up a new window for the examination of the neural mechanisms of empathy in human relationships (Chapter 3). With the technical advancements in functional brain imaging, it is now possible to observe and record the neurophysiological indicators of empathy. This exciting new discovery should prove to be extremely valuable in future research designed to identify the structural (neuroanatomical) and functional (neurophysiological) aspects of empathy in the human brain.

In addition, based on the studies cited in Chapter 3, both the limbic system and neocortex areas of the brain have often been implicated in neuroanatomical studies of empathy. However, future research must make a distinction between empathy (described in this book as cognitive empathy), and sympathy (or so called emotional empathy) and examine whether different areas of the brain are activated by empathic or sympathetic responses. As I suggested in Chapter 3, intuitively one can speculate that the neocortex is more likely to be activated in cognitive empathy and the limbic system is more likely to be implicated in sympathy, but this speculation needs empirical verification.

Concluding Remarks

We embarked on the journey to the terrain of empathy with the hope of exploring the roads leading to empathy (antecedents) and the paths leading from empathy (outcomes). Like the wings that evolved to allow birds to fly high on search of food, or like the long necks that evolved to allow giraffes to feed on leaves so high on the trees that other species could not reach, empathy, we learned, has evolutionary roots that sprouted for the purpose of survival.

Similarly, we learned that empathy—like hearing, vision, and language—has neuroanatomical and neurophysiological underpinnings. Empathy, like human love, connects people more closely, reduces interpersonal space, and fulfills the human need for affiliation, support, and understanding. In the context of patient care, empathy is no longer a vague concept because an operational definition offered in this book has clarified its meaning and it is no longer an abstract entity because it can be quantified with a valid and reliable instrument discussed in this book.

Empathy can increase altruistic, prosocial, and helping behaviors; reduce aggressive behavior; encourage avoidance of conflict; improve conflict management; and promote understanding (Larson & Yao, 2005). In the context of patient care, empathy can eliminate the constraints of the clinician–patient relationship. It can bridge the gap between givers and receivers of help and contribute to the physical, mental, and social well-being of both patient and clinician. Like height, weight, eye color, and type of hair, empathy varies among humans. However, a sense of unity can emerge from variation among human beings once empathic understanding prevails, once one can view the world from the other person's perspective, once one can stand in another person's shoes.

The following saying has been attributed to Albert Einstein: "A person starts to live when he can live outside himself." Empathic engagement takes a person outside himself or herself and allows the person to hear others with the third ear and to view the world of others with the mind's eye. Empathic engagement brings unity from diversity, making all of us akin regardless of sex, age, race, culture, religion, and other divisive factors. So, that is why any attempt toward empathic understanding of a fellow human being is a step toward building a civilization. Thus, the lesson to be learned is that implementation of remedies for enhancement of empathy—not just declaration of their desirability—is a mandate that must be acted upon, not only by teachers and healers of human infirmity, but by all members of the human race for the sake of healing human ills unto eternity. Because a person cannot hate "the other" once empathy bonds them together, empathy can be viewed as a remedy for the psyche and soul of humankind. And maybe it can serve as a means of achieving a global peace here, there, everywhere on earth because, as the Persian poet Saadi stated in a verse cited in the Preface, "all human beings are in truth akin."

Appendices

A

Jefferson Scale of Physician Empathy (JSPE) (HP-Version)

Instructions: Please indicate the extent of your agreement or disagreement with *each* of the following statements by marking the appropriate circle to the right of each statement.

Please use the following 7-point scale *(a higher number on the scale indicates more agreement):*
Mark <u>one and only one</u> response for each statement.

1———2———3———4———5———6———7
Strongly disagree ***Strongly agree***

	1	2	3	4	5	6	7
1. My understanding of how my patients and their families feel does not influence medical or surgical treatment.......	○	○	○	○	○	○	○
2. My patients feel better when I understand their feelings....	○	○	○	○	○	○	○
3. It is difficult for me to view things from my patients' perspectives..	○	○	○	○	○	○	○
4. I consider understanding my patients' body language as important as verbal communication in caregiver–patient relationships..	○	○	○	○	○	○	○
5. I have a good sense of humor that I think contributes to better clinical outcomes..................................	○	○	○	○	○	○	○
6. Because people are different, it is difficult for me to see things from my patients' perspectives......................	○	○	○	○	○	○	○
7. I try not to pay attention to my patients' emotions in history taking or in asking about their physical health......	○	○	○	○	○	○	○
8. Attentiveness to my patients' personal experiences does not influence treatment outcomes	○	○	○	○	○	○	○
9. I try to imagine myself in my patients' shoes when providing care to them	○	○	○	○	○	○	○
10. My patients value my understanding of their feelings, which is therapeutic in its own right	○	○	○	○	○	○	○
11. Patients' illnesses can be cured only by medical or surgical treatment; therefore, emotional ties to my patients do not have a significant influence on medical or surgical outcomes..	○	○	○	○	○	○	○
12. Asking patients about what is happening in their personal lives is not helpful in understanding their physical complaints...	○	○	○	○	○	○	○
13. I try to understand what is going on in my patients' minds by paying attention to their nonverbal cues and body language	○	○	○	○	○	○	○
14. I believe that emotion has no place in the treatment of medical illness	○	○	○	○	○	○	○

15. Empathy is a therapeutic skill without which success in treatment is limited.................................... ○ ○ ○ ○ ○ ○ ○
16. An important component of the relationship with my patients is my understanding of their emotional status as well as that of their families............................... ○ ○ ○ ○ ○ ○ ○
17. I try to think like my patients in order to render better care ○ ○ ○ ○ ○ ○ ○
18. I do not allow myself to be influenced by strong personal bonds between my patients and their family members ..... ○ ○ ○ ○ ○ ○ ○
19. I do not enjoy reading nonmedical literature or the arts.... ○ ○ ○ ○ ○ ○ ○
20. I believe that empathy is an important therapeutic factor in medical or surgical treatment..................... ○ ○ ○ ○ ○ ○ ○

B

Jefferson Scale of Physician Empathy (JSPE) (S-Version)

Instructions: Please indicate the extent of your agreement or disagreement with *each* of the following statements by marking the appropriate circle to the right of each statement.

Please use the following 7-point scale *(a higher number on the scale indicates more agreement):*
Mark one and only one response for each statement.

1——2——3——4——5——6——7
Strongly disagree ***Strongly agree***

	1	2	3	4	5	6	7
1. Physicians' understanding of their patients' feelings and the feelings of their patients' families does not influence medical or surgical treatment	○	○	○	○	○	○	○
2. Patients feel better when their physicians understand their feelings	○	○	○	○	○	○	○
3. It is difficult for a physician to view things from patients' perspectives	○	○	○	○	○	○	○
4. Understanding body language is as important as verbal communication in physician–patient relationships	○	○	○	○	○	○	○
5. A physician's sense of humor contributes to better clinical outcomes	○	○	○	○	○	○	○
6. Because people are different, it is difficult to see things from patients' perspectives	○	○	○	○	○	○	○
7. Attention to patients' emotions is not important in history taking	○	○	○	○	○	○	○
8. Attentiveness to patients' personal experiences does not influence treatment outcomes	○	○	○	○	○	○	○
9. Physicians should try to stand in their patients' shoes when providing care to them	○	○	○	○	○	○	○
10. Patients value a physician's understanding of their feelings, which is therapeutic in its own right	○	○	○	○	○	○	○
11. Patients' illnesses can be cured only by medical or surgical treatment; therefore, physicians' emotional ties with their patients do not have a significant influence in medical or surgical treatment	○	○	○	○	○	○	○
12. Asking patients about what is happening in their personal lives is not helpful in understanding their physical complaints	○	○	○	○	○	○	○
13. Physicians should tr to understand what is going on in their patients' minds by paying attention to their nonverbal cues and body language	○	○	○	○	○	○	○

14. I believe that emotion has no place in the treatment of medical illness .... ○ ○ ○ ○ ○ ○ ○
15. Empathy is a therapeutic skill without which the physician's success is limited................................. ○ ○ ○ ○ ○ ○ ○
16. Physicians' understanding of the emotional status of their patients, as well as that of their families is one important component of the physican–patient relationship.. ○ ○ ○ ○ ○ ○ ○
17. Physician should try to think like their patients in order to render better care.................................. ○ ○ ○ ○ ○ ○ ○
18. Physicians should not allow themselves to be influenced by strong personal bonds between their patients and their family members.......................... ○ ○ ○ ○ ○ ○ ○
19. I do not enjoy reading nonmedical literature or the arts.... ○ ○ ○ ○ ○ ○ ○
20. I believe that empathy is an important therapeutic factor in medical treatment................................. ○ ○ ○ ○ ○ ○ ○

C

Jefferson Scale of Patient's Perceptions of Physician Empathy (JSPPPE)

Instructions: We would like to know the extent of your agreement or disagreement with *each* of the following statements *about your doctor named below.* Please use the following 7-point scale and write your rating number from 1 to 7 on the underlined space before each statement (1 means that you strongly disagree, and 7 means you strongly agree with the statement; a higher number indicates more agreement).

1——2——3——4——5——6——7
Strongly disagree ***Strongly agree***

Dr. (Name of the physician in here)____________________

1. __Can view things from my perspective (see things as I see them).
2. __Asks about what is happening in my daily life.
3. __Seems concerned about me and my family.
4. __Understands my emotions, feelings, and concerns.
5. __Is an empathic doctor.

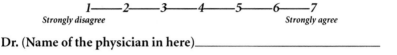

References

Association of American Medical Colleges. (2004). Medical School Objectives Project. Available at: http://www.aamc.org/meded/msop.

Abbott, L. C. (1983). A study of humanism in family physicians. *The Journal of Family Practice, 16*, 1141–1146.

American Board of Internal Medicine. (1983). Evaluation of humanistic qualities in the internist. *Annals of Internal Medicine, 99*, 720–724.

Ackoff, R. L., & Emery, F. E. (1981). *On purposeful systems.* Seaside, CA: Intersystems.

Acuna, L. E. (2000). Dont' cry for us Argentinians: Two decades of teaching medical humanities. *Journal of Medical Ethics: Medical Humanities, 26*, 66–70.

Adams, G. R., Jones, R. M., Schvaneveldt, J. D., & Jenson, G. O. (1982). Antecedents of affective role-taking behaviour: Adolescent perceptions of parental socialization styles. *Journal of Adolescence, 5*, 259–265.

Adler, H. M. (1997). The history of the present illness as treatment: Who's listening, and why does it matter? *The Journal of the American Board of Family Practice, 10*, 28–35.

Adler, H. M. (2002). The sociophysiology of caring in the doctor-patient relationship. *Journal of General Internal Medicine, 17*, 874–882.

Adler, H. M., & Mammett, V. B. O. (1973). The doctor-patient relationship revisited: An analysis of the placebo effect. *Annals of Internal Medicine, 78*, 595–598.

Adolphs, R., Tranel, D., Damasio, H., & Damasio, A. R. (1994). Impaired recognition of emotion in facial expression following bilateral damage to human amygdala. *Nature, 372*, 669–672.

Agosta, C. (1984). Empathy and intersubjectivity. In J. Lichtenberg, M. Borenstein, & D. Silver (Eds.), *Empathy II* (pp. 43–61). Hillsdale, NJ: Analytic Press.

Ainsworth, M. D. S. (1985a). Attachment across the life span. *Bulletin of the New York Academy of Medicine, 61*, 792–812.

Ainsworth, M. D. S. (1985b). Patterns of infant-mother attachment: Antecedents and effects on development. *Bulletin of the New York Academy of Medicine, 61*, 771–791.

Ainsworth, M. D. S., Blehar, M. C., Waters, E., & Wall, S. (1978). *Patterns of attachment: A psychological study of the strange situation.* Hillsdale, NJ: Erlbaum.

Alcorta-Garza, A., Gonzalez-Guerrero, J. F., Tavitas-Herrera, S. E., Rodrigues-Lara, F. J., & Hojat, M. (2005). Validacion de la Escala de Empatia Medica de Jefferson en estudiantes de medicina mexicanos [Validation of the Jefferson Scale of Physician Empathy in Mexican medical students]. *Salud Mental [Mental Health], 28*, 57–63.

Ali, N. S., Khalil, H. Z., & Yousef, W. (1993). A comparison of American and Egyptian cancer patients' attitudes and unmet needs. *Cancer Nursing, 16*, 193–203.

Allport, F. H. (1924). *Social psychology.* Boston: Houghton Mifflin.

Allport, G. W. (1960). The open system in personality theory. *Journal of Abnormal and Social Psychology, 61*, 301–310.

Amini, F., Lewis, T., Lannon, R., Louie, A., Baumbacher, G., McGuinness, T., & Schiff, E. Z. (1996). Affect, attachment, memory: Contributions toward psychobiologic integration. *Psychiatry, 59*, 213–239.

Anastasi, A. (1976). *Psychological testing.* New York: Macmillan.

Anthony, A. A., & Wain, H. J. (1971). An investigation of the outcome of empathy training for medical corpsmen. *Psychological Aspects of Disability, 18*, 86–88.

Archer, J. (2004). Sex differences in aggression in real-world settings: A meta-analytic review. *Review of General Psychology, 8*, 291–322.

Aring, C. D. (1958). Sympathy and empathy. *Journal of the American Medical Association, 167*, 448–452.

Arnkoff, D. B., Glass, C. R., & Shapiro, S. (2002). Expectations and preferences. In J. C.Norcross (Ed.), *Psychotherapy relationships at work: Therapist contributions and responsiveness to patients* (pp. 335–356). Oxford: Oxford University Press.

Arnold, L. (2002). Assessing professional behavior: Yesterday, today, and tomorrow. *Academic Medicine, 77,* 28–37.

Arnold, L., Calkins, E. V., & Willoughby, T. L. (1997). Antecedent and concurrent correlates of primary care practice. *Teaching and Learning in Medicine, 9,* 192–199.

Aronfreed, J. (1970). The socialization of altruistic and sympathetic behavior: Some theoretical and experimental analyses. In J. Macauley & L. Berkowitz (Eds.), *Altruistic and helping behavior* (pp. 103–126). New York: Academic Press.

Aronson, E., & Patnoe, S. (1997). *Jigsaw classroom.* New York: Longman.

Ashcroft, J., & Straus, A. (1993). *Families first: Report of the National Commission on America's Urban Families.* Washington, DC: National Commission on America's Urban Families.

Ashworth, C. D., Williamson, P., & Montano, D. (1984). A scale to measure physician beliefs about psychosocial aspects of patient care. *Social Science & Medicine, 19,* 1235–1238.

Astin, H. S. (1967). Assessment of empathic ability by means of a situational test. *Journal of Counseling Psychology, 14,* 57–60.

Avery, J. K. (1985). Lawyers tell what turns some patients litigious. *Medical Malpractice Review, 2,* 35–37.

Ax, A. F. (1964). Goals and methods of psychophysiology. *Psychophysiology, 1,* 8–25.

Ayra, D. K. (1993). To empathize or to dissociate—a physician's dilemma. *Journal of the Royal Society of Medicine, 86,* 3.

Bacharach, M. H. (1976). Empathy: We know what we mean, but what do we measure? *Archives of General Psychiatry, 33,* 35–38.

Baggaley, A. R. (1983). Deciding on the ratio of number of subjects to number of variables in factor analysis. *Multivariate Experimental Clinical Research, 6,* 81–86.

Bailey, B. A. (2001). Empathy in medical students: Assessment and relationship to specialty choice. *Dissertation Abstracts International, 62* (6-A), p. 2024.

Balint, M. (1957). *The doctor, his patient and the illness.* New York: International Universities Press.

Ballou, J. W. (1978). *The psychology of pregnancy.* Lexington, MA: Lexington Books.

Bandura, A. (1977). *Social learning theory.* Englewood Cliffs, NJ: Prentice Hall.

Banks, J. A. (1997). *Educating citizens in a multicultural society.* New York: Teachers College Press.

Barnett, M. A., Howard, J. A., King, L. M., & Dino, G. A. (1980). Antecedents of empathy: Retrospective accounts of early socialization. *Personality & Social Psychology Bulletin, 6,* 361–365.

Barnett, M. A. (1987). Empathy and related responses to children. In N. Eisenberg & J. Strayer (Eds.), *Empathy and its development* (pp. 146–162). New York: Cambridge University Press.

Barnett, M. A., Feighny, K. M., & Esper, J. A. (1983). Effect of anticipated victim responsiveness and empathy upon volunteering. *The Journal of Social Psychology, 119,* 211–218.

Barnett, R. C., Biener, L., & Baruch, G. K. (1987). *Gender and stress.* New York: Free Press.

Barnsley, J., Williams, A. P., Cockerill, R., & Tanner, J. (1999). Physician characteristics and the physician-patient relationship: Impact of sex, year of graduation, and specialty. *Canadian Family Physician, 45,* 935–942.

Baron-Cohen, S. (2003). *The essential difference: The truth about the male and female brain.* New York: Basic Books.

Baron-Cohen, S., & Wheelwright, S. (2004). The empathy quotient: An investigation of adults with Asperger syndrome or high functioning autism, and normal sex differences. *Journal of Autism and Developmental Disorders, 34,* 163–175.

Barondess, J. A. (2003). Medicine and professionalism. *Archives of Internal Medicine, 163,* 145–149.

Barrett-Lennard, G. T. (1962). Dimensions of therapist response as causal factors in therapeutic change. *Psychological Monographs, 76,* 1–36.

Barrett-Lennard, G. T. (1986). The relationship inventory now: Issues and advances in theory, method and use. In L. S. Greenberg & W. M. Pinsof (Eds.), *The psychotherapeutic process: A research handbook* (pp. 439–476). New York: Guilford.

Barsky, A. J. (1981). Hidden reasons some patients visit doctors. *Annals of Internal Medicine, 94*, 492–498.
Bartholomew, K., & Horowitz, L. (1991). Attachment styles among adults: A test of four-category model. *Journal of Personality and Social Psychology, 61*, 226–244.
Basch, M. F. (1983). Empathic understanding: A review of the concept and some theoretical considerations. *Journal of the American Psychoanalytic Association, 31*, 101–126.
Basch, M. F. (1996). Affect and defense. In D. L. Nathanson (Ed.), *Knowing feeling: Affect, script, and psychotherapy* (pp. 257–269). New York: W. W. Norton.
Bateson, G. (1971). A systems approach. *International Journal of Psychiatry, 9*, 242–244.
Batson, C. D. (1991). *The altruism question: Toward a social psychological answer.* Hillsdale, NJ: Erlbaum.
Batson, C. D., & Coke, J. S. (1981). Empathy: A source of altruistic motivation for helping? In J. P. Rushton & R. M. Sorrentino (Eds.), *Altruism and helping behavior: Social personality, and developmental perspectives* (pp. 167–211). Hillsdale, NJ: Erlbaum.
Batson, C. D., Coke, J. S., & Pych, V. (1983). Limits on the two-stage model of empathic mediation of helping: A reply to Archer, Diaz-Loving, Gollwitzer, Davis, and Foushee. *Journal of Personality and Social Psychology, 45*, 895–898.
Batson, C. D., Polycarpou, M. P., Harmon-Jones, E., Imhoff, H. J., Mitchener, E. C., Bednar, L. L., Klein, T. R., & Highberger, L. (1997a). Empathy and attitudes: Can feeling for a member of a stigmatized group improve feelings toward the group? *Journal of Personality and Social Psychology, 72*, 105–118.
Batson, C. D., Sager, K., Garst, E., Kang, M., Rubchinsky, K., & Dawson, K. (1997b). Is empathy-induced helping due to self-other merging? *Journal of Personality and Social Psychology, 73*, 495–509.
Baumann, A. O., Deber, R. B., Silverman, B. E., & Mallette, C. M. (1998). Who cares? Who cures? The ongoing debate in the provision of health care. *Journal of Advanced Nursing, 28*, 1040–1045.
Bavelas, J. B., Black, A., Lemery, C. R., & Mullett, J. (1986). "I show how you feel": Motor mimicry as a communicative act. *Journal of Personality and Social Psychology, 50*, 322–329.
Bayes, M. A. (1972). Behavioral cues of interpersonal warmth. *Journal of Consulting and Clinical Psychology, 39*, 333–339.
Becker, H., & Sands, D. (1988). The relationship of empathy to clinical experience among male and female nursing students. *Journal of Nursing Education, 27*, 198–203.
Becker, H. S., & Geer, B. (1958). The fate of idealism in medical school. *American Sociological Review, 23*, 50–56.
Beckman, H. B., & Frankel, R. M. (1984). The effect of physician behavior on the collection of data. *Annals of Internal Medicine, 101*, 692–696.
Beckman, H. B., Markakis, K. M., Suchman, A. L., & Frankel, R. M. (1994). The doctor-patient relationship and malpractice: Lessons from plaintiff depositions. *Archives of Internal Medicine, 154*, 1365–1370.
Beddoe, A. E., & Murphy, S. O. (2004). Does mindfulness decrease stress and foster empathy among nursing students? *Journal of Nursing Education, 43*, 305–312.
Beecher, H. K. (1955). The powerful placebo. *Journal of the American Medical Association, 159*, 1602–1606.
Beisecker, A. E., & Beisecker, T. D. (1990). Patient information-seeking behaviors when communicating with doctors. *Medical Care, 28*, 19–28.
Bellet, P. S., & Maloney, M. J. (1991). The importance of empathy as an interviewing skill in medicine. *Journal of the American Medical Association, 266*, 1831–1832.
Bellini, L. M., Baime, M., & Shea, J. A. (2002). Variation of mood and empathy during internship. *Journal of the American Medical Association, 287*, 3143–3146.
Bellini, L. M., & Shea, J. A. (2005). Mood change and empathy decline persist during three years of internal medicine training. *Academic Medicine, 80*, 164–167.
Belsky, J. (1988). The "effects" of infant day care reconsidered. *Childhood Research Quarterly, 3*, 235–272.
Bem, S. L. (1974). The measurement of psychological androgyny. *Journal of Consulting and Clinical Psychology, 42*, 155–162.
Benbassat, J., & Baumal, R. (2004). What is empathy, and how can it be promoted during clinical clerkships? *Academic Medicine, 79*, 832–839.

Benedict, R. H. B., Priore, R. L., Miller, C., Munschauser, F., & Jacobs, L. (2001). Personality disorder in multiple sclerosis correlates with cognitive impairment. *Journal of Neuropsychiatry & Clinical Neurosciences, 13*, 70–76.

Bennett, J. A. (1995). "Methodological notes on empathy": Further considerations. *Advances in Nursing Science, 18*, 36–50.

Bennett, M. J. (2001). *The empathic healer: An endangered species.* San Diego, CA: Academic Press.

Benton, A. L. (1991). The prefrontal region: Its early history. In H. Levin, H. M. Eisenberg, & A. L. Benton (Eds.), *Frontal lobe function and dysfunction* (pp. 3–32). New York: Oxford University Press.

Beres, D., & Arlow, J. A. (1974). Fantasy and identification in empathy. *Psychoanalytic Quarterly, 43*, 26–40.

Berger, D. M. (1987). *Clinical empathy.* Northvale, NJ: Jason Aronson.

Berger, S. M. (1962). Conditioning through vicarious instigation. *Psychological Review, 69*, 450–466.

Berkman, L., & Syme, S. (1979). Social networks, host resistance, and mortality: A nine-year follow-up of Alameda County residents. *American Journal of Epidemiology, 109*, 186–204.

Berkman, L. F. (1995). The role of social relations in health promotion. *Psychosomatic Medicine, 57*, 245–254.

Berkman, L. F. (2000). Which influences cognitive function: Living alone or being alone? *Lancet, 355*, 1291–1292.

Berkman, L. F., Glass, T., Brissette, I., & Seeman, T. E. (2000). From social integration to health: Durkheim in the new millennium. *Social Science & Medicine, 51*, 843–857.

Berkman, L. F., Leo-Summers, L., & Horwitz, R. I. (1992). Emotional support and survival after myocardial infarction. *Annals of Internal Medicine, 117*, 1003–1009.

Bertakis, K. D., Helms, L. J., Callahan, E. J., Azari, R., & Robbins, J. A. (1995). The influence of gender on physician practice style. *Medical Care, 33*, 407–416.

Bertakis, K. D., Roter, D., & Putman, S. M. (1991). The relationship of physician medical interview style to patient satisfaction. *Journal of Family Practice, 32*, 175–181.

Beutler, L. E., Johnson, D. T., Neville, C. W., & Workman, S. N. (1973). Some sources of variance in "Accurate Empathy" ratings. *Journal of Consulting and Clinical Psychology, 40*, 167–169.

Beven, J. P., O'Brien-Malone, A., & Hall, G. (2004). Using the Interpersonal Reactivity Index to assess empathy in violent offenders. *International Journal of Forensic Psychology, 1*, 33–41.

Bickel, J. (1994). Special needs and affinities of women medical students. In E. S. More & M. A. Milligan (Eds.), *The empathic practitioner: Empathy, gender, and medicine* (pp. 237–249). New Brunswick, NJ: Rutgers University Press.

Bjorklund, D. F., & Kipp, K. (1996). Parental investment theory and gender differences in the evolution of inhibition mechanism. *Psychological Bulletin, 100*, 163–188.

Black, D. M. (2004). Sympathy reconfigured: Some reflections on sympathy, empathy and the discovery of values. *International Journal of Psychoanalysis, 85*, 579–595.

Black, H., & Phillips, S. (1982). An intervention program for the development of empathy in student teachers. *Journal of Psychology: Interdisciplinary & Applied, 112*, 159–168.

Blackman, N., Smith, K., Brokman, R., & Stern, J. (1958). The development of empathy in male schizophrenics. *Psychiatric Quarterly, 32*, 546–553.

Blackwell, B. (1973). Drug therapy, patient compliance. *New England Journal of Medicine, 289*, 249–252.

Bland, C. J., Meurer, L. N., & Maldonado, G. (1995). Determinants of primary care specialty choice: A non-statistical meta-analysis of the literature. *Academic Medicine, 70*, 620–641.

Blanton, S. (1960). *The healing power of poetry.* New York: Crowell.

Blass, C. D., & Hech, E. J. (1975). Accuracy of accurate empathy ratings. *Journal of Counseling Psychology, 22*, 243–246.

Blazer, D. G. (1982). Social support and mortality in an elderly community population. *American Journal of Epidemiology, 115*, 684–694.

Block, J. H. (1976). Assessing sex differences: Issues, problems, and pitfalls. *Merrill-Palmer Quarterly, 22*, 283–308.

Bloom, B. L., Asher, S. J., & White, S. W. (1978). Marital disruption as a stressor: A review analysis. *Psychological Bulletin, 85*, 867–894.
Blumenthal, J. A., Burg, M. M., Barefoot, J., Williams, R. B., Haney, T., & Zimet, G. (1987). Social support, type A behavior, and coronary artery disease. *Psychosomatic Medicine, 49*, 331–340.
Blumgart, H. L. (1964). Caring for the patient. *New England Journal of Medicine, 270*, 449–456.
Bohart, A. C., Elliot, R., Greenberg, L. S., & Watson, J. C. (2002). Empathy. In J. C. Norcross (Ed.), *Psychotherapy relationships that work: Therapist contributions and responsiveness to patients* (pp. 89–108). Oxford, UK: Oxford University Press.
Bolognini, S. (1997). Empathy and "empathism." *International Journal of Psychoanalysis, 78*, 279–293.
Book, H. E. (1988). Empathy: Misconceptions and misuses in psychotherapy. *American Journal of Psychiatry, 145*, 420–424.
Book, H. E. (1991). Is empathy cost efficient? *American Journal of Psychotherapy, 45*, 21–30.
Borgenicht, L. (1984). Richard Selzer and the problem of detached concern. *Annals of Internal Medicine, 100*, 923–934.
Borke, H. (1971). Interpersonal perception of young children: Ego-centrism or empathy. *Developmental Psychology, 5*, 263–269.
Boruch, R. F. (1982). Evidence and inference in research on mass psychogenic illness. In M. J. Colligan, J. W. Pennebaker, & L. R. Murphy (Eds.), *Mass psychogenic illness: A social psychological analysis* (pp. 101–125). Hillsdale, NJ: Erlbaum.
Bowers, M. R., Swan, J. E., & Koehler, W. F. (1994). What attributes determine quality and satisfaction with health care delivery? *Health Care Management Review, 19*, 49–55.
Bowlby, J. (1973). *Attachment and loss (Vol. 2): Separation: Anxiety and anger*. New York: Basic Books.
Bowlby, J. (1980). *Attachment and loss (Vol. 3):Loss: Sadness and depression*. New York: Basic Books.
Bowlby, J. (1982). *Attachment and loss (Vol. 1): Attachment*. New York: Basic Books.
Bowlby, J. (1988). *A secure base: Parent-child attachment and healthy human development*. New York: Basic Books.
Boyd, R. W., & DiMascio, A. (1957). Social behavior and automatic physiology: A sociophysiological study. *Journal of Nervous and Mental Disease, 120*, 207–212.
Branch, W. T. (2000). The ethics of caring and medical education. *Academic Medicine, 75*, 127–132.
Branch, W. T., & Malik, T. K. (1993). Using windows of opportunities in brief interviews to understand patients' concerns. *Journal of the American Medical Association, 169*, 1667–1668.
Branch, W. T., Pels, R. J., & Hafler, J. P. (1998). Medical students' empathic understanding of their patients. *Academic Medicine, 73*, 360–362.
Bretherton, I. (1987). New perspectives on attachment relations: Security, communication, and internal working models. In J. Osofsky (Ed.), *Handbook of infant development* (pp. 1061–1100). New York: John Wiley & Sons.
Bridgman, D. L. (1981). Enhanced role taking through cooperative interdependence: A field study. *Child Development, 52*, 1231–1238.
Brislin, R. W. (1970). Back-translation for cross-cultural research. *Journal of Cross-Cultural Psychology, 1*, 185–216.
Brislin, R. W. (1980). Translation and content analysis of oral and written material. In H. C.Triandis & R. W. Brislin (Eds.), *Handbook of cross-cultural psychology/social psychology* (pp. 389–444). Boston: Allyn & Bacon.
Brock, C. D., & Salinsky, J. V. (1993). Empathy: An essential skill for understanding the physician-patient relationship in clinical practice. *Family Medicine, 25*, 245–248.
Brody, H. (1985). Placebo effect: An examination of Grunbaum's definition. In L. White, B. Tursky, & G. E. Schwartz (Eds.), *Placebo: Theory, research, and mechanisms* (pp. 37–58). New York: Guilford Press.
Brody, H. (1997). Placebo response, sustained partnership, and emotional resilience in practice. *Journal of the American Board of Family Practice, 10*, 72–74.
Brothers, L. (1989). A biological perspective on empathy. *American Journal of Psychiatry, 146*, 10–19.

Brown, J., & Dunn, J. (1996). Continuities in emotional understanding from 3 to 6 years. *Child Development, 67,* 789–802.
Brownell, A. K., & Cote, L. (2001). Senior residents' views on the meaning of professionalism and how they learn about it. *Academic Medicine, 76,* 734–737.
Bruner, J. (1990). *Acts of meaning.* Cambridge, MA: Harvard University Press.
Bryant, B. K. (1982). An index of empathy for children and adolescents. *Child Development, 53,* 413–425.
Buccino, G., Binkofski, F., Fink, G. R., Fadiga, L., Fogassi, L., Gallese, V., Seitz, R. J., Zilles, K., Rizzolatti, G., & Freund, H. J. (2001). Action observation activates premotor and parietal areas in a somatotypic manner: An fMRI study. *European Journal of Neuroscience, 13,* 400–404.
Buchheimer, A. (1963). The development of ideas about empathy. *Journal of Counseling Psychology, 10,* 61–70.
Buck, R. (1984). *The communication of emotion.* New York: Guilford Press.
Buck, R., & Ginsberg, B. (1997a). Communicative genes and the evolution of empathy: Selfish and social emotions as voices of selfish and social genes. *Annals of the New York Academy of Sciences, 807,* 481–483.
Buck, R., & Ginsburg, B. (1997b). Communicative genes and the evolution of empathy. In W. Ickes (Ed.), *Empathic accuracy* (pp. 17–43). New York: Guilford.
Buck, R., Miller, R. E., & Caul, W. F. (1974). Sex, personality, and physiological variables in the communication of affect via facial expression. *Journal of Personality and Social Psychology, 30,* 587–596.
Buck, R. W., Savin, V. J., Miller, R. E., & Caul, W. F. (1972). Communication of affect through facial expressions in humans. *Journal of Personality and Social Psychology, 23,* 362–371.
Burack, J. H., Irby, D. M., Carline, J. D., Ambrozy, D. M., Ellsbury, K. E., & Stritter, F. T. (1997). A study of medical students' specialty-choice pathways: Trying on possible selves. *Academic Medicine, 72,* 534–541.
Burdi, M. D., & Baker, L. C. (1999). Physicians' perceptions of autonomy and satisfaction in California. *Health Affairs, 18,* 134–145.
Burlingham, D. (1967). Empathy between infant and mother. *Journal of the American Psychoanalytic Association, 15,* 764–780.
Burns, D. D., & Nolen-Hoeksema, S. (1992). Therapeutic empathy and recovery from depression in cognitive-behavioral therapy: A structural equation model. *Journal of Consulting and Clinical Psychology, 60,* 441–449.
Burnstein, A. G., Loucks, S., Kobos, J., Johnson, G., Talbert, R. L., & Stanton, B. (1980). A longitudinal study of personality characteristics of medical students. *Journal of Medical Education, 55,* 786–787.
Bush, L. K., Barr, C. L., McHugo, G. J., & Lanzetta, J. T. (1989). The effects of facial control and facial mimicry on subjective reactions to comedy routines. *Motivation and Emotion, 13,* 31–52.
Buss, D. M. (1995). Psychological sex differences: Origins through sexual selection. *American Psychologist, 50,* 164–168.
Buss, D. M. (2003). *The evolution of desire: Strategies of human mating.* New York: Basic Books.
Buss, D. M., & Schmitt, D. P. (1993). Sexual strategies theory: An evolutionary perspective on human mating. *Psychological Review, 100,* 204–232.
Butow, P. N., Maclean, M., Dunn, S. M., Tattersall, M. H. N., & Boyer, M. J. (1997). The dynamics of change: Cancer patients' preferences for information, involvement and support. *Annals of Oncology, 8,* 857–863.
Bylund, C. L., & Makoul, G. (2002). Empathic communication and gender in the physician-patient encounter. *Patient Education and Counseling, 48,* 207–216.
Bylund, C. L., & Makoul, G. (2005). Examining empathy in medical encounters: An observational study using the empathic communication coding system. *Health Communication, 18,* 123–140.
Cacioppo, J. T., Hawkley, L. C., Crawford, E., Ernst, J. M., Burleson, M. H., Kowalewski, R. B., Malarkey, W. B., Cauter, E. V., & Berntson, G. G. (2002). Loneliness and health: Potential mechanisms. *Psychosomatic Medicine, 64,* 401–417.
Cahill, L. (2005). His brain, her brain. *Scientific American, 292,* 40–47.
Calhoun, J. B. (1962). Population density and social pathology. *Scientific American, 206,* 3–10.

Calman, K. C., Downie, R. S., Duthie, M., & Sweeney, B. (1988). Literature and medicine: A short course for medical students. *Medical Education, 22*, 265–269.

Campbell, D. T. & Fiske, D. W. (1959). Convergent and discriminant validation by the multitrait-multimethod matrix. *Psychological Bulletin, 56*, 81–105.

Campos, J., & Sternberg, C. (1981). Perception, appraisal and emotion in the onset of social referencing. In M. E. Lamb & L. R. Sherrod (Eds.), *Infant social cognition* (pp. 273–314). Hillsdale, NJ: Erlbaum.

Campus-Outcalt, D., Senf, J., Watkins A. J., & Bastacky, S. (1995). The effects of medical school curricula, faculty role models, and biomedical research on choice of generalist physician career: A review and quality assessment of the literature. *Academic Medicine, 70*, 611–619.

Cannon, W. (1957). "Voodoo" death. *Psychosomatic Medicine, 19*, 182–190.

Carkhuff, R. (1969). *Helping and human relations: Selection and training* (Vol. 1). New York: Holt, Rinehart & Winston.

Carmel, S., & Glick, S. M. (1996). Compassionate-empathic physicians: Personality traits and social-organizational factors that enhance or inhibit this behavior pattern. *Social Science and Medicine, 43*, 1253–1261.

Carr, L., Iacoboni, M., Dubeau, M. C., Mazziotta, J. C., & Lenzi, G. L. (2003). Neural mechanisms of empathy in humans: A relay from neural systems for imitation to limbic areas. *Proceedings of the National Academy of Sciences of the U.S.A., 100*, 5497–5502.

Carr, P. L., Ash, A. S., & Friedman, E. H. (1998). Relation of family responsibilities and gender to the productivity and career satisfaction of medical faculty. *Annals of Internal Medicine, 129*, 532–538.

Carter, F. (1976). *The education of Little Tree.* Albuquerque: University of New Mexico Press.

Case, R. B., Moss, A. J., Case, N., McDermott, M., & Eberly, S. (1992). Living alone after myocardiac infarction: Impact on prognosis. *Journal of the American Medical Association, 267*, 515–519.

Caspi, A., & Silva, P. A. (1995). Temperamental qualities at age three predict personality traits in young adulthood: Longitudinal evidence from a birth cohort. *Child Development, 66*, 486–492.

Castiglioni, A. (1941). *A history of medicine.* New York: Knopf.

Cataldo, K. P., Peeden, K., Geesey, M. E., & Dickerson, L. (2005). Association between Balint training and physician empathy and work satisfaction. *Family Medicine, 37*, 328–331.

Cattle, R. B. (1966). The scree test for the number of factors. *Multivariate Behavioral Research, 1*, 245–276.

Charon, R. (1993). The narrative road to empathy. In H. Spiro, M. G. McCrea Curnen, E. Peschel, & D. St. James (Eds.), *Empathy and the practice of medicine* (pp. 147–159). New Haven: Yale University Press.

Charon, R. (2000). Medicine, the novel, and the passage of time. *Annals of Internal Medicine, 132*, 63–68.

Charon, R. (2001a). Narrative medicine: A model for empathy, reflection, profession, and trust. *Journal of the American Medical Association, 286*, 1897–1902.

Charon, R. (2001b). Narrative medicine: Form, function, and ethics. *Annals of Internal Medicine, 134*, 83–87.

Charon, R., Greene, M. G., & Adelman, R. (1994). Woman readers, woman doctors: A feminist reader-response theory of medicine. In E. S. More & M. A. Milligan (Eds.), *The empathic practitioner: Empathy, gender, and medicine* (pp. 205–221). New Brunswick, NJ: Rutgers University Press.

Charon, R., & Montello, M. (2002). *Stories matter: The role of narrative in medical ethics.* New York: Routledge.

Charon, R., Trautmann Banks, J., Connelly, J. E., Hunsaker Hawkins, A., Montgomery Hunter, K., Hudson Jones, A., Montello, M., & Poirer, S. (1995). Literature in medicine: Contribution to clinical practice. *Annals of Internal Medicine, 122*, 599–606.

Chartrand, T. L., & Bargh, J. A. (1999). The chameleon effect: The perception-behavior link and social interaction. *Journal of Personality and Social Psychology, 76*, 893–910.

Chessick, R. D. (1992). *What constitutes the patient in psychotherapy: Alternative approaches to understanding humans.* Northvale, N.J.: Jason Aronson.

Chinsky, J. M., & Rappaport, J. (1970). Brief critique of the meaning and reliability of "Accurate Empathy" ratings. *Psychological Bulletin, 73*, 379–382.

Chismar, D. (1988). Empathy and sympathy: The important difference. *Journal of Value Inquiry, 22*, 257–266.
Chlopan, B. E., McCain, M. L., Carbonell, J. L., & Hagen, R. L. (1985). Empathy: Review of available measures. *Journal of Personality and Social Psychology, 48*, 635–653.
Chodorow, N. (1978). *The reproduction of mothering: Psychoanalysis and sociology of gender.* Berkeley, CA: University of California Press.
Chow, K. L., Riesen, A. H., & Newell, F. W. (1957). Degeneration of retinal ganglion cells in infant chimpanzees reared in darkness. *Journal of Comparative Neurology, 107*, 27–42.
Christenfeld, N., & Gerin, W. (2000). Social support and cardiovascular reactivity. *Biomedicine and Pharmacotherapy, 54*, 251–257.
Christodoulou, G. N., Lykousras, L. P., Mountaokalakis, T., Voulgari, A., & Stefanis, C. N. (1995). Personalities of psychiatric versus other medical trainers. *Journal of Nervous and Mental Disease, 183*, 330–340.
Ciechanowski, P. S., Russo, J. E., Katon, W. J., & Walker, F. A. (2004). Attachment theory in health care: The influence of relationship style on medical students' specialty choice. *Medical Education, 38*, 262–270.
Clark, K. B. (1980). Empathy—a neglected topic in psychological research. *American Psychologist, 35*, 187–190.
Clearly, P. D., & McNeil, B. J. (1988). Patient satisfaction as an indicator of quality care. *Inquiry, 25*, 25–36.
Cleghorn, S. M. (1978). Empathy: Listening with the third ear. *Tennessee Education, 8*, 7–11.
Cliffordson, C. (2002). The hierarchical structure of empathy: Dimensional organization and elations to social functioning. *Scandinavian Journal of Psychology, 43*, 49–59.
Clouser, K. D. (1990). Humanities in medical education: Some contributions. *Journal of Medical Philosophy, 15*, 289–301.
Cohen, J. (1987). *Statistical power analysis for the behavioral sciences.* Hillsdale, NJ: Erlbaum.
Cohen, S. (1988). Psychological models for the role of social support in the etiology of physical disease. *Health Psychology, 7*, 269–297.
Cohen, S. (2004). Social relationship and health. *American Psychologist, 59*, 676–684.
Cohen, S., & Matthews, K. A. (1987). Social support, type A behavior, and coronary artery disease. *Psychosomatic Medicine, 49*, 325–330.
Coke, J. S., Batson, C. D., & McDavis, K. (1978). Empathic mediation of helping: A two-stage model. *Journal of Personality and Social Psychology, 36*, 752–766.
Cole, D. A., Martin, N. C., & Steiger, J. H. (2005). Empirical and conceptual problems with longitudinal trait-state models: Introducing a trait-state-occasion model. *Psychological Methods, 10*, 3–20.
Coleridge, S. T. (1802). Letter to William Sotheby, July 13th. In E. L.Griggs (Ed.), *Collected letters of Samuel Taylor Coleridge* (Vol. 2). Oxford, UK: Oxford University Press. (Reprinted in 1956.)
Coles, R. (1989). *Call of stories: Teaching and moral imagination.* Boston: Houghton-Mifflin.
Collier, V. U., MaCue, J. D., Markus, A., & Smith, L. (2002). Stress in medical residency: status quo after a decade or reform? *Annals of Internal Medicine, 136*, 384–390.
Colligan, M. J., & Murphy, L. R. (1982). A review of mass psychogenic illness in work settings. In M.J.Colligan, J. W. Pennebaker, & L. R. Murphy (Eds.), *Mass psychogenic illness: A social psychological analysis* (pp. 33–52). Hillsdale, NJ: Erlbaum.
Colligan, M. J., Pennebaker, J. W., & Murphy, L. R. (1982). *Mass psychogenic illness: A social psychological analysis.* Hillsdale, NJ: Erlbaum.
Collins, F. S. (1999). Shattuck lecture—medical and societal consequences of the human genome project. *New England Journal of Medicine, 341*, 28–37.
Colliver, J. A., Willis, M. S., Robbs, R. S., Cohen, D. S., & Swartz, M. H. (1998). Assessment of empathy in a standardized-patient examination. *Teaching and Learning in Medicine, 10*, 8–10.
Colman, A. M. (2001). *A dictionary of psychology.* London, UK: Oxford University Press.
Comas-Diaz, L., & Jacobsen, F.M. (1991). Ethnocultural transference and countertransference in the therapeutic dyad. *American Journal of Orthopsychiatry, 61*, 392–402.
Comstock, L. M., Hooper, E. M., Goodwin, J. M., & Goodwin, J. S. (1982). Physician behaviors that correlate with patient satisfaction. *Journal of Medical Education, 57*, 105–112.
Connellan, J., Baron-Cohen, S., Wheelwright, S., Batki, A., & Ahluwalia, J. (2000). Sex differences in human neonatal social perception. *Infant Behavior & Development, 23*, 113–118.

Cooper-Patrick, L., Gallo, J. J., & Gonzales, J. J. (1999). Race, gender and partnership in the patient-physician relationship. *Journal of the American Medical Association, 282,* 583–589.

Costa, P. T., Jr., & McCrea, R. B. (1992). *Revised NEO Personality Inventory (NEO PI-R) and NEO Five Factor Inventory (NEO-FFI): Professional manual.* Odessa, FL: Psychological Assessment Resources.

Coulehan, J. L., & Williams, P. (2001). Vanquishing virtue: The impact of medical education. *Academic Medicine, 76,* 598–605.

Cousins, N. (1985). How patients appraise physicians. *New England Journal of Medicine, 313,* 1422–1424.

Coutts-van Dijk, L. C., Bray, J. H., Moore, S., & Rogers, J. (1997). Prospective study of how students' humanism and psychosocial beliefs relate to specialty matching. *Academic Medicine, 72,* 1106–1108.

Coutts, L. C., & Rogers, J. C. (2000). Humanism: Is its evaluation captured in commonly used performance measures? *Teaching and Learning in Medicine, 12,* 28–32.

Crabb, W. T., Moracco, J. C., & Bender, R. C. (1983). A comparative study of empathy training with programmed instruction for lay helpers. *Journal of Counseling Psychology, 30,* 221–226.

Cristy, B. L. (2001). Wounded healer: The impact of a therapist's illness on the therapeutic situation. *Journal of the American Academy of Psychoanalysis, 29,* 33–42.

Cronbach, L. J. (1951). Coefficient alpha and the internal structure of tests. *Psychometrika, 16,* 297–334.

Cross, D. G., & Sharpley, C. F. (1982). Measurement of empathy with the Hogan Empathy Scale. *Psychological Reports, 50,* 62.

Crouse, B. B., & Mehrabian, A. (1977). Affiliation of opposite-sex strangers. *Journal of Research in Personality, 11,* 38–47.

Cummings, S. A., Savitz, L. A., & Konrad, T. R. (2001). Reported response rates to mailed physician questionnaires. *Health Sciences Research, 35,* 1347–1355.

Cyphert, F. R., & Gant, W. L. (1970). The Delphi technique: A tool for collecting opinions in teacher education. *The Journal of Teacher Education, 21,* 417–425.

Dalton, R., Sunblad, L., & Hylbert, S. (1976). Using principles of social learning in training for communication in empathy. *Journal of Counseling Psychology, 23,* 454–457.

Damasio, A. (2003). *Looking for Spinoza: Joy, sorrow and the feeling brain.* New York: Harcourt Brace.

Damasio, H., Grabowski, T., Frank, R., Galaburda, A. M., & Damasio, A. R. (1994). The return of Phineas Gage: Clues about the brain from the skull of a famous patient. *Science, 264,* 1102–1105.

Darwin, C. (1965). *The expression of emotion in man and animals.* New York: St. Martin's Press. (Originally published in 1872.)

Darwin, C. (1981). *The descent of man, and selection in relation to sex.* Princeton University Press. (Originally published in 1871.)

DasGupta, S., & Charon, R. (2004). Personal illness narratives: Using reflective writing to teach empathy. *Academic Medicine, 79,* 351–356.

Davis, M. H. (1983). Measuring individual differences in empathy: Evidence for a multidimensional approach. *Journal of Personality and Social Psychology, 44,* 113–126.

Davis, M. H. (1994). *Empathy: A social psychological approach.* Boulder, CO Westview.

Davis, M. H., & Franzoi, S. L. (1991). Stability and change in adolescent self-consciousness and empathy. *Journal of Research in Personality, 25,* 70–87.

Davis, M. H., Luce, C., & Kraus, S. J. (1994). The heritability of characteristics associated with dispositional empathy. *Journal of Personality, 62,* 369–391.

Davis, M. R. (1985). Perception of affective reverberation component. In A. P.Goldstein & G. Y. Michaels (Eds.), *Empathy: Development, training, and consequences* (pp. 62–108). Hillsdale, NJ: Erlbaum.

Davis, M. S. (1968). Physiological, psychological and demographic factors in patient compliance with doctor's orders. *Medical Care, 6,* 115–122.

Davison, A. N., & Peters, A. (1970). *Myelination.* Springfield, IL: Charles C Thomas.

Dawes, R. M. (1999). A message from psychologists to economists: Mere predictability doesn't matter like it should (without a good story appended to it). *Journal of Economic Behavior & Organization, 39,* 20–40.

Dawkins, R. (1999). *The selfish gene.* Oxford, UK: Oxford University Press.

Dawson, G. (1994). Development of emotional expression and emotion regulation in infancy: Contribution of the frontal lobe. In G. Dawson & K. W. Fischer (Eds.), *Human behavior and the developing brain* (pp. 346–379). New York: Guilford.

Day, S. C., Norcini, J. J., Shea, J. A., & Benson, J. A. Jr. (1989). Gender differences in clinical competence of residents in internal medicine. *Journal of General Internal Medicine, 4*, 309–312.

de Quervain, D. J. F., Fischbacher, U., Treyer, V., Schellhammer, M., Schnyder, U., Buck, A., & Fehr, E. (2004). The neutral basis of altruistic punishment. *Science, 305*, 1254–1258.

Deardroff, P. A., Finch, A. J. Jr., Kendall, P. C., Liran, F., & Indrisano, V. (1975). Empathy and socialization in repeat offenders, first offenders, and normals. *Journal of Counseling Psychology, 22*, 453–455.

Deardroff, P. A., Kendall, P. C., Finch, A. J., Jr., & Sitartz, A. M. (1977). Empathy, locus and control and anxiety in college students. *Psychological Reports, 40*, 1236–1238.

DeCasper, A. J., & Fifer, W. P. (1980). Of human bonding: Newborns prefer their mothers' voices. *Science, 208*, 1174–1176.

DeCasper, A. J., & Prescott, P. A. (1984). Human newborn's perception of male voices' preference, discrimination, and reinforcing value. *Developmental Psychology, 17*, 481–491.

Decety, J., & Jackson, P. L. (2004). The functional architecture of human empathy. *Behavior and Cognitive Neuroscience Review, 3*, 71–100.

Decety, J., & Jackson, P. L. (2006). A social-neuroscience perspective on empathy. *Current Directions in Psychological Science, 15*, 54–58.

DeKruif (1926). *Microb hunters*. New York: Harcourt, Brace.

Demos, E. V. (1988). Affect and the development of self: A new frontier. In A.Goldberg (Ed.), *Frontiers in self psychology: Progress in self psychology (Vol. 3*, pp. 27–33). Hillsdale, NJ: Analytic Press.

D'Orazio, D. M. (2004). Letter to the editor. *Sexual Abuse: A Journal of Research and Treatment, 16*, 173–174.

DeValck, C., Bensing, J., Bruynooghe, R., & Batenburg, V. (2001). Cure-oriented versus care-oriented attitudes in medicine. *Patient Education and Counseling, 45*, 119–126.

Di Blasi, Z., Harkness, E. E., Georgiou, A., & Kleijnen, J. (2001). Influence of context effect on health outcomes: A systematic review. *Lancet, 357*, 762.

Dillard, J. P., & Hunter, J. E. (1989). On the use and interpretation of the Emotional Empathy Scale, the Self-Consciousness Scale, and the Self-Monitoring Scale. *Communication Research, 16*, 104–129.

DiLollo, V., & Berger, S. M. (1965). Effect of apparent pain in others on observers' reaction time. *Journal of Personality and Social Psychology, 2*, 573–575.

DiMascio, A., Boyd, R. W., & Greenblatt, M. (1957). Physiological correlates of tension and antagonism during psychotherapy: A study of "interpersonal physiology." *Psychosomatic Medicine, 19*, 99–104.

DiMatteo, M. R. (1979). A social-psychological analysis of physician-patient rapport toward a science of the art of medicine. *Journal of Social Issues, 35*, 12–33.

DiMatteo, M. R., Hays, R. D., & Prince, L. M. (1986). Relationship of physicians' nonverbal communication skills to patient satisfaction, appointment noncompliance, and physician workload. *Health Psychology, 5*, 581–594.

DiMatteo, M. R., Prince, I. M., & Taranta, A. (1979). Patients' perceptions of physicians' behavior: Determinants of patient commitment to the therapeutic relationship. *Journal of Community Health, 4*, 280–290.

DiMatteo, M. R., Sherbourne, C. D., Hays, R. D., Ordway, L., Kravitz, R. L., McGlynn, E. A., Kaplan, S., & Rogers, W. H. (1993). Physicians' characteristics influence patients' adherence to medical treatment: Results from the Medical Outcomes Study. *Health Psychology, 12*, 93–102.

DiMatteo, M. R., Taranta, A., Friedman, H. S., & Prince, L. M. (1980). Predicting patient satisfaction from physicians' nonverbal communication skills. *Medical Care, 17*, 376–387.

Diseker, R. A., & Michielutte, R. (1981). An analysis of empathy in medical students before and following clinical experience. *Journal of Medical Education, 56*, 1004–1010.

Divinagarcia, R. M., Harkin, T. J., Bonk, S., & Schluger, N. W. (1998). Screening by specialists to reduce unnecessary test ordering in patients evaluated for tuberclosis. *Chest, 114*, 664–666.

Downie, R. S. (1991). Literature and medicine. *Journal of Medical Ethics, 17*, 93–96.
Dubnicki, C. (1977). Relationship among therapist empathy and authoritarianism. *Journal of Counseling and Clinical Psychology, 45*, 958–959.
Duff, P. (2002). Professionalism in medicine: An A-Z primer. *Obstetrics and Gynecology, 99*, 1127–1128.
Dunstone, D. C., & Reames, H. R. J. (2001). Physician satisfaction revisited. *Social Science & Medicine, 52*, 825–837.
Durkheim, E. (1951). *Suicide: A study in sociology, (J. A. Spauling & G. Simpson, Trans.)*. Glencoe, IL: Free Press.
Dymond, R. F. (1949). A scale for the measurement of empathic ability. *Journal of Consulting Psychology, 13*, 127–133.
Dymond, R. F. (1950). Personality and empathy. *Journal of Counseling Psychology, 14*, 343–350.
Eagly, A. H. (1995). The science and politics of comparing women and men. *American Psychologist, 50*, 145–158.
Eagly, A. H., & Crowley, M. (1986). Gender and helping behavior: A meta-analytic review of the social psychological literature. *Psychological Bulletin, 100*, 283–308.
Eagly, A. H., & Steffen, V. J. (1986). Gender and aggressive behavior: A meta-analytic review of the social psychological literature. *Psychological Bulletin, 100*, 309–330.
Edwards, A. L. (1957). *The social desirability variable in personality assessment and research*. New York: Dryden.
Edwards, M. T., & Zimet, C. N. (1976). Problems and concerns among medical students. *Journal of Medical Education, 51*, 619–625.
Egan, G. (1975). *The skilled helper*. Monterey, CA: Brooks/Cole.
Egolf, B., Lasker, J., Wolf, S., & Potvin, L. (1992). Featuring health risks and mortality: The Rosato effect, a 50–year comparison of mortality rates. *American Journal of Public Health, 82*, 1089–1092.
Ehrlich, C. H., & Jaffe, C. (2002). Social support for dying. In J. D., Morgan (Ed.), *Social support: A reflection of humanity* (pp. 17–31). Amityville, NY: Baywood Publishing.
Eibel-Eibesfeldt, I. (1979). *The biology of peace and war*. New York: Viking.
Eisenberg-Berg, N., & Lennon, R. (1980). Altruism and the assessment of empathy in the preschool years. *Child Development, 51*, 552–557.
Eisenberg-Berg, N., & Mussen, P. (1978). Empathy and moral development in adolescence. *Developmental Psychology, 14*, 185–186.
Eisenberg, N. (1989). *Empathy and related emotional responses* (Vol. 44). San Francisco: Jossey-Bass.
Eisenberg, N. (1983). The relation between empathy and altruism: Conceptual and methodological issues. *Academic Psychology Bulletin, 5*, 195–208.
Eisenberg, N., & Lennon, R. (1983). Sex differences in empathy and related capacities. *Psychological Bulletin, 94*, 100–131.
Eisenberg, N., & Miller, P. A. (1987). The relation of empathy to prosocial and related behaviors. *Psychological Bulletin, 101*, 91–119.
Eisenberg, N., & Strayer, J. (1987a). Critical issues in the study of empathy. In N.Eisenberg & J. Strayer (Eds.), *Empathy and its development* (pp. 3–13). Cambridge, UK: Cambridge University Press.
Eisenberg, N., & Strayer, J. (1987b). *Empathy and its development*. Cambridge, UK: Cambridge University Press.
Eisenthal, S. E., Emery, R., Lazare, A., & Udin, H. (1979). Adherence and negotiated approach in patienthood. *Archives of General Psychiatry, 36*, 393–398.
Ekman, P. (1992). An argument for basic emotions. *Cognition and Emotion, 6*, 169–200.
Ekman, P., & Friesen, W. V. (1974). Detecting deception from the body or face. *Journal of Personality and Social Psychology, 29*, 288–298.
Elizur, A., & Rosenheim, E. (1982). Empathy and attitudes among medical students: The effects of group experience. *Journal of Medical Education, 57*, 675–683.
Engel, G. L. (1977). The need for a new medical model: A challenge for biomedicine. *Science, 196*, 129–136.
Engel, G. L. (1990). The essence of the biopsychosocial model: From 17th to 20th century science. In H. Balner (Ed.), *A challenge for biomedicine?* (pp. 13–18). Amsterdam and Rockland, MA: Swets & Zeitlinger, Inc.

Engler, C. M., Saltzman, G. A., Walker, M. L., & Wolf, F. M. (1981). Medical student acquisition and retention of communication and interviewing skills. *Journal of Medical Education, 56*, 572–579.
Entman, S. S., Glass, C. A., Hickson, G. B., Githens, P. B., Whetten-Goldstein, K., & Sloan, F. A. (1994). The relationship between malpractice claims history and subsequent obstetric care. *Journal of the American Medical Association, 272*, 1588–1591.
Erera, P. I. (1997). Empathy training for helping professionals: Model and evaluation. *Journal of Social Work Education, 33*, 245–260.
Eron, L. D. (1958). The effect of medical education on attitudes: A follow-up study. *Journal of Medical Education, 33*, 25–33.
Eslinger, P. J. (1998). Neurological and neuropsychological bases of empathy. *European Neurology, 93*, 193–199.
Eslinger, P. J., Satish, U., & Grattan, L. M. (1996). Alterations in cognitive- and affective-based empathy after cerebral damage. *Journal of International Neuropsychological Society, 2*, 15–16.
Evans, B. J., Stanley, R. O., & Burrows, G. D. (1993). Measuring medical students' empathy skills. *British Journal of Medical Psychology, 66*, 121–133.
Fahrbach, S. E., Morrell, I. I., & Pfaff, D. W. (1985). Role of oxytocin in the onset of estrogen-facilitated maternal behavior. In J. A. Amico & A. G. Robinson (Eds.), *Oxytocin: Clinical and laboratory studies* (pp. 372–388). Amsterdam: Elsevier.
Falvo, D., & Tippy, P. (1988). Communicating information to patients. Patient satisfaction and adherence as associated with resident skill. *Journal of Family Medicine*, 643–647.
Farber, N. J., Novack, D. H., & O'Brien, M. K. (1997). Love, boundaries, and the patient-physician relationship. *Archives of Internal Medicine, 157*, 2291–2294.
Feighny, K. M., Arnold, L., Monaco, M., Munro, S., & Earl, B. (1998). In pursuit of empathy and its relation to physician communication skills: Multidimensional empathy training for medical students. *Annals of Behavioral Science and Medical Education, 5*, 13–21.
Feldman, C., & Kornfield, J. (1991). *Stories of the spirit, stories of the heart.* New York: Harper Collins.
Fenichel, O. (1945). *The psychoanalytic theory of neurosis.* New York: W. W. Norton.
Feshbach, N. D. (1982). Sex differences in empathy and social behavior in children. In N. Eisenberg (Ed.), *The development of prosocial behavior* (pp. 315–338). New York: Academic Press.
Feshbach, N. D. (1989). Empathy training and prosocial behavior. In J. Groebel & R. A. Hinde (Eds.), *Aggression and war: Their biological and social bases* (pp. 101–111). Cambridge, UK: Cambridge University Press.
Feshbach, N. D., & Roe, K. (1968). Empathy in six and seven year olds. *Child Development, 39*, 133–145.
Festinger, L. (1964). *Conflict, decision, and dissonance.* Stanford, CA: Stanford University Press.
Feudtner, C., Christakis, D. A., & Christakis, N. A. (1994). Do clinical clerks suffer ethical erosion? Students' perception of their ethical environment and personal development. *Academic Medicine, 69*, 670–679.
Ficklin, F. L., Browne, V. L., Powell, R. C., & Carter, J. E. (1988). Faculty and house staff members as role models. *Journal of Medical Education, 63*, 392–396.
Fifer, W. P., & Moon, C. M. (1994). The role of mother's voice in the organization of brain function in the newborn. *Acta Pædiatrica Scandinavica, 397*, 86–93.
Fine, V. K., & Therrien, M. E. (1977). Empathy in the doctor-patient relationship: Skill training for medical students. *Journal of Medical Education, 52*, 752–757.
Fishbein, M., & Ajzen, I. (1975). *Belief, attitude, intention, and behavior: An introduction to theory and research.* Reading, MA: Addison-Wesley.
Fishbein, R. H. (1999). Scholarship, humanism, and the young physician. *Academic Medicine, 74*, 646–651.
Flagler, E. (1997). Narrative ethics: A means to enrich medical education. *Annals of the Royal College of Physicians & Surgeons of Canada, 30*, 217–220.
Flores, G. (2002). Mad scientists, compassionate healers, and greedy egotists: The portrayal of physicians in the movies. *Journal of the American Medical Association, 94*, 635–658.
Flores, G., Gee, D., & Kastner, B. (2000). The teaching of cultural issues in US and Canadian medical schools. *Academic Medicine, 75*, 451–455.
Fonagy, P. (2001). *Attachment theory and psychoanalysis.* New York: Other Press.

Fonagy, P., & Target, M. (1996). Playing with reality: I. Theory of mind and the normal development of psychic reality. *International Journal of Psychoanalysis, 77*, 217–233.
Forsythe, M., Calnan, M., & Wall, B. (1999). Doctors as patients: Postal survey examining consultants and general practitioners adherence to guidelines. *British Medical Journal, 319*, 605–608.
Fox, C. M., Harper, A. P., Hyner, G. C., & Lyle, R. M. (1994). Loneliness, emotional expression, marital quality and major life events in women who developed breast cancer. *Journal of Community Health, 19*, 467–482.
Frances, A., First, M. B., & Pincus, H. A. (1995). *DSM-IV guidebook.* Washington, DC: American Psychiatric Association.
Francis, V., & Morris, M. (1969). Gaps in doctor-patient communication: Patients' response to medical advice. *The New England Journal of Medicine, 280*, 535–540.
Frank, E., & Harvey, L. K. (1996). Preventive advice rates of women and men physicians. *Archives of Family Medicine, 5*, 215–219.
Fratiglioni, L., Wang, H. X., Ericsson, K., Maytan, M., & Winblad, B. (2000). Influence of social network on occurrence of dementia: A community-based longitudinal study. *Lancet, 355*, 1315–1319.
Free, N. K., Green, B. L., Grace, M. C., Chernus, L. A., & Whitman, R. M. (1985). Empathy and outcome in brief focal dynamic therapy. *American Journal of Psychiatry, 142*, 917–921.
Freemon, B., Negrete, V. F., Davis, M., & Korsch, B. M. (1971). Gaps in doctor-patient communication: Doctor-patient interaction analysis. *Pediatric Research, 5*, 298–311.
Frenk, J. (1998). Medical care and health improvement: The critical link. *Annals of Internal Medicine, 129*, 419–420.
Fretz, B. R. (1966). Postural movement in a counseling dyad. *Journal of Counseling Psychology, 13*, 343.
Freud, S. (1955). Group psychology and the analysis of the ego. In J. Strachey (Ed. & Trans.), *The standard edition of the complete psychological works of Sigmund Freud* (Vol. 18). London: Hogarth Press and the Institute of Psychoanalysis. (Original work published in 1921.)
Freud, S. (1958a). Recommendation to physicians practicing psychoanalysis. In J. Strachey (Ed. & Trans.), *The standard edition of the complete psychological works of Sigmund Freud* (Vol. 12, pp. 109–120). London: Hogarth Press and the Institute of Psychoanalysis. (Original work published in 1912.)
Freud, S. (1958b). *On beginning the treatment.* In J. Starchey (Ed. & Trans.). *The standard edition of the complete psychological works of Sigmund Freud.* (Vol. 12, pp. 121–144). London: Hogarth Press and the Institute of Psychoanalysis. *(Original work published in 1913.)*
Freud, S. (1960). Jokes and their relation to the unconscious. In J. Strachey (Ed. & Trans.). *The standard edition of the complete psychological works of Sigmund Freud* (Entire Vol. 8). London: Hogarth Press and the Institute of Psychoanalysis. (Original work published in 1905.)
Freud, S. (1964). An outline of psychoanalysis. In J. Strachey, J. (Ed. & Trans.), *The standard edition of the complete psychological works of Sigmund Freud* (Vol. 23, pp. 139–301), London: Hogarth Press and the Institute of Psychoanalysis. (Original work published in 1938.)
Friedman, E. (1990). The perlis of detachment. *Health Care Forum Journal, 33*, 9–10.
Friedman, H. S., Prince, L. M., Riggio, R. E., & DiMatteo, M. R. (1980). Understanding and assessing nonverbal expressiveness: The affective communication test. *Journal of Personality and Social Psychology, 39*, 333–351.
Frodi, A., & Macauley, J. (1977). Are women always less aggressive than men? A review of the experimental literature. *Psychological Bulletin, 84*, 634–660.
Fruen, M., Rothman, A., & Steiner, J. (1974). Comparisons of characteristics of male and female medical school applicants. *Journal of Medical Education, 49*, 137–145.
Fussel, F. W. & Bonney, W. C. (1990). A comparative study of childhood experience of psychotherapists and physicists: Implications for clinical practice. *Psychotherapy, 27*, 505–512.
Gabbard, G. O. (1994). On love and lust in erotic transference. *Journal of the American Psychoanalytic Association, 42*, 385–403.
Gabbard, G. O., & Nadelson, C. (1995). Professional boundaries in the physician-patient relationship. *Journal of the American Medical Association, 273*, 1445–1449.

Galanter, M., Talbott, D., Gallegos, K., & Rubenstone, E. (1990). Combined alcoholics anonymous and professional care for addicted physicians. *American Journal of Psychiatry, 147*, 64–68.
Gallese, V. (2001). The 'shared manifold' hypothesis: From mirror neurons to empathy. *Journal of Conscious Studies, 8*, 33–50.
Gallese, V. (2003). The roots of empathy: The shared manifold hypothesis and the neural basis of intersubjectivity. *Psychopathology, 36*, 171–180.
Gallese, V., Fadiga, L., Fogassi, L., & Rizzolatti, G. (1996). Action cognition in the premotor cortex. *Brain, 119*, 593–609.
Gallese, V., Keysers, C., & Rizzolatti, G. (2004). A unifying view of the basis of social cognition. *Trends in Cognitive Sciences, 8*, 394–403.
Gartrell, N., Herman, J., Olarte, S., Feldstein, M., & Localio, R. (1986). Psychiatrist-patient sexual contact: Results of a national survey. I: Prevalence. *American Journal of Psychiatry, 143*, 1126–1131.
Gaufberg, E. H., Joseph, R. C., Pels, R. J., Wyshak, G., Wieman, D., & Nadelson, C. C. (2001). Psychosocial training in U.S. internal medicine and family practice residency programs. *Academic Medicine, 76*, 738–742.
Geisinger, K. F. (1994). Cross-cultural normative asssessment: Translation and adaptation issues influencing the normative interpretation of assessment instruments. *Psychological Assessment, 6*, 304–312.
Geller, G., Tambor, E. S., Chase, G. A., & Holtzman, N. A. (1993). Measuring physicians' tolerance for ambiguity and its relationship to their reported practices regarding genetic testing. *Medical Care, 31*, 989–1001.
Gendreau, P., Burke, D. M., & Grant, B. A. (1980). A second evaluation of the Rideau inmate volunteer program. *Canadian Journal of Criminology, 22*, 66–77.
Gianakos, D. (1996). Empathy revisited. *Archives of Internal Medicine, 156*, 135–136.
Gibson, E. J., & Walk, R. D. (1960). The visual cliff. *Scientific American, 202*, 64–71.
Gillberg, C. (1992). The Emanuel Miller memorial lecture 1991: Autism and autistic-like conditions: Subclasses among disorders of empathy. *Journal of Child Psychology and Psychiatry, 33*, 813–842.
Gillberg, C. (1996). The long-term outcome of childhood empathy disorders. *European Child, and Adolescent Psychiatry, 5* (Suppl.), 52–56.
Gilligan, C. (1982). *In a different voice: Psychological theory and women's development.* Cambridge, MA: Harvard University Press.
Girgis, A., & Sanson-Fisher, R. W. (1995). Breaking bad news: Consensus guidelines for medical practitioners. *Journal of Clinical Oncology, 13*, 2449–2456.
Gladding, S. T. (1978). Empathy, gender, and training as factors in the identification of normal infant cry-signals. *Perceptual & Motor Skills, 47*, 267–270.
Gladstein, G. A. (1977). Empathy and counseling outcome: An empirical and conceptual review. *The Counseling Psychologist, 6*, 70–79.
Gladstein, G. & Feldstein, J. (1983). Using film to increase counselor empathic experiences. *Counselor Education and Supervision, 23*, 125–131.
Gladstein, G. A., and associates (1987). *Empathy and counseling: Explorations in theory and research.* New York: Springer-Verlag.
Glaser, K., Hojat, M., Veloski, J. J., Blacklow, R. S., & Goepp, C. E. (2004). Science, verbal, or quantitative skills: Which is the most important predictor of physician competence? *Educational and Psychological Measurement, 52*, 395–406.
Glaser, K., Markham, F. W., Adler, H. M., McManus, P. R., & Hojat, M. (2005). Patients' perceptions of their physicians' empathy and physicians' scores on the Jefferson Scale of Physician Empathy. Manuscript submitted for publication.
Glynn, L. M., Christenfeld, N., & Gerin, W. (1999). Gender, social support, and cardiovascular response to stress. *Psychosomatic Medicine, 61*, 234–242.
Goldberg, P. E. (2000). The physician-patient relationship: Three psychodynamic concepts that can be applied to primary care. *Archives of Family Medicine, 9*, 1164–1168.
Golden, L. (1992). *Aristotle on tragic and comic mimesis.* Atlanta, GA: Scholars Press.
Golden, T. (2002). Acknowledging the masculine and feminine in offering support. In J. D. Morgan (Ed.), *Social support: A reflection of humanity* (pp. 73–84). Amityville, NY: Baywood Publishing.

Goldstein, A. P., & Michaels, G. Y. (1985). *Empathy: Development, training, and consequences.* Hillsdale, NJ: Erlbaum.
Goleman, D. (1995). *Emotional intelligence: Why it can matter more than I.Q.* New York: Bantam Books.
Gonnella, J. S., & Hojat, M. (2001). Biotechnology and ethics in medical education of the new millennium: Physician roles and responsibilities. *Medical Teacher, 23,* 371–377.
Gonnella, J. S., Hojat, M., Erdmann, J. B., & Veloski, J. J. (1993a). What have we learned, and where do we go from here? *Academic Medicine,* (Suppl.) *68,* S79–S87.
Gonnella, J. S., Hojat, M., Erdmann, J. B., & Veloski, J. J. (1993b). What have we learned, and where do we go from here? In J. S. Gonnella, M. Hojat, J. B. Erdmann, & J. J. Veloski (Eds.), *Assessment measures in medical school, residency, and practice: The connections* (pp. 155–173). New York: Springer.
Good, R. S. (1972). After office hours: The third ear. *Obstetrics & Gynecology, 40,* 760–762.
Goodchild, C. E., Skinner, T. C., & Parkin, T. (2005). The value of empathy in dietetic consultation: A pilot study to investigate its effect on satisfaction, autonomy and agreement. *Journal of Human Nutrition and Diet, 18,* 181–185.
Goodwin, J. S., Hunt, W. C., Key, C. R., & Samet, J. M. (1987). The effect of marital status on stage, treatment, and survival of cancer patients. *Journal of the American Medical Association, 258,* 3125–3130.
Gorsuch, R. L. (1974). *Factor analysis.* Philadelphia: W. B.Saunders.
Goubert, L., Craig, K. D., Vervoort, T., Morley, S., Sullivan, M. J. L., Williams, A. C. C., Cano, A., & Crombez, G. (2005). Facing others in pain: The effects of empathy. *Pain, 118,* 285–288.
Gough, H. G., & Hall, W. B. (1977). A comparison of physicians who did or did not respond to a postal questionnaire. *Journal of Applied Psychology, 62,* 777–780.
Gould, S. J. (1981). The *mismeasurement of man.* New York: W. W. Norton.
Grant, J. P. (1991). *The state of the world's children.* Oxford, UK: Oxford University Press.
Grattan, L. M., & Eslinger, P. J. (1989). Higher cognitive and social behavior: Changes in cognitive flexibility and empathy after lesions. *Nueropsychology, 3,* 185.
Greenberg, L. S., Watson, J. C., Elliot, R., & Bohart, A. C. (2001). Empathy. *Psychotherapy, 38,* 380–384.
Greenson, R. R. (1960). Empathy and its vicissitudes. *International Journal of Psychoanalysis, 41,* 418–424.
Greenson, R. (1967). *The techniques and practice of psychoanalysis.* New York: International University Press.
Greif, E. B., & Hogan, R. (1973). The theory and measurement of empathy. *Journal of Counseling Psychology, 20,* 280–284.
Gross, E. B. (1992). Gender difference in physician stress. *Journal of the American Medical Women's Association, 29,* 57–68.
Gruen, R. J., & Mendelsohn, G. (1986). Emotional responses to affective displays in others: The distinction between empathy and sympathy. *Journal of Personality and Social Psychology, 51,* 609–614.
Gruin, P., Peng, T., Lopez, G., & Nagda, B. A. (1999). Context, identity, and intergroup relations. In D. A. Prentice & D. T. Miller (Eds.), *Cultural divides: Understanding and overcoming group conflict* (pp. 133–172). New York: Russell Sage Foundation.
Guillemin, F., Bombardier, C., & Beaton, D. (1993). Cross-cultural adaptation of health-related quality of life measures: Literature review and proposed guidelines. *Journal of Clinical Epidemiology, 46,* 1417–1432.
Gulanick, N., & Schmeck, R. (1977). Modeling praise and criticism in teaching empathic responding. *Counselor Education and Supervision, 16,* 284–290.
Gustafson, J. P. (1986). *The complex secret of brief psychotherapy.* New York: W. W. Norton.
Guttman, H., & Laporte, L. (2002). Alexithymia, empathy, and psychological symptoms in family context. *Comprehensive Psychiatry, 43,* 448–455.
Guzzetta, R. A. (1976). Acquisition and transfer of empathy by the parents of early adolescents through structured learning training. *Journal of Community Psychology, 23,* 449–453.
Hall, E. T. (1966). *The hidden dimension.* Garden City, NJ: Doubleday.
Hall, J. A. (1978). Gender effects in decoding nonverbal cues. *Psychological Bulletin, 85,* 845–857.
Hall, J. A. (1985). *Nonverbal sex differences.* Baltimore: Johns Hopkins University Press.

Hall, J. A., & Dornan, M. C. (1988). Meta-analysis of satisfaction with medical care: Description of research domain and analysis of overall satisfaction level. *Social Science & Medicine, 27*, 637–644.

Hall, J. A., Irish, J. T., Roter, D. L., Ehrlic, C. M., & Miller, L. H. (1994). Gender in medical encounters: An analysis of physician and patient communication in a primary care setting. *Health Psychology, 13*, 384–392.

Hall, J. A., Roter, D. L., & Katz, N. R. (1988). Meta-analysis of correlates of provider behavior in medical encounters. *Medical Care, 26*, 657–675.

Halpern, J. (2001). *From detached concern to empathy: Humanizing medical practice.* New York: Oxford University Press.

Hamilton, N. G. (1984). Empathic understanding. In J. Lichtenberg, M. Bornstein, & D. Silver (Eds.), *Empathy II* (pp. 217–222). Hillsdale, NJ: The Analytic Press.

Hamilton, W. D. (1964). The genetic evolution of social behavior. *Journal of Theoretical Biology, 7*, 1–52.

Haney, C., Banks, C., & Zimbardo, P. (1973). Interpersonal dynamics in a simulated prison. *International Journal of Criminology and Penology, 1*, 69–97.

Hari, R., Forss, N., Avikainen, S., Kirveskari, E., Salenius, S., & Rizzolatti, G. (1998). Activation of human primary motor cortex during action observation: A neuromagnetic study. *Proceedings of the National Academy of Science, 95*, 15061–15065.

Harrigan, J. A., & Rosenthal, R. (1983). Physicians' head and body position as determinants of perceived rapport. *Journal of Applied Social Psychology, 13*, 496–509.

Harsch, H. H. (1989). The role of empathy in medical students' choice of specialty. *Academic Psychiatry, 13*, 96–98.

Hartup, W. W., & Stevens, N. (1999). Friendships and adaptation across the life span. *American Psychological Society, 8*, 76–79.

Hass, J. S., Cook, E. F., Puopolo, A. L., Burnstin, H. R., Clearly, P. D., & Brennan, T. A. (2000). Is professional satisfaction of general internists associated with patient satisfaction? *Journal of General Internal Medicine, 15*, 122–128.

Hasse, R. F., & Tepper, D. T., Jr. (1972). Nonverbal components of empathic communication. *Journal of Counseling Psychology, 19*, 417–424.

Hatcher, S. L., Nadeau, M. S., Walsh, L. K., Reynolds, M., Gala, J., & Marz, K. (1994). The teaching of empathy for high school and college students: Testing Rogerian methods with the Interpersonal Reactivity Index. *Adolescence, 29*, 961–974.

Hebb, D. (1946). *The organization of behaviour.* New York: John Wiley & Sons.

Heilman, K. M., Scholes, R., & Watson, R.T. (1975). Auditory affective agnosia: Disturbed comprehension of affective speech. *Journal of Neurology, Neurosurgery and Psychiatry, 38*, 69–72.

Hekmat, H., Khajavi, F., & Mehryar, A. H. (1974). Psychoticism, neuroticism, and extraversion: The personality determinants of empathy. *Journal of Clinical Psychology, 30*, 559–561.

Hekmat, H., Khajavi, F., & Mehryar, A. H. (1975). Some personality correlates of empathy. *Journal of Counseling and Clinical Psychology, 43*, 89.

Henderson, J. T., & Weisman, C. S. (2001). Physician gender effects on preventive screening and counseling: An analysis of male and female patients' health care experiences. *Medical Care, 39*, 1281–1292.

Henderson, S. (1974). Care-eliciting behavior in man. *The Journal of Nervous and Mental Disease, 159*, 172–181.

Hennen, B. K. (1975). Continuity of care in family practice. *The Journal of Family Practice, 2*, 371–372.

Henry-Tillman, R., Deloney, L. A., Savidge, M., Graham, C. J., & Klimberg, S. (2002). The medical student as patient navigator as an approach to teaching empathy. *The American Journal of Surgery, 183*, 659–662.

Herman, J. (2000). Reading for empathy. *Medical Hypotheses, 54*, 167–168.

Hess, U., Blairy, S., & Phillippot, P. (1999). Facial mimicry. In P. Phillippot, R. Feldman, & E. Coats (Eds.), *The social context of nonverbal behavior* (pp. 213–241). Cambridge, UK: Cambridge University Press.

Hickson, G. B., Clayton, E. W., Entman, S. S., Miller, C. S., Githens, P. B., Whetten-Goldstein, K., & Sloan, F. A. (1994). Obstetricians' prior malpractice experience and patients' satisfaction with care. *Journal of the American Medical Association, 272*, 1583–1587.

Hickson, G. B., Clayton, E. W., Githens, P. B., & Sloan, F. A. (1992). Factors that prompted families to file medical malpractice claims following perinatal injuries. *Journal of the American Medical Association, 267,* 1359–1363.

Hinshelwood, R. (1989). *A dictionary of Kleinian thought.* London: Free Association Press.

Hirshberg, C., & Barasch, M. I. (1995). *Remarkable recovery.* New York: Riverside Books.

Hislop, T. G., Waxler, N. E., Coldman, A. J., Elwood, J. M., & Kan, L. (1987). The prognostic significance of psychosocial factors in women with breast cancer. *Journal of Chronic Diseases, 40,* 729–735.

Hittelman, J. H., & Dickes, R. (1979). Sex differences in neonatal eye contact time. *Merrill-Pamler Querterly, 25,* 171–184.

Hodges, S. D., & Wegner, D. M. (1997). Automatic and controlled empathy. In W. Ickes (Ed.), *Empathic accuracy* (pp. 311–339). New York: Guilford.

Hoffman, M. L. (1977). Sex differences in empathy and related behaviors. *Psychological Bulletin, 84,* 712–722.

Hoffman, M. L. (1978). Psychological and biological perspectives on altruism. *International Journal of Behavioral Development, 1,* 323–339.

Hoffman, M. L. (1981). The development of empathy. In J. Rushton & R. Sorrentino (Eds.), *Altruism and helping behavior: Social personality and developmental perspectives* (pp. 41–63). Hillsdale, NJ: Erlbaum.

Hoffman, M. L. (1982). The measurement of empathy. In C. E. Izard (Ed.), *Measuring emotions in infants and children* (pp. 279–296). Cambridge, UK: Cambridge University Press.

Hogan, R. (1969). Development of an empathy scale. *Journal of Consulting and Clinical Psychology, 33,* 307–316.

Hogan, R. (1976). Moral conduct and moral character: A psychological perspective. *Psychological Bulletin, 79,* 217–232.

Hogan, R., & Dickstein, E. (1972). A measure of moral value. *Journal of Consulting and Clinical Psychology, 39,* 210–214.

Hogan, R., & Mankin, D. (1970). Determinants of interpersonal attraction: A clarification. *Psychological Reports, 26,* 235–238.

Hogan, R., & Weiss, D. S. (1974). Personality correlates of superior academic achievement. *Journal of Consulting Psychology, 21,* 144–151.

Hojat, M. (1982a). Loneliness as a function of selected personality variables. *Journal of Clinical Psychology, 38,* 137–141.

Hojat, M. (1982b). Psychometric characteristics of the UCLA Loneliness Scale. *Educational and Psychological Measurement, 42,* 917–925.

Hojat, M. (1983). Comparison of transitory and chronic loners on selected personality variables. *British Journal of Psychology, 74,* 199–202.

Hojat, M. (1992). Social and economic factors in patients with coronary disease. *Journal of the American Medical Association, 268,* 195–196.

Hojat, M. (1993). The world's declaration of the rights of the child: Anticipated challenges. *Psychological Reports, 72,* 1011–1022.

Hojat, M. (1995). Developmental pathways to violence: A psychodynamic paradigm. *Peace Psychology Review, 1,* 177–196.

Hojat, M. (1996). Perception of maternal availability in childhood and selected psychosocial characteristics in adulthood. *Genetic, Social, and General Psychology Monographs, 122* , 425–450.

Hojat, M. (1997). The U.N. Convention: Lost in the clash of adverse opinions. *American Psychologist, 52,* 1384–1385.

Hojat, M. (1998). Satisfaction with early relationships with parents and psychosocial attributes in adulthood: Which parent contributes more? *Journal of General Psychology, 159,* 203–220.

Hojat, M., Borenstein, B. D., & Shapurian, R. (1990). Perception of childhood dissatisfaction with parents and selected personality traits in adulthood. *The Journal of Genetic Psychology, 117,* 241–253.

Hojat, M., & Crandall, R. (Eds.) Hojat, M. & Crandall, R. (1989). *Loneliness: Theory, research, and applications.* Newbury, CA: Sage.

Hojat, M., Erdmann, J. B., Veloski, J. J., Nasca, T. J., Callahan, C., Julian, E., & Peck, J. (2000a). A validity study of the writing sample section of the Medical College Admission Test. *Academic Medicine, 75,* S25–S27.

Hojat, M., Fields, S. K., Rattner, S. L., Griffiths, M., Cohen, M. J. M., & Plumb, J. (1997). Attitudes toward the physician-nurse alliance: Comparisons of medical and nursing students. *Academic Medicine, 72*, 1–3.

Hojat, M., Glaser, K., Xu, G., Veloski, J. J., & Christian, E. B. (1999). Gender comparisons of medical students' psychosocial profile. *Medical Education, 33*, 342–349.

Hojat, M., Glaser, K. M., & Veloski, J. J. (1996). Associations between selected psychosocial attributes and ratings of physician competence. *Academic Medicine, 71*, S103–S105.

Hojat, M., Gonnella, J. S., Erdmann, J. B., Rattner, S. L., Veloski, J. J., Glaser, K., & Xu, G. (2000b). Gender comparisons of income expectations in the USA at the beginning of medical school during the past twenty-eight years. *Social Science & Medicine, 50*, 1665–1672.

Hojat, M., Gonnella, J. S., Erdmann, J. B., Veloski, J. J., Louis, D. Z., Nasca, T. J., & Rattner, S. L. (2000c). Physicians' perceptions of the changing health care system: Comparisons by gender and specialties. *Journal of Community Health, 25*, 455–471.

Hojat, M., Gonnella, J. S., Erdmann, J. B., & Vogel, W. H. (2003). Medical students' cognitive appraisal of stressful life events as related to personality, physical well-being, and academic performance: A longitudinal study. *Personality and Individual Differences, 35*, 219–235.

Hojat, M., Gonnella, J. S., Mangione, S., Nasca, T. J., & Magee, M. (2003a). Physician empathy in medical education and practice: Experience with the Jefferson Scale of Physician Empathy. *Seminars in Integrative Medicine, 1*, 25–41.

Hojat, M., Gonnella, J. S., Mangione, S., Nasca, T. J., Veloski, J. J., Erdmann, J. B., Callahan, E. J., & Magee, M. (2002a). Empathy in medical students as related to academic performance, clinical competence, and gender. *Medical Education, 36*, 522–527.

Hojat, M., Gonnella, J. S., Nasca, T. J., Mangione, S., Veloski, J. J., & Magee, M. (2002b). The Jefferson Scale of Physician Empathy: Further psychometric data and differences by gender and specialty at item level. *Academic Medicine, 77*, S58–S80.

Hojat, M., Gonnella, J. S., Nasca, T. J., Mangione, S., Veloski, J. J., & Magee, M. (2002c). The Jefferson Scale of Physician Empathy: Further psychometric data and differences by gender and specialty at item level. *Academic Medicine, 77*, S58–S60.

Hojat, M., Gonnella, J. S., Nasca, T. J., Mangione, S., Vergare, M., & Magee, M. (2002d). Physician empathy: Definition, components, measurement, and relationship to gender and specialty. *American Journal of Psychiatry, 159*, 1563–1569.

Hojat, M., & Herman, M. W. (1985). Developing an instrument to measure attitudes toward nurses: Preliminary psychometric findings. *Psychological Reports, 56*, 571–579.

Hojat, M., Mangione, S., Gonnella, J. S., Nasca, T. J., Veloski, J. J., & Kane, G. (2001a). Empathy in medical education and patient care [Letter to the editor]; *Academic Medicine, 76*, 669–670.

Hojat, M., Mangione, S., Kane, G., & Gonnella, J. S. (2005a). Relationships between scores of the Jefferson Scale of Physician Empathy (JSPE) and the Interpersonal Reactivity Index (IRI). *Medical Teacher, 27*, 625–628.

Hojat, M., Mangione, S., Nasca, T. J., Cohen, M. J. M., Gonnella, J. S., Erdmann, J. B., Veloski, J. J., & Magee, M. (2001b). The Jefferson Scale of Physician Empathy: Development and preliminary psychometric data. *Educational and Psychological Measurement, 61*, 349–365.

Hojat, M., Mangione, S., Nasca, T. J., Rattner, S. L., Erdmann, J. B., Gonnella, J. S., & Magee, M. (2004). An empirical study of decline of empathy in medical school. *Medical Education, 38*, 934–941.

Hojat, M., Nasca, T. J., Magee, M., Feeney, K., Pascual, R., Urbano, F., & Gonnella, J. S. (1999a). A comparison of the personality profiles of internal medicine residents, physician role models, and the general population. *Academic Medicine, 74*, 54–60.

Hojat, M., Robeson, M., Damjanov, I., Veloski, J. J., Glaser, K., & Gonnella, J. S. (1993). Students' psychosocial characteristics as predictors of academic performance in medical school. *Academic Medicine, 68*, 635–637.

Hojat, M., Robeson, M., Veloski, J. J., Blacklow, R. S., Xu, G., & Gonnella, J. S. (1994). Gender comparisons prior to, during, and after medical school using two decades of longitudinal data at Jefferson Medical College. *Evaluation and the Health Professions, 17*, 290–306.

Hojat, M., Samuel, S., & Thompson, T. L. (1995). Searching for the lost key under the light of biomedicine: A triangular biopsychosocial paradigm may cast additional light on

medical education, research and patient care. In S. K. Majumdar, L. M. Rosenfeld, D. B. Nash, & A. M. Audet (Eds.), *Medicine & health care into the 21st century* (pp. 310–325). Easton, PA: Pennsylvania Academy of Science.
Hojat, M., & Shapurian, R. (1986). Anxiety and its measurement: A study of psychometric characteristics of a short form of the Taylor Manifest Anxiety Scale in Iranian students. *Journal of Social Behavior and Personality, 1*, 621–630.
Hojat, M., Shapurian, R., Foroughi, D., Nayerahmadi, H., Farzaneh, M., Shafieyan, M., & Parsi, M. (2000). Gender differences in traditional attitudes toward marriage and the family: An empirical study of Iranian immigrants in the United States. *Journal of Family Issues, 21*, 419–434.
Hojat, M., Shapurian, R., Nayerahmadi, H., Farzaneh, M., Foroughi, D., Parsi, M., & Azizi, M. (1999). Premarital sexual, childrearing, and family attitudes of Iranian men and women in the United States and in Iran. *Journal of Psychology, 133*, 19–31.
Hojat, M., Shapurian, R., & Mehryar, A. H. (1986). Psychometric properties of a Persian version of the short form of the Beck Depression Inventory. *Psychological Reports, 59*, 331–338.
Hojat, M., Veloski, J. J., Louis, D. Z., Xu, G., Ibarra, D., Gottlieb, J. E., & Erdmann, J. B. (1999b). Perceptions of medical seniors of the current changes in the United States health care system. *Evaluation and the Health Professions, 22*, 169–183.
Hojat, M., Veloski, J. J., & Zeleznik, C. (1985). Predictive validity of the MCAT for students with two sets of scores. *Journal of Medical Education, 60*, 911–918.
Hojat, M., & Vogel, W. H. (1989). Socioemotional bonding and neurobiochemistry. *Journal of Social Behavior and Personality, 2*, 135–144.
Hojat, M., Vogel, W. H., Zeleznik, C., & Borenstein, B. D. (1988). Effects of academic and psychosocial predictors of performance in medical school on coefficients of determination. *Psychological Reports, 63*, 383–394.
Hojat, M., & Xu, G. (2004). A visitor's guide to effect sizes: Statistical versus practical (clinical) importance of research findings. *Advances in Health Sciences Education, 9*, 241–249.
Hojat, M., Zuckerman, M., Gonnella, J. S., Mangione, S., Nasca, T. J., Vergare, M., & Magee, M. (2005b). Empathy in medical students as related to specialty interest, personality, and perceptions of mother and father. *Personality and Individual Differences, 39*, 1205–1215.
Holland, J. C. (2001). Improving the human side of cancer care: Psycho-oncology's contribution. *Cancer Journal, 7*, 458–471.
Holland, J. C., Geary, N., Marchini, A., & Tross, S. (1987). An international survey of physician attitudes and practice in regard to revealing the diagnosis of cancer. *Cancer Investigation, 5*, 151–154.
Holleman, W. L. (2000). The play's the thing: Using literature and drama to teach about death and dying. *Family Medicine, 32*, 523–524.
Hollowell, E. E., & De Ville, K. A. (2003). Physicians: Avoid treating family members. Available at: *http://www.nchealthlaw.com/mla10.html.*
Holmes, C. A. (1992). The wounded healer. *International Journal of Communicative Psychoanalysis & Psychotherapy, 6*, 33–36.
Hooper, E. M., Comstock, L. M., Goodwin, J. M., & Goodwin, J. S. (1982). Patient characteristics that influence physician behavior. *Medical Care, 20*, 630–638.
Hoover, R. N. (2000). Cancer: Nature, nurture, or both. *The New England Journal of Medicine, 343*, 135–136.
Hornblow, A. R., Kidson, M. A., & Ironside, W. (1988). Empathic processes: Perception by medical students of patients' anxiety and depression. *Medical Education, 22*, 15–18.
Hornblow, A. R., Kidson, M. A., & Jones, K. V. (1977). Measuring medical students' empathy: A validation study. *Medical Education, 11*, 7–12.
Hornstein, H. A. (1978). Promotive tension and prosocial behavior: A Lewinian analysis. In L. Wispe (Ed.), *Altruism, sympathy, and helping: Psychological and sociological principles* (pp. 177–207). New York: Academic Press.
House, J. S., Landis, K. R., & Umberson, D. (1988). Social relationships and health. *Science, 241*, 540–544.
House, J. S., Robbins, C., & Metzner, H. L. (1982). The association of social relationships and activities with mortality: Prospective evidence from the Tecumseh Community Health Study. *American Journal of Epidemiology, 116*, 123–140.
Houston, W. R. (1938). The doctor himself as a therapeutic agent. *Annals of Internal Medicine, 11*, 1416–1425.

Howell, E. A., Gardiner, B., & Concato, J. (2002). Do women prefer female obstetricians? *Obstetrics and Gynecology, 100*, 827–828.
Hróbjartsson, A., & Gøtzsche, P. C. (2001). Is the placebo powerless? An analysis of clinical trials comparing placebo with no treatment. *The New England Journal of Medicine, 344*, 1594–1632.
Hubel, D. H. (1967). Effect of distortion of sensory input on the visual system of kittens. *The Physiologist, 10*, 17–54.
Hubel, D. H., & Wiesel, T. N. (1963). Receptive fields of cell in striate cortex of young ,visually inexperienced kittens. *Journal of Neurophysiology, 26*, 994–1002.
Hubel, D. H., & Wiesel, T. N. (1970). The period of susceptibility to the physiological effects of unilateral eye closure in kittens. *Journal of Physiology, 206*, 419–436.
Hudson, G. R. (1993). Empathy and technology in the coronary care unit. *Intensive and Critical Care Nursing, 9*, 55–61.
Humphrey, N. (1983). *Consciousness regained.* Oxford: Oxford University Press.
Hunsdahl, J. B. (1967). Concerning Einfiühlung (empathy): A concept analysis of its origin and early development. *Journal of History of the Behavioral Sciences, 3*, 180–191.
Hunt, E., & Agnoli, F. (1991). The Whorfian hypothesis: A cognitive psychology perspective. *Psychological Review, 98*, 337–389.
Hurwitz, B. (2000). Narrative and the practice of medicine. *Lancet, 365*, 2086–2089.
Hyde, J. S. (2005). The gender similarities hypothesis. *American Psychologist, 60*, 581–592.
Hyde, J. S. (1984). How large are gender differences in aggression? *Developmental Psychology, 20*, 722–736.
Hyyppa, M. T., Kronholm, E., & Mattlar, C. (1991). Mental well-being of good sleepers in a random sample population. *British Journal of Medical Psychology, 64*, 25–34.
Iacoboni, M., Woods, R. P., Brass, M., Bekkering, H., Mazziotta, J. C., & Rizzolatti, G. (1999). Cortical mechanisms of human imitation. *Science, 286*, 2526–2528.
Ickes, W. (1997). *Empathic accuracy.* New York: Guilford Press.
Ingelfinger, F. J. (1980). Arrogance. *The New England Journal of Medicine, 303*, 1507–1511.
Insel, T. R. (2000). Toward a neurology of attachment. *Review of General Psychology, 4*, 176–185.
Isabella, R. A., & Belsky, J. (1991). Interaction synchrony and the origin of infant-mother attachment: A replication study. *Child Development, 62*, 373–384.
Ishikawa, H., Takayama, T., Yamazaki, Y., Skei, Y., & Katsumata, N. (2002). Physician-patient communication and patient satisfaction in Japanese cancer consultation. *Social Science & Medicine, 55*, 301–311.
Issac, M. D., & Michael, W. B. (1981). *Handbook of research and evaluation.* San Diego, CA: Edits.
Ivey, A. (1971). *Microcounseling: Innovations in interviewing training.* Springfield, Ill: Charles C Thomas.
Ivey, A. E. (1974). Microcounseling and media therapy: State of the art. *Counselor Education and Supervision, 4*, 173–183.
Jack, D. C. (1993). *Silencing the self: Women and depression.* Cambridge, MA: Harvard University Press.
Jackson, P. L., Meltzoff, A. N., & Decety, J. (2005). How do we perceive the pain of others? A window into the neural process involved in empathy. *Neuroimage, 24*, 771–779.
Jackson, S. W. (1992). The listening healer in the history of psychological healing. *American Journal of Psychiatry, 149*, 1623–1632.
Jackson, S. W. (2001). The wounded healer. *Bulletin of the History of Medicine, 75*, 1–36.
Jaffe, D. S. (1986). Empathy, counteridentification, counter transference: A review with some personal perspectives on the "analytic instrument." *Psychoanalytic Quarterly, 15*, 215–243.
Jamison, R., & Johnson, J. E. (1975). Empathy and therapeutic orientation in paid and volunteer crisis phone workers, professional therapists, and undergraduate college students. *Journal of Community Psychology, 3*, 269–274.
Janssens, J. M. A. M., & Gerris, J. R. M. (1992). Child rearing, empathy and prosocial development. In J. M. A. M. Janssens & J. R. M. Gerris (Eds.), *Child rearing: Influence on prosocial development* (pp. 57–75). Amsterdam: Swets & Zeitlinger.
Jarski, R. W., Gjerde, C. L., Bratton, B. D., Brown, D. D., & Matthes, S. S. (1985). A comparison of four empathy instruments in simulated patient-medical student interactions. *Journal of Medical Education, 60*, 545–551.

Jensen, N. (1994). The empathic physician. *Archives of Internal Medicine, 154,* 108.
Johnson, J. A., Cheek, J. M., & Smither, R. (1983). The structure of empathy. *Journal of Personality and Social Psychology, 45,* 1299–1312.
Johnston, M. A. C. (1992). A model program to address insensitive behaviors toward medical students. *Academic Medicine, 67,* 236–237.
Jones, A. H. (1987). Reflections, projections, and the future of literature-and-medicine. In D. Wear, M. Kohn, & S. Stocker (Eds.), *Literature and medicine: A claim for a discipline* (pp. 29–40). McLean, VA: Society for Health and Human Values.
Jones, A. H. (1997). Literature and medicine: Narrative ethics. *Lancet, 349,* 1243–1246.
Jose, P. E. (1989). The role of gender and gender role similarity in readers' identification with story characters. *Sex Roles, 21,* 697–713.
Jung, C. G. (1964). *Man and his symbols.* Garden City, NY: Doubleday.
Kaiser, H. (1960). The application of electronic computer factor analysis. *Educational and Psychological Measurement, 20,* 141–151.
Kalisch, B. J. (1971). An experiment in the development of empathy in nursing students. *Nursing Research, 20,* 202–211.
Kalisch, B. J. (1973). What is empathy? *American Journal of Nursing, 73,* 1548–1552.
Kalliopuska, M. (1992a). Attitudes towards health, health behavior, and personality factors among school students very high on empathy. *Psychological Reports, 70,* 1119–1122.
Kalliopuska, M. (1992b). Self-esteem and narcissism among the most and least empathetic Finnish baseball players. *Perceptual & Motor Skills, 75,* 945–946.
Kalliopuska, M. (1994). Empathy related to living in towns versus the countryside. *Psychological Reports, 74,* 896–898.
Kandel, E. R. (1998). A new intellectual framework for psychiatry. *American Journal of Psychiatry, 155,* 457–469.
Kane, G. C., Gotto, J. L., Mangione, S., West, S., & Hojat, M. (2005). Relationships between patient's perceptions of resident empathy and the ABIM patient rating of communication skills, humanistic qualities and professionalism: A pilot study. Manuscript submitted for publication.
Kaplan, G. A., Salonem, J. T., & Cohen, R. D. (1988). Social connections and mortality from all causes and from cardiovascular disease: Prospective evidence from eastern Finland. *American Journal of Epidemiology, 128,* 370–380.
Kaplan, N. B., & Bloom, S. W. (1960). The use of sociological and social psychological concepts in physiological research. *Journal of Nervous and Mental Disease, 131,* 128–134.
Kaplan, R. M., & Simon, H. J. (1990). Compliance in medical care: Reconsideration of self-predictions. *Annals of Behavioral Medicine, 12,* 66–71.
Karen, R. (1994). *Becoming attached.* New York: Warner Books.
Karniol, R., Gabay, R., Ochion, Y., & Harari, Y. (1998). Is gender or gender-role orientation a better predictor of empathy in adolescence? *Sex Roles, 39,* 45–59.
Kassebaum, D. G., & Szenas, P. L. (1994). Factors influencing the specialty choice of 1993 medical school graduates. *Academic Medicine, 69,* 164–170.
Kassirer, J. P. (1998). Doctor discontent. *New England Journal of Medicine, 339,* 1543–1545.
Katz, J. (1984). *The silent world of doctor and patient.* New York: Free Press.
Katz, R. L. (1963). *Empathy: Its nature and uses.* New York: Free Press.
Kause, D. R., Robbins, A., Heidrich, R., Abrassi, I. B., & Anderson, L. A. (1980). The long-term effectiveness of interpersonal skills training in medical school. *Journal of Medical Education, 55,* 595–601.
Kay, J. (1990). Traumatic deidealization and the future of medicine. *Journal of the American Medical Association, 263,* 572–573.
Keller, S., Shiflett, S. C., Schleifer, S. J., & Bartlett, J. A. (1994). *Human stress and immunity.* San Diego, CA: Academic Press.
Kelman, H. C. (1958). Compliance, identification, and internalization: Three processes of attitude change. *Conflict Resolution, 2,* 51–60.
Kendall, P. C., & Wilcox, C. E. (1980). Cognitive behavioral treatment for impulsivity: Concrete versus conceptual training in non-self-controlled problem children. *Journal of Counseling and Clinical Psychology, 48,* 80–91.
Kennedy, S., Kiecolt-Glaser, J. K., & Glaser, R. (1988). Immunological consequences of acute and chronic stressors: Mediating role of interpersonal relationships. *British Journal of Medical Psychology, 61,* 77–85.

Kenny, D. T. (1995). Determinants of patient satisfaction with the medical consultation. *Psychology and Health, 10*, 427–437.

Kerr, R. F., & Speroff, B. J. (1954). Validation and evaluation of the Empathy Test. *Journal of General Psychology, 50*, 269–276.

Kerr, W. A. (1947). *The Empathy Test: Form A* . Chicago: Psychometric Affiliates.

Kestenbaum, R., Farber, E. A., & Sroufe, L. A. (1989). Individual differences in empathy among preschoolers: Relation to attachment history. In N. Eisenberg (Ed.), *Empathy and related emotional responses* (pp. 51–64). San Francisco: Jossey-Bass.

Ketterer M. W., & Buckholtz, C. D. (1989). Somatization disorder. *Journal of the American Osteopathic Association, 89*, 489–490.

Keverne, E. B., Nevison, C. M., & Martel, F. L. (1997). Early learning and social bond. *Annals of the New York Academy of Sciences, 807*, 329–339.

Keysers, C., Kohler, E., Umilta, M. A., Nanetti, L., Fogassi, L., Gallese, & Gallese, V. (2003). Audiovisual mirror neurons and action recognition. *Experimental Brain Research, 153*, 628–663.

Keysers, C., & Perrett, D. I. (2004). Demystifying social cognition: A Hebbian perspective. *Trends in Cognitive Sciences, 8*, 501–507.

Keysers, C., Wicker, B., Gazzola, V., Anton, J. L., Fogassi, L., & Gallese, V. (2004). A touching sight: SII/VP activation during the observation and experience of touch. *Neuron, 42*, 335–346.

Kiecolt-Glaser, J. K., Garner, W., Speicher, C. E., Penn, G. M., Holiday, J.E., & Glaser, R. (1984). Psychosocial modifiers of immunocompetence in medical students. *Psychosomatic Medicine, 46*, 7–14.

Kim, S. S., Kaplowitz, S., & Johnston, M. V. (2004). The effects of physician empathy on patient satisfaction and compliance. *Evaluation and the Health Professions, 27*, 237–251.

Kipper, D. A., & Ben-Ely, Z. (1979). The effectiveness of the psychodramatic double method, the reflection method, and lecturing in the training of empathy. *Journal of Clinical Psychology, 35*, 370–375.

Klaus, M., & Kennell, J. H. (1970). Mothers separated from their newborn infants. *Pediatric Clinics of North America, 17*, 1015–1037.

Klaus, M. H., Jerauld, R., Kreger, N. S., McAlpine, W., Steffa, M., & Kennell, J. H. (1972). Maternal attachment: Importance of the first post-partum days. *New England Journal of Medicine, 286*, 460–463.

Kleinman, A. (1988). *The illness narratives: Suffering, healing, and the human condition*. New York: Basic Books.

Kleinman, A. (1995). *Writing at the margin: Discourse between anthropology and medicine*. Berkeley, CA: University of California Press.

Kleinman, A., Eisenberg, L., & Good, B. (1978). Culture, illness, and care: Clinical lessons from anthropologic and cross-cultural research. *Annals of Internal Medicine, 88*, 251–258.

Kliszcz, J., Hebanowski, M., & Rembowski, J. (1998). Emotional and cognitive empathy in medical schools. *Academic Medicine, 73*, 541.

Knapp, B. L. (1984). *A Jungian approach to literature*. Carbondale, IL: Southern Illinois University.

Knight, J. A. (1981). *Doctor-to-be: Coping with trials and triumphs of medical school*. New York: Appleton-Century.

Koenig, H. G. (2002). *Spirituality in patient care*. Philadelphia: Templeton Foundation Press.

Kohler, E., Keysers, C., Umilta, M. A., Fogassi, L., Gallese, V., & Rizzolatti, G. (2002). Hearing sounds, understanding actions: Action representation in mirror neurons. *Science, 297*, 846–848.

Kohn, L. T., Corrigan. J. M., & Donaldson, M. S. (2000). *To err is human: Building a safe health system*. Washington, DC: National Academy Press.

Kohut, H. (1959). Introspection, empathy and psychoanalysis. *Journal of American Psychoanalysis, 7*, 459–483.

Kohut, H. (1971). *Analysis of the self: A systematic approach to the psychoanalytic treatment of narcissistic personality disorders*. New York: International Universities Press.

Kohut, H. (1984). Introspection, empathy, and the semicircle of mental health. In J. Lichtenberg, M. Bornstein, & D. Silver (Eds.), *Empathy (Vol. 1, pp. 81–100)*. Hillsdale, NJ: Erlbaum.

Kolb, B., & Taylor, L. (1981). Affective behavior in patients with localized cortical excisions: Role of lesion site and side. *Science, 214,* 81–89.
Konner, M. (2004). The ties that bind.[Comment.] *Nature, 429,* 705.
Korsch, B. M., Gozzi, E. K., & Francis, V. (1968a). Gaps in doctor-patient interaction and patient satisfaction. *Pediatrics, 42,* 855–871.
Korsch, B. M., Gozzi, E. K., & Francis, V. (1968b). Gaps in doctor-patient communication: I. Doctor-patient interaction and patient satisfaction. *Pediatrics, 42,* 855–871.
Kramer, C. (1974). Folk linguistics. *Psychology Today, 8,* 82–85.
Kramer, D., Ber, R., & Moore, M. (1987). Impact of workshop on students' and physicians' rejecting behaviors in patient interviews. *Journal of Medical Education, 62,* 904–910.
Kramer, D., Ber, R., & Moores, M. (1989). Increasing empathy among medical students. *Medical Education, 23,* 168–173.
Krebs, D. (1975). Empathy and altruism. *Journal of Personality and Social Psychology, 32,* 1134–1146.
Kremer, J. F., & Dietzen, L. L. (1991). Two approaches to teaching accurate empathy to undergraduates: Teacher-intensive and self-directed. *Journal of College Student Development, 32,* 69–75.
Kunyk, D., & Olson, J. K. (2001). Clarification of conceptualizations of empathy. *Journal of Advanced Nursing, 35,* 317–325.
Kupfer, D. J., Drew, F. L., Curtis, E. K., & Rubinstein, D. N. (1978). Personality style and empathy in medical students. *Journal of Medical Education, 53,* 507–509.
Kurtines, W., & Hogan, R. (1972). Sources of conformity in unspecialized college students. *Journal of Abnormal Psychology, 80,* 49–51.
Kurtz, R. R., & Grummon, D. L. (1972). Different approaches to the measurement of therapist empathy and their relationship to therapy outcomes. *Journal of Consulting and Clinical Psychology, 39,* 106–115.
LaFrance, M., Hecht, M. A., & Levy Paluck, E. (2003). The contingent smile: A meta-analysis of sex differences in smiling. *Psychological Bulletin, 129,* 305–334.
LaMonica, E. L. (1981). Construct validity of an empathy instrument. *Research in Nursing & Health, 4,* 389–400.
LaMonica, E. L., Carew, D. K., Winder, A. E., Haase, A. M., & Blanchard, K. H. (1976). Empathy training as the major thrust of a staff development program. *Nursing Research, 25,* 447–451.
Lamont, L. M., & Lundstrom, W. J. (1977). Identifying successful industrial salesmen by personality and personal characteristics. *Journal of Marketing Research, 14,* 517–529.
Lancaster, T., Hart, R., & Gardner, S. (2002). Literature and medicine: Evaluating a special study module using the nominal group technique. *Medical Education, 36,* 1071–1076.
Lane, F. E. (1986). Utilizing physician empathy with violent patients. *American Journal of Psychotherapy, 40,* 448–456.
Lanzetta, J. T., & Englis, B. G. (1989). Expectation of cooperation and competition and their effects on observers' vicarious emotional response. *Journal of Personality and Social Psychology, 56,* 543–554.
Lanzetta, J. T., & Kleck, R. E. (1970). Encoding and decoding nonverbal affect in humans. *Journal of Personality and Social Psychology, 16,* 12–19.
LaRocco, J. M., House, J. S., & French, J. R. P. (1980). Social support, occupational stress, and health. *Journal of Health and Social Behavior, 21,* 202–218.
Larson, D. (1993). *The helpers journey: Working with people facing grief, loss, and life-threatening illness.* Champaign, IL: Research Press.
Larson, E. B., & Yao, X. (2005). Clinical empathy as emotional labor in the patient-physician relationship. *Journal of the American Medical Association, 293,* 1100–1106.
Laskowski, C., & Pellicore, K. (2002). The wounded healer archetype: Applications to palliative care practice. *American Journal of Hospice & Palliative Care, 19,* 403–407.
Lawrence, E. J., Shaw, P., Baker, D., Baron-Cohen, S., & David, A. S. (2004). Measuring empathy: Reliability and validity of the Empathy Quotient. *Psychological Medicine, 34,* 911–924.
Layton, J. M. (1979). The use of modeling to teach empathy to nursing students. *Research in Nursing & Health, 2,* 163–176.
Layton, J. M., & Wykle, M. H. (1990). A validity study of four empathy instruments. *Research in Nursing & Health, 13,* 319–325.

Lazarus, R. S. (1982). Thoughts on the relations between emotion and cognition. *American Psychologist, 37*, 1019–1024.

Leiper, R. & Casares, P. (2000). An investigation of the attachment organization of clinical psychologists and its relationship to clinical practice. *British Journal of Medical Psychology, 73*, 449–464.

Lerner, A. (1978). *Poetry in the therapeutic experience*. Elmsford, NY: Pergamon Press.

Lerner, A. (2001). Poetry therapy. In R. J. Corsini (Ed.), *Handbook of innovative therapies* (pp. 472–479). New York: John Wiley & Sons.

Lerner, M. J., & Meindl, J. R. (1981). Justice and altruism. In J. P. Rushton & J. R. Sorrentino (Eds.), *Altruism and helping behavior: Social, personality, and developmental perspectives* (pp. 213–232). Hillsdale, NJ: Erlbaum.

Letourneau, C. (1981). Empathy and stress: How they affect parental aggression. *Social Work, 26*, 383–389.

Levasseur, J., & Vance, A. R. (1993). Doctors, nurses, and empathy. In H. M. Spiro, M. G. Mccrea Curnen, E. Peschel, & D. St. James (Eds.), *Empathy and practice of medicine* (pp. 76–84). New Haven: Yale University Press.

Levenson, R. W., & Ruef, A. M. (1992). Empathy, a physiological substrate. *Journal of Personality and Social Psychology, 63*, 234–246.

Levine, L. E., & Hoffman, M. L. (1975). Empathy and cooperation in 4-year olds. *Developmental Psychology, 4*, 533–534.

Levinson, W. (1994). Physician-patient communication: A key to malpractice prevention. *Journal of the American Medical Association, 272*, 1619–1620.

Levinson, W., Gorawara-Bhat, R., & Lamb, J. (2000). A study of patient clues and physician responses in primary care and surgical settings. *Journal of the American Medical Association, 284*, 1021–1027.

Levinson, W., Roter, D., Mullooly, J. P., Dull, V. T., & Frankel, R. (1997). Physician-patient communication: The relationship with malpractice claims among primary care physicians and surgeons. *Journal of the American Medical Association, 277*, 553–559.

Levy, D. (Ed.) (1999). *Medical milestones from the National Heart, Lung, and Blood Institute's Framingham Heart Study*. Center for Bio-Medical Communication.

Levy, J. (1997). A note on empathy. *New Ideas in Psychology, 15*, 179–184.

Lewin, K. (1936). *A dynamic theory of personality*. New York: McGraw-Hill.

Lewinsohn, R. (1998). Medical theories, science, and the practice of medicine. *Social Science & Medicine, 46*, 1261–1270.

Lewis, J. M. (1998). For better or worse: Interpersonal relationships and individual outcome. *American Journal of Psychiatry, 155*, 582–589.

Lewis, T., Amini, F., & Lannon, R. (2000). *A general theory of love*. New York: Vintage Books.

Lichtenstein, P., Holm, N. V., Verkasalo, P. K., Iliadou, A., Kaprio, J., Koskenvuo, M., Pukkala, E., Skytthe, A., & Hemminki, K. (2000). Environmental and heritable factors in the causation of cancer: Analyses of cohort twins from Sweden, Denmark, and Finland. *New England Journal of Medicine, 343*, 78–85.

Lief, H. I., & Fox, R. C. (1963). Training for "detached concerns" in medical students. In H. I. Lief, V. F. Lief, & N. R. Lief (Eds.), *The psychological basis of medical practice* (pp. 12–35). New York: Harper & Row.

Lief, H. I., Lief, V. F., & Lief, N. R. (Eds.). (1963). *The psychological basis of medical practice*. New York: Harper & Row.

Likert, R. (1932). A technique for the measurement of attitudes. *Archives of Psychology, 140*, 5–35.

Lilienfeld, R. (1978). *The rise of systems theory: An ideological analysis*. New York: John Wiley & Sons.

Linn, L. S. (1974). Care vs. cure: How the nurse practitioner views the patient. *Nursing Outlook, 22*, 641–644.

Linn, L. S. (1975). A survey of the "care-cure" attitudes of physicians, nurses, and their students. *Nursing Forum, 14*, 145–161.

Linn, L. S., Cope, D. W., & Leake, B. (1984). The effect of gender and training of residents on satisfaction ratings by patients. *Journal of Medical Education, 59*, 964–966.

Linn, L. S., DiMatteo, M. R., Cope, D. W., & Robbins, A. (1987). Measuring physicians' humanistic attitudes, values, and behaviors. *Medical Care, 25*, 504–515.

Linn, L. S., Yager, J., Cope, D., & Leake, B. (1985). Health status, job satisfaction, job stress, and life satisfaction among academic and clinical faculty. *Journal of the American Medical Association, 254,* 2775–2782.
Lipner, R. S., Blank, L. L., Leas, B. F., & Fortna, G. S. (2002). The value of patient and peer ratings in recertification. *Academic Medicine, 77,* S64–S66.
Litvack-Miller, W., McDougall, D., & Romney, D. M. (1997). The structure of empathy during middle childhood and its relationship to prosocial behavior. *Genetic, Social, and General Psychology Monographs, 123,* 303–324.
Lopez, G. E., Gurin, P., & Nagda, B. A. (1998). Education and understanding structural causes for group inequalities. *Political Psychology, 19,* 305–329.
Lott, D. A. (1998). Brain development, attachment and impact on psychic vulnerability *Psychiatric Times, 15.* Retrieved December 20, 2004, from http://www.psychiatrictimes.com.
Lounsburg, M. L., & Bates, J. E. (1982). The cries of infants of differing levels of perceived temperamental difficultness: Acoustic properties and effects on listeners. *Child Development, 53,* 677–686.
Lu, M. C. (1995). Why it was hard for me to learn compassion as a third-year medical student. *Cambridge Quarterly of Healthcare Ethics, 4,* 454–458.
Luborsky, L., Chandler, M., Auerbach, A. H., Cohen, J., & Bacharach, H. M. (1971). Factors influencing the outcome of psychotherapy: A review of quantitative research. *Psychological Bulletin, 75,* 145–185.
Ludmerer, K. M. (1999). Time to heal. American medical education from the turn of the century to the era of managed care. New York, Oxford University Press.
Luscher, T. F., & Vetter, W. (1990). Adherence to medication. *Journal of Human Hypertension, 4 (Suppl. 1),* 43–46.
Lutchmaya, S., Baron-Cohen, S., & Raggatt, P. (2002). Foetal testosterone and vocabulary size in 18 and 24-month old infants. *Infant Behavior & Development, 24,* 418–424.
Lynch, J. J. (1977). *The broken heart: The consequences of loneliness.* New York: Basic books.
Maccoby, E. E., & Jacklin, C. N. (1974). *The psychology of sex differences.* Stanford, CA: Stanford University press.
MacKay, R., Hughes, J. R., & Carver, E. J. (Eds.). (1990). *Empathy in the helping relationship.* New York: Springer.
MacLean, P. D. (1967). The brain in relation to empathy and medical education. *Journal of Nervous and Mental Disease, 144,* 374–382.
MacLean, P. D. (1990). *The triune brain evolution.* New York: Plenum Press.
Macmillan, M. B. (2000). Restoring Phineas Gage: A 150th retrospective. *Journal of History of Neurosciences, 9,* 42–62.
MacPherson, H., Mercer, S. W., Scullion, T., & Thomas, K. J. (2003). Empathy, enablement, and outcome: An exploratory study on acupuncture patient's perceptions. *Journal of Alternative & Complementary Medicine, 9,* 869–876.
Magee, M., & Hojat, M. (1998). Personality profiles of male and female positive role models in medicine. *Psychological Reports, 82,* 547–559.
Magee, M., & Hojat, M. (2001). Impact of health care system on physicians' discontent. *Journal of Community Health, 26,* 357–365.
Maheux, B., Beaudoin, C., Berkson, L. C. L., Des Marchais, J., & Jean, P. (2000). Medical faculty as humanistic physicians and teachers: The perceptions of students at innovative and traditional medical schools. *Medical Education, 34,* 630–634.
Maheux, B., & Beland, F. (1989). Students' perceptions of values emphasized in three medical schools. *Journal of Medical Education, 61,* 308–316.
Maheux, B., Duford, F., Beland, F., Jacques, A., & Levesque, A. (1990). Female medical practitioners: More preventive and patient oriented? *Medical Care, 28,* 87–92.
Main, M., & Solomon, J. (1990). Procedures for identifying infants as disorganized/disoriented during the Ainsworth strange situation. In M. Greenberg, D. Cicchetti, & E. M. Cummings (Eds.), *Attachment in the preschool years: Theory, research and intervention* (pp. 121–160). Chicago: University of Chicago Press.
Makoul, G. (1998). Perpetuating passivity: Reliance and reciprocal determinism in physician-patient interaction. *Journal of Health Communication, 3,* 233–259.
Makoul, G. (2001). Essential elements of communication in medical encounters: The Kalamazoo consensus statement. *Academic Medicine, 76,* 390–393.

Makoul, G., & Strauss, A. (2003). Building therapeutic relationships during patient visits. *Journal of General Internal Medicine, 18 (Suppl. 1)*, 275.

Malno, R. B., Boag, T. J., & Smith, A. A. (1957). Physiological study of personal interaction. *Psychosomatic Medicine, 19*, 105–119.

Mangione, S., Kane, G., Caruso, J. W., Gonnella, J. S., Nasca, T. J., & Hojat, M. (2002). Assessment of empathy in different years of internal medicine training. *Medical Teacher, 24*, 371–374.

Mandell, H., & Spiro, H. (1987). *When doctors get sick.* New York: Plenum.

Mann, L., Wise, T. N., Trinidad, A., & Kohanski, R. (1994). Alexithymia, affect recognition, and the five-factor model of personality in normal subjects. *Psychological Reports, 74*, 563–567.

Mansen, T. J. (1993). Role-taking abilities of nursing education administrators and their perceived leadership effectiveness. *Journal of Professional Nursing, 9*, 347–357.

Marcus, E. R. (1999). Empathy, humanism, and the professionalization process of medical education. *Academic Medicine, 74*, 1211–1215.

Markham, B. (1979). Can a behavioral science course change medical students' attitudes? *Journal of Psychiatric Education*, *3*, 44–54.

Markus, H. R., & Kitayama, S. (1991). Culture and the self: Implications for cognition, emotion, and motivation. *Psychological Review, 98*, 224–253.

Marmot, M. G., & Syme, S. L. (1976). Acculturation and coronary heart disease in Japanese-Americans. *American Journal of Epidemiology, 104*, 225–247.

Marshall, P. A., & O'Keefe, J. P. (1994). Medical students' first person narrative of a patient's story of AIDS. *Social Science & Medicine, 40*, 67–76.

Marshall, W. L., & Maric, A. (1996). Cognitive and emotional components of generalized empathy deficits in child molesters. *Journal of Child Sexual Abuse, 5*, 101–111.

Martin, G. B., & Clark, R. D. (1982). Distress crying in neonates: Species and peer specificity. *Developmental Psychology, 18*, 3–9.

Marx, B. P., Heidt, J. M., & Gold, S. D. (2005). Perceived uncontrollability and unpredictability, self-regulation, and sexual revictimization. *Review of General Psychology, 9*, 67–90.

Matthews, D. A., & Feinstein, A. R. (1989). A new instrument for patients' rating of physician performance in the hospital setting. *Journal of General Internal Medicine, 4*, 14–22.

Matthews, D. A., Suchman, A. L., & Branch, W. T. (1993). Making "connexions": Enhancing the therapeutic potential of patient-clinician relationships. *Annals of Internal Medicine, 118*, 973–977.

Matthews, K. A., Batson, C. D., Horn, J., & Rosenman, R. H. (1981). Principles in his nature which interest him in the fortune of others . . . ": The heritability of empathic concern for others. *Journal of Personality, 49*, 237–247.

Mayerson, E. W. (1976). *Putting the ill at ease.* New York: Harper & Row.

Mays, L. C., Carter, A. S., Eggar, H. L., & Pajer, K. A. (1991). Reflection on stillness: Mother's reaction to the still-face situation. *Journal of Academy of Child and Adolescent Psychiatry, 30*, 22–28.

McClintock, M. K. (1971). Menstrual synchrony and suppression. *Nature, 229*, 244–245.

McEwen, B. S. (1998). Protective and damaging effects of stress mediators. *New England Journal of Medicine, 338*, 171–179.

McKellar, P. (1957). *Imagining and thinking: A psychological analysis.* New York: Basic Books.

McKinlay, J. B., & McKinlay, S. M. (1981). Medical measures and the decline of mortality. In P. Conrad & R. Kern (Eds.), *The sociology of health and illness: Critical perspectives* (pp. 12–30). New York: St. Martin's Press.

Mclean, M. (2004). The choice of role models by students at a culturally diverse South African medical school. *Medical Teacher, 26*, 133–141.

McLellan, J. D., Jansen-McWilliams, L., Comer, D. M., Gardner, W. P., & Kelleher, K. J. (1999). The Physician Belief Scale and psychosocial problems in children: A report from the pediatric research in office settings and the ambulatory sentinel practice network. *Journal of Developmental & Behavioral Pediatrics, 20*, 24–30.

McLellan, M. F., & Husdon Jones, A. (1996). Why literature and medicine? *Lancet, 348*, 109–111.

McManus, I. C. (1995). Humanity and the medical humanities. *Lancet, 346*, 1143–1145.

McMillan, J. R., Clifton, A. K., McGrath, D., & Gale, W. S. (1977). Women's language: Uncertainty or interpersonal sensitivity and emotionality. *Sex Roles, 3*, 545–559.

McVey, L. J., Davis, D. E., & Cohen, H. J. (1989). The aging game: An approach to education in geriatrics. *Journal of the American Medical Association, 262,* 1507–1509.
Mead, G. H. (1934). *Mind, self and society.* Chicago: University of Chicago Press.
Means, J. J. (2002). Mighty prophet/wounded healer. *Journal of Pastoral Care, 56,* 41–49.
Meeuwesen, L., Schaap, C., & Van der Staak, C. (1991). Verbal analysis of doctor-patient communication. *Social Science & Medicine, 32,* 1143–1150.
Mehrabian, A. (1969). Significance of posture and position in the communication of attitude and status relationships. *Psychological Bulletin, 71,* 359–372.
Mehrabian, A., & Epstein, N. A. (1972). A measure of emotional empathy. *Journal of Personality, 40,* 525–543.
Mehrabian, A., & O'Reilly, E. (1980). Analysis of personality measures in terms of basic dimensions of temperament. *Journal of Personality and Social Psychology, 38,* 492–503.
Mehrabian, A., Young, A. L., & Sato, S. (1988). Emotional empathy and associated individual differences. *Current Psychology: Research & Reviews, 7,* 221–240.
Mello, M. M., Studdert, D. M., DesRoches, C. M., Peugh, J., Zapert, K., Brennan, T. A., & Sage, W. M. (2004). Caring for patients in a malpractice crisis: Physician satisfaction and quality of care. *Health Affairs, 23,* 42–53.
Meltzoff, A. N., & Moore, M. K. (1977). Imitation of facial and manual gestures by human neonates. *Science, 198,* 75–78.
Meltzoff, A. N., & Moore, M. K. (1983). Newborn infants imitate adult facial gestures. *Child Development, 54,* 702–709.
Meltzoff, J., & Kornreich, M. (1970). *Research in psychotherapy.* New York: Atherton.
Mengel, M. B. (1987). Physician ineffectiveness due to family-of-origin issues. *Family Systems Medicine, 5,* 176–190.
Mercer, S. W., & Reynolds, W. J. (2002). Empathy and quality of care. *British Journal of General Practice, 52,* S9–S12.
Mercer, S. W., Watt, G. C. M., & Reilly, D. (2001). Empathy is important for enablement. *British Medical Journal, 322,* 865.
Merlyn, S. (1998). Improving doctor-patient communicationity: Not an option, but a necessity. *British Medical Journal, 316,* 1922.
Meyers, A. R. (1987). Lumping it: The hidden denomination of the medical malpractice crisis. *American Journal of Public Health, 77,* 1544–1548.
Milgram, S. (1963). Behavioral study of obedience. *Journal of Abnormal and Social Psychology, 67,* 371–378.
Milgram, S. (1968). Some conditions of obedience and disobedience to authority. *Human Relations, 6* , 259–276.
Miller, K. (2002). *Communication theories: Perspective, processes, and context.* Boston: McGraw-Hill.
Miller, M. N., & McGowen, K. R. (2000). The Painful truth: Physicians are not invincible. *Southern Medical Journal, 91,* 966–972.
Miller, P. A., & Eisenberg, N. (1988). The relation of empathy to aggressive and externalizing/antisocial behavior. *Psychological Bulletin, 103,* 324–344.
Milner, K., Squire, L. R., & Kanel, E. R. (1998). Cognitive neuroscience and the study of memory. *Neuron, 20,* 445–468.
Montgomery Hunter, K., Charon, R., & Coulehan, J. L. (1995). The study of literature in medical education. *Academic Medicine, 70,* 787–794.
Moore, B. E., & Fine, B. D. (1968). *A glossary of psychoanalytic terms and concepts.* New York: American Psychoanalytic Association.
Moore, D. B. (1996). Illegal action-official reaction: Affect theory, criminology, and the criminal justice system. In D. L. Nathanson (Ed.), *Knowing feeling: Affect, script, and psychotherapy* (pp. 346–378). New York: W. W. Norton.
Moore, P. J., Adler, N. E., & Robertson, P. A. (2000). Medical malpractice: The effect of doctor-patient relations on medical patient perceptions and malpractice intentions. *Western Journal of Medicine, 173,* 244–250.
Moreno, J. L. (1934). *Who shall survive?* Washington, DC: Nervous and Mental Disease Publishing Co.
Morgan, J. D. (Ed.). (2002). *Social support: A reflection of humanity.* Amityville, New York: Baywood Publishing Company.

Mori, M. S., Vigh, A., Miayata, T., & Yoshihara, S. (1990). Oxytocin is the major prolactin releasing factor in the posterior pituitary. *Endocrinology, 125*, 1009–1013.

Morse, J. M., Anderson, G., Bottorff, J. L., Yonge, O., O'Brien, B., Solberg, S. M., & McIlveen, K. H. (1992). Exploring empathy: A conceptual fit for nursing practice? *Image: Journal of Nursing Scholarship, 24*, 273–280.

Moser, R. S. (1984). Perceived role-taking behavior and course grades in junior year college nursing students. *Journal of Nursing Education, 23*, 294–297.

Moss, H. A. (1967). Sex, age, and state as determinants of mother-infant interaction. *Merrill-Palmer Quarterly, 13*, 19–36.

Mumford, L. (1967). *The myth of the machine*. New York: Harcourt, Brace & World.

Murray, H. A. (1938). *Explorations in personality*. Englewood Cliffs, NJ: Prentice-Hall.

Mussen, P., & Eisenberg-Berg, N. (1977). *Roots of caring, sharing, and helping: The development of prosocial behavior in children*. San Francisco: W. H. Freeman.

Naftulin, D. H., Ware, J. E., Jr., & Donnelly, F. A. (1973). The Doctor Fox lecture: A paradigm of educational seduction. *Journal of Medical Education, 48*, 630–635.

Nathanson, D. L. (Ed.). (1996). *Knowing feeling: Affect, script, and psychotherapy*. New York: W. W. Norton.

Nauta, W. J. H., & Feirtag, M. (1986). *Fundamental neuroanatomy*. New York: W. H. Freeman.

Nelson, D. W., & Baumgarte, R. (2004). Cross-cultural misunderstandings reduce empathic responding. *Journal of Applied Social Psychology, 34*, 391–401.

Neubauer, R. B., & Neubauer, A. (1990). *Nature's thumbprint: The new genetics of personality*. Reading, MA: Addison-Wesley.

Neuwirth, Z. E. (1997). Physician empathy—should we care? *Lancet, 350*, 606.

Newman, T. B. (2003). The power of stories over statistics. *British Medical Journal, 327*, 1224–1427.

Newton, B. W., Savidge, M. A., Barber, L., Cleveland, E., Clardy, J., Beeman, G., & Hart, T. (2000). Differences in medical students' empathy. *Academic Medicine, 75*, 1215.

Newton, N., Feeler, D., & Rawlins, C. (1968). Effect of lactation on maternal behavior in mice with comparative data on humans. Lying-in. *Journal of Reproductive Medicine, 1*, 257–262.

Newton, N., & Newton, M. (1967). Psychologic aspects of lactation. *New England Journal of Medicine, 277*, 1179–1188.

Nicholas, D. (2002). Social support of the bereaved: Some practical suggestions. In J. D.Morgan (Ed.), *Social support: A reflection of humanity* (pp. 33–43). Amityville, NY: Baywood Publishing.

Nightingale, S. D., Yarnold, P. R., & Greenberg, M. S. (1991). Sympathy, empathy, and physician resource utilization. *Journal of General Internal Medicine, 6*, 420–423.

Nolte, J. (1993). *The human brain: An introduction to its functional anatomy* (3rd ed.). St. Louis: Mosby.

Novack, D. H. (1987). Therapeutic aspects of the clinical encounter. *Journal of General Internal Medicine, 2*, 346–355.

Novack, D. H., Epstein, R. M., & Paulsen, R. H. (1999). Toward creating physician-healers: Fostering medical students' self-awareness, personal growth, and well-being. *Academic Medicine, 74*, 516–520.

O'Conner, J. P., Nash, D. B., Buehler, M. L., & Bard, M. (2002). Satisfaction higher for physician executives who treat patients, survey finds. *Physician Executive, 28*, 16–21.

Oatley, K. (2004). Scripts, transformation, and suggestiveness of emotions in Shakespeare and Chekhov. *Review of General Psychology, 8*, 323–340.

Olinick, S. L. (1984). A critique of empathy and sympathy. In J. Lichtenbergh, M. Borenstein, & D. Silver (Eds.), *Empathy I* (pp. 137–166). Hillsdale, N.J.: Analytic Press.

Oliver, J. (1939). An ancient poem on the duties of a physician, Part 1. *Bulletin of the History of Medicine, 7*, 315.

Olson, J., & Hanchett, E. (1997). Nurse-expressed empathy, patient outcomes, and development of a middle-range theory. *Image—The Journal of Nursing Scholarship, 29*, 71–76.

Ong, L. M., DeHaes, J. M., Hoos, A. M., & Lammies, F. B. (1995). Doctor-patient communication: A review of the literature. *Social Science & Medicine, 40*, 903–918.

Oppenheim, A. (1992). *Questionnaire design: Interviewing and attitude measurement*. London: Printer Publishing.

Orlando, I. (1961). *The dynamic nurse-patient relationship*. New York: Putman.

Orlando, I. (1972). *The discipline and teaching of nursing process*. New York: Putman.

Ornish, D. (1998). *Love and survival: The scientific basis for the healing power of intimacy.* New York: Harper Collins.
Orth-Gomer, K., & Johnson, J. V. (1987). Social network integration and mortality: A six year follow-up study of random sample of the Swedish population. *Journal of Chronic Diseases, 40,* 949–957.
Ortmeyer, C. F. (1974). Variations in mortality, morbidity, and health care by marital status. In L. L. Erhardt & J. E. Beln (Eds.), *Mortality and morbidity in the United States* (pp. 159–184). Cambridge, MA: Harvard University Press.
Osler, W. (1932). *Aequanimitas with other addresses to medical schools, nurses, and practitioners of medicine.* Philadelphia, PA: Blakiston.
Osofsky, J. D., & O'Connell, E. J. (1977). Patterning of newborn behavior in an urban population. *Child Development, 48,* 532–536.
Pacala, J. T., Boult, C., Bland, C., & O'Brien, J. (1995). Aging game improves medical students caring for elderly. *Gerontology and Geriatrics Education, 15,* 45–57.
Page, K. M., & Novak, M. A. (2002). Empathy leads to fairness. *Bulletin of Mathematical Biology, 64,* 1101–1116.
Papadakis, M. A., Teherani, A., Banach, M. A., Knettler, T. R., Rattner, S. L., Stern, D. T., Veloski, J. J., & Hodgson, C. S. (2005). Disciplinary action by ethical boards and prior behavior in medical school. *New England Journal of Medicine, 353,* 2673–2682.
Papousek, M., Papousek, H., & Symmes, D. (1991). The meaning of melodies in motherese in tone and stress languages. *Infant Behavior & Development, 14,* 415–440.
Parlow, J., & Rothman, A. (1974). Attitudes toward social issues in medicine of five health science facilities. *Social Science & Medicine, 8,* 351–358.
Pascalis, O., DeSchonen, S., Morton, J., Deruella, C., & Fabre-Grenet, M. (1995). Mother's face recognition by neonates: A replication and extension. *Infant Behavior & Development, 18,* 79–85.
Patterson, C. H. (1984). Empathy, warmth, and genuineness in psychotherapy: A review of reviews. *Psychotherapy, 21,* 431–438.
Peabody, F. W. (1984). The care of the patient. *Journal of the American Medical Association, 252,* 813–818.
Pecukonis, E. V. (1990). A cognitive/affective empathy training program as a function of ego development in aggressive adolescent females. *Adolescence, 25,* 59–76.
Pedersen, C. A., Ascher, J. A., Monroe, Y. L., & Prange, A. J. J. (1982). Oxytocin induces maternal behavior in virgin female rats. *Science, 216,* 648–649.
Pedersen, C. A., & Prange, A. J. J. (1979). Induction of maternal behavior in virgin rats after intracerebroventicular administration of oxytocin. *Proceedings of the National Academy of Sciences, 76,* 6661–6665.
Pellegrino, E. (1979). *Humanism and the physician.* Knoxville, TN: University of Tennessee Press.
Pennebaker, J. W. (1990). *Opening up: The healing power of confining in others.* New York: William Morrow.
Pennebaker, J. W., Kiecolt-Glaser, J. K., & Glaser, K. (1988). Disclosure of traumas and immune function: Health implications for psychotherapy. *Journal of Consulting and Clinical Psychology, 56,* 239–245.
Penninx, B. W., van Tilburg, T., & Kriegsman, D. M. (1997). Effects of social support and personal coping resources on mortality in older age: The Longitudinal Aging Study, Amsterdam. *American Journal of Epidemiology, 146,* 510–519.
Pennington, R. E., & Pierce, W. L. (1985). Observations of empathy of nursing-home staff: A predictive study. *International Journal of Aging and Human Development, 21,* 281–291.
Perry, R. J., Rosen, H. R., Kramer, J. H., Beer, J. S., Levenson, R. L., & Miller, B. L. (2001). Hemispheric dominance for emotions, empathy and social behaviour: Evidence from right and left handeds with frontotemporal dementia. *Neurocase, 7,* 145–160.
Peschel, E. R. (1980). *Medicine and literature.* New York: Neale Watson.
Peter, E., & Gallop, R. (1994). The ethic of care: A comparison of nursing and medical students. *Image—The Journal of Nursing Scholarship, 26,* 47–50.
Piaget, J. (1967). *Six psychological studies .* New York: Random House.
Pigman, G. W. (1995). Freud and the history of empathy. *International Journal of Psychoanalysis., 76,* 237–256.

Platek, S. M., Critton, S. R., Myers, T. E., & Gallup, G. G. (2003). Contagious yawning: The role of self awareness and mental state attribution. *Cognitive Brain Research, 17,* 223–227.
Platek, S. M., Keenan, J. P., Gallup, G. G., & Mohamed, F. B. (2004). Where am I? The neurological correlates of self and other. *Cognitive Brain Research, 19,* 114–122.
Platek, S. M., Mohamed, F. B., & Gallup, G. G. (2005). Contagious yawning and the brain. *Cognitive Brain Research, 23,* 448–452.
Platt, F. W., & Keller, V. F. (1994). Empathic communication: A teachable and learnable skill. *Journal of General Internal Medicine, 9,* 222–226.
Plutchik. R. (1987). Evolutionary bases of empathy. In N. Eisenberg & J. Strayer (Eds.), *Empathy and its development* (pp. 38–46). New York: Cambridge University Press.
Polgar, C., & Thomas, S. (1988). *Introduction to research in health sciences.* Edinburgh: Churchill Livingston.
Pollak, O. (1976). *Human behavior and the helping professions.* New York: Spectrum Publications.
Poole, A. D., & Sanson-Fisher, R. W. (1980). Long-term effects of empathy training on the interview skills of medical students. *Patient Counseling and Health Education, 2,* 125–127.
Powell, A. S., Boakes, J. P., & Slater, P. (1988). Hostility and the medical student: How a trait measure influences perception of medical specialties. *Medical Education, 22,* 222–230.
Preston, S. D., & deWaal, F. B. M. (2002). Empathy: It's ultimate and proximate bases. *Behavioral and Brain Sciences, 25,* 1–20.
Prinz, W. (1997). Perception and action planning. *European Journal of Cognitive Psychology, 9,* 129–154.
Pumilia, C. V. (2002). Psychological impact of the physician-patient relationship on compliance: A case study and clinical strategies. *Progress in Transplantation, 12,* 10–16.
Radley, C. (1992). Imagining ethics: Literature and practice of ethics. *Journal of Clinical Ethics, 3,* 38–45.
Rankin, K. P., Kramer, J. H., & Miller, B. L. (2005). Patterns of cognitive and emotional empathy in frontotemporal lobar degeneration. *Cognitive Behavioral Neurology, 18,* 28–36.
Raudonis, B. M. (1993). The meaning and impact of empathic relationships in hospice nursing. *Cancer Nursing, 16,* 304–309.
Ray, O. (2004). How the mind hurts and heals the body. *American Psychologist, 59,* 29–40.
Raynolds, P., Boyd, P. T., & Blacklow, R. S. (1994). The relationships between social ties and survival among black and white breast cancer patients: National Cancer Institute, Cancer Survival Study Group. *Cancer Epidemiology, Biomarkers & Prevention, 3,* 253–259.
Reed, V. A., Jernstedt, C., & Reber, E. S. (2001). Understanding and improving medical student specialty choice: Synthesis of the literature using decision theory as a referent. *Teaching and Learning in Medicine, 13,* 117–129.
Reik, T. (1948). *Listening with the third ear: The inner experience of a psychoanalyst.* New York: Farrar, Straus.
Reiser, M. F., Reeves, R. B., & Armington, J. (1955). Effects of variation in laboratory procedure and experimenter upon the ballistoeargram, blood pressure, and heart rate in healthy young men. *Psychosomatic Medicine, 17,* 185–199.
Reisetter, B. C. (2003). *Relationship between psychosocial physician characteristic and physician price awareness.* Doctoral dissertation, University of Mississippi, Dissortation Abstracts International, 63 (10–B), P. 4620.
Reiter-Palmon, R., & Connelly, M. S. (2000). Item selection counts: A comparison of empirical key and rational scale validities in theory-based and non-theory-based item pools. *Journal of Applied Psychology*, *85,* 143–151.
Rempel, J. K., Holmes, J. G., & Zanna, M. P. (1985). Trust in close relationships. *Journal of Personality and Social Psychology, 49,* 95–112.
Reverby, S. (1987). A caring dilemma: Womanhood and nursing in historical perspective. *Nursing Research, 36,* 1–5.
Reynolds, W. J. (2000). *The measurement and development of empathy in nursing.* Burlington, VT: Ashgate.
Richard, F. D., Bond, C. F., Jr., & Stokes-Zoota, J. J. (2003). One hundred years of social psychology quantitatively described. *Review of General Psychology, 7,* 331–363.
Richard, G. V., Nakamoto, D. M., & Lockwood, J. H. (2001). Medical career choices: Traditional and new possibilities. *Journal of the American Medical Association, 285,* 2249–2250.

Richter, C. P. (1957). On the phenomenon of sudden death in animals and man. *Psychosomatic Medicine, 19*, 191–198.

Ridley, M., & Dawkins, R. (1981). The natural selection of altruism. In J. P. Rushton & R. M. Sorrentino (Eds.), *Altruism and helping behavior: Social, personality, and developmental perspectives* (pp. 19–39). Hillsdale, NJ: Erlbaum.

Riggio, R. E., Tucker, J., & Coffaro, D. (1989). Social skills and empathy. *Personality and Individual Differences, 10*, 93–99.

Rizzolatti, G., Fadiga, L., Gallese, V., & Fogassi, L. (1996). Premotor cortex and the recognition of motor action. *Cognitive Brain Research, 3*, 131–141.

Roberts, B. W., & DelVecchio, W. F. (2000). The rank-order consistency of personality traits from childhood to old age: A quantitative review of longitudinal studies. *Psychological Bulletin, 126*, 3–25.

Robinson, J. L., Zahn-Waxler, C., & Emde, R. N. (1994). Patterns of development in early empathic behavior: Environmental and child constitutional influences. *Social Development, 3*, 125–145.

Robinson, J. P. (1978). General attitudes toward people. In J. P. Robinson & P. R. Shaver (Eds.), *Measures of social psychological attitudes* (pp. 587–627). Ann Arbor, MI: Institute for Social Research.

Rodriguez, M. S., & Cohen, S. (1998). Social support. In H. S. Friedman (Ed.), *Encyclopedia of mental health* (pp. 535–544). San Diego, CA: Academic Press.

Roe, A. (1957). Early determinants of vocational choice. *Journal of Consulting Psychology, 4*, 212–217.

Roe, K. V. (1977). A study of empathy in young Greek and U.S. children. *Journal of Cross-Cultural Psychology, 8*, 493–502.

Rogers, C. R. (1959). A theory of therapy: Personality and interpersonal relationships as developed in the client-centered framework. In S. Koch (Ed.), *Psychology, a study of science: Foundations of the person and the social context* (pp. 184–256). New York: McGraw Hill.

Rogers, C. R. (1975). Empathic: An unappreciated way of being. *Counseling Psychologist, 5*, 2–11.

Rogers, C. R., Gendlin, E., Kiesler, D., & Truax, C. B. (1967). *The therapeutic relationship and its impact.* Madison: University of Wisconsin Press.

Rokeach, M. (1973). *The nature of human values.* New York: Free Press.

Romano, J. M., Jensen, M. P., Turner, J. A., Good, A. B., & Hops, H. (2000). Chronic pain patient-partner interactions: Further support for a behavioral model of chronic pain. *Behavior Therapy, 31*, 415–440.

Rosenberg, D. A., & Silver, H. K. (1984). Medical student abuse—an unnecessary and preventable cause of stress. *Journal of the American Medical Association, 251*, 739–742.

Rosenberg, M. (1965). *Society and adolescent self-image.* Princeton, NJ: Princeton University Press.

Rosenberg, M. (1957). *Occupation and values.* Glencoe, IL: Free Press.

Rosenberg, M. J., & Hovland, C. I. (1960). Cognitive, affective, and behavioral components of attitudes. In M. J. Hovland & M. J. Rosenberg (Eds.), *Attitude organization and change* (pp. 1–14). New Haven, CT: Yale University Press.

Rosenfeld, H. M. (1965). Effect of an approval-seeking induction on interpersonal proximity. *Psychological Reports, 17*, 120–122.

Rosenhan, D. L. (1973). On being sane in insane places. *Science, 179*, 250–258.

Rosenow, E. C. (1999). The challenge of becoming a distinguished clinician. *Mayo Clinic Proceedings, 74*, 635–637.

Rosenthal, R., Hall, J. A., DiMatteo, M. R., Rogers, P. L., & Archer, D. (1979). *Sensitivity to non-verbal communication: The PONS test.* Baltimore, MD: Johns Hopkins University Press.

Ross, E. D., & Mesulam, M. M. (1979). Dominant language functions of the right hemisphere? Prosody and emotional gesturing. *Archives of Neurology, 36*, 144–148.

Ross, J. B., & McLaughlin, M. M. (1949). *The portable medieval reader.* New York: Vikins Press.

Roter, D., Lipkin, M., & Korsgaard, A. (1991). Sex differences in patients' and physicians' communication during primary care medical visits. *Medical Care, 29*, 1088–1093.

Roter, D. L., & Hall, J. A. (1997). Gender differences in patient-physician communication. In S. J. Gallant, G. P. Keita, & R. Royak-Schater (Eds.), *Health care for women: Psychological, social, and behavioral influences* (pp. 57–71). Washington, DC: American Psychological Association.

Roter, D. L., Hall, J. A., & Aoki, Y. (2002). Physician gender effects in medical communication. *Journal of the American Medical Association, 288*, 756–764.
Roter, D. L., Hall, J. A., Kern, D. E., Baker, L. R., Cole, K. A., & Roca, R. P. (1995). Improving physicians' interviewing skills and reduction in patients' emotional distress: A randomized clinical trail. *Archives of Internal Medicine, 155*, 1877–1884.
Roter, D. L., Hall, J. A., Merisca, R., Nordstrom, B., Cretin, D., & Svarstad, B. (1998). Effectiveness of interventions to improve patient compliance: A meta-analysis. *Medical Care, 36*, 1138–1161.
Rovezzi-Carroll, S., & Fitz, P. A. (1984). Predicting allied health major fields of study with selected personality characteristics. *College Student Journal, 18*, 43–51.
Rushton, J. P. (1981). The altruistic personality. In P. J. Rushton & R. M. Sorrentino (Eds.), *Altruism and helping behavior: Social, personality, and developmental perspectives* (pp. 251–266). Hillsdale, NJ: Erlbaum.
Rushton, J. P., Chrisjohn, R. D., & Fekker, G. C. (1981). The altruistic personality and the self-report Altruism Scale. *Personality and Individual Differences, 2*, 293–302.
Rushton, J. P., Fulker, D. W., Neale, M. C., Nias, D. K. B., & Eysenck, H. J. (1986). Altruism and aggression: The heritability of individual differences. *Journal of Personality and Social Psychology, 50*, 1192–1198.
Russek, L. G., & Schwartz, G. E. (1997). Perceptions of parental caring predict health status in midlife: A 35-year follow up of the Harvard Mastery of Stress study. *Psychosomatic Medicine, 59*, 144–149.
Russell, D., Peplau, L. A., & Cutrona, C. B. (2004). The revised UCLA Loneliness Scale. *Journal of Personality and Social Psychology, 39*, 472–480.
Rutter, M., Caspi, A., Fergusson, D., Horwood, L. J., Goodman, R., Maughan, B., Moffitt, T. E., Melzer, H., & Carroll, J. (2005). Sex differences in developmental reading ability: New findings from 4 epidemiological studies. *Journal of the American Medical Association, 291*, 2007–2012.
Sackett, D. H., & Haynes, R. B. (1976). *Compliance with therapeutic regimens*. Baltimore, MD: Johns Hopkins University Press.
Sage, W. M. (2002). Putting the patient in patient safety: Linking patient complaints and malpractice risk. *Journal of the American Medical Association, 287*, 3003–3005.
Sagi, A., & Hoffman, M. L. (1976). Empathic distress in newborns. *Developmental Psychology, 12*, 175–176.
Salovey, P., & Mayer, J. D. (1990). Emotional intelligence. *Imagination, Cognition, and Personality, 9*, 185–211.
Sandler, G. (1980). The importance of the history in the medical clinic and the cost of unnecessary tests. *American Heart Journal, 100*, 928–931.
Sandoval, A. M., Hancock, D., Poythress, N., Edens, J. F., & Lilienfeld, S. (2000). Construct validity of the Psychopathic Personality Inventory in a correctional sample. *Journal of Personality Assessment, 74*, 262–281.
Sanson-Fisher, R., & Maguire, P. (1980). Should skills in communication with patients be taught in medical schools? *Lancet, 2*, 523–526.
Sanson-Fisher, R. W., & Poole, A. D. (1978). Training medical students to empathize: An experimental study. *Medical Journal of Australia, 1*, 473–476.
Schachter, S. (1959). *The psychology of affiliation*. Stanford, CA: Stanford University Press.
Schafer, R. (1959). Generative empathy in the treatment situation. *Psychoanalytic Quarterly, 28*, 342–373.
Schaflen, A. E. (1964). The significance of posture in communication systems. *Psychiatry, 27*, 316–331.
Schlesinger, M. (2002). A loss of faith: The sources of reduced political legitimacy for the American medical profession. *Milbank Quarterly, 80*, 185–235.
Schmidt, C. W., & Baker, L. R. (1986). Psychotherapy in ambulatory practice. In L. R. Barker, J. R. Burton, & P. D. Zieve (Eds.), *Principles of ambulatory medicine* (pp. 133–139). Baltimore: Williams & Wilkins.
Schneiderman, L. J. (2002). Empathy and the literary imagination. *Annals of Internal Medicine, 137*, 627–629.
Schoenbach, V., Kaplan, B. H., Fredman, L., & Kleinbaum, D. G. (1986). Social ties and mortality in Evans County, Georgia. *American Journal of Epidemiology, 123*, 577–591.

Schore, A. N. (1996). *Affect regulation and the origin of the self: The neurobiology of emotional development.* Hillsdale, NJ: Erlbaum.

Schroeder, T. (1925). The psycho-analytic method of observation. *International Journal of Psychoanalysis, 6,* 155–170.

Schutte, N. S., Malouff, J. M., Bobik, C., Coston, T. D., Greeson, C., Jedulicka, C., Rhodes, E., & Wendorf, G. (2001). Emotional intelligence and interpersonal relations. *Journal of Social Psychology, 141,* 523–536.

Schwaber, E. (1981). Empathy: A mode of analytic listening. *Psychoanalytic Inquiry, 1,* 357–392.

Scourfield, J., Martin, N., Lewis, G., & McGuffin, P. (1999). Heritability of social cognitive skills in children and adolescents. *British Journal of Psychiatry, 175,* 564.

Seaberg, D. C., Godwin, S. A., & Perry, S. J. (1999). Teaching empathy in an emergency medicine residency. *Academic Emergency Medicine, 6,* 485.

Seaberg, D. C., Godwin, S. A., & Perry, S. J. (2000). Teaching patient empathy: the ED visit program. *Academic Emergency Medicine, 7,* 1433–1436.

Seeman, T. E., Berkman, L. F., & Kohout, F. (1993). Intercommunity variation in the association between social ties and mortality in elderly: A comparative analysis of three communities. *Annals of Epidemiology, 3,* 325–335.

Seeman, T. E., & Syme, L. (1987). Social network and coronary artery disease: A comparison of the structure and function of social relations and predictors of disease. *Psychosomatic Medicine, 49,* 341–354.

Self, D. J., Schrader, D. E., Baldwin, D. C. Jr., & Wolinsky, F. D. (1993). The moral development of medical students: A pilot study of the possible influence of medical education. *Medical Education, 27,* 26–34.

Shamasundar, M. R. C. (1999). Reflections: Understanding empathy and related phenomena. *American Journal of Psychotherapy, 53,* 232–245.

Shamay-Tsoory, S. G., Tomer, R., Goldsher, D., Berger, B. D., & Aharon-Peretz, J. (2004). Impairment in cognitive and affective empathy in patients with brain lesions: Anatomical and cognitive correlates. *Journal of Clinical and Experimental Neuropsychology, 26,* 1113–1127.

Shapiro, D. E., Boggs, S. R., Melamed, B. G., & Graham-Pole, J. (1992). The effect of varied physician affect on recall, anxiety, and perceptions in women at risk of breast cancer: An analogue study. *Health Psychology, 11,* 61–66.

Shapiro, A. K., & Shapiro, E. (1984). Patient-provider relationships and the placebo effect. In J. D. Matarazzo, S. M. Weiss, J. A. Herd, N. E. Miller, & S. M. Weiss (Eds.), *Behavioral health: A handbook of health enhancement and disease prevention* (pp. 371–383). New York: Wiley-Intersceince.

Shapiro, J. (2002). How do physicians teach empathy in the primary care setting? *Academic Medicine, 77,* 323–328.

Shapiro, J., & Hunt, L. (2003). All the world's a stage: The use of theatrical performance in medical education. *Medical Education, 37,* 922–927.

Shapiro, R. S., Simpson, D. E., & Lawrence, S. L. (1989). Survey of sued and non-sued physicians and suing patients. *Annals of Internal Medicine, 149,* 2190–2196.

Shapiro, T. (1974). The development and distortions of empathy. *Psychoanalytic Quarterly, 43,* 4–25.

Shapurian, R., & Hojat, M. (1985). Psychometric characteristics of a Persian version of the Eysenck Personality Questionnaire. *Psychological Reports, 57,* 631–639.

Shaver, P., & Hazan, C. (1989). Being lonely, falling in love: Perspectives from attachment theory. In M. Hojat & R. Crandall (Eds.), *Loneliness: Theory, research, and applications* (pp. 105–124). Newbury, CA: Sage.

Sheehan, K. H., Sheehan, D. V., White, K., Leibowitz, A., & Baldwin, D. C. Jr. (1990). A pilot study of medical student 'abuse': Student perceptions of mistreatment and misconduct in medical school. *Journal of the American Medical Association, 263,* 533–537.

Shelton, W. (1999). Can virtue be taught? *Academic Medicine, 74,* 671–674.

Sherif, C. W., Sherif, M., & Nebergall, R. E. (1965). *Attitudes and attitude change: The social judgment-involvement approach.* Philadelphia: W. B. Saunders.

Sherman, J. J., & Cramer, A. (2005). Measurement of changes in empathy during dental school. *Journal of Dental Education, 69,* 338–345.

Shorey, H.S, & Snyder, C.R. (2006). The role of adult attachment styles in psychopathologyand psychotherapy outcomes. *Review of General Psychology, 10,* 1–20.

Shorter, E. (1986). *Bedside manners: The troubled history of doctors and patients.* Harmondsworth, UK: Viking.
Siegel, D. J. (1999). *The developing mind: How relationships and the brain interact to shape who we are.* New York: Guilford.
Sierles, F. S., Vergare, M., Hojat, M., & Gonnella, J. S. (2004). Academic performance of psychiatrists compared other specialists before, during, and after medical school. *American Journal of Psychiatry, 161,* 1477–1482.
Silver, H. K. (1982). Medical students and medical school. *Journal of the American Medical Association, 247,* 309–310.
Silver, H. K., & Glicken, A. D. (1990). Medical student abuse: Incidence, severity, and significance. *Journal of the American Medical Association, 263,* 527–532.
Simmons, J. M. P., Robie, P. W., Kendrick, S. B., Schumacher, S., & Roberge, L. P. (1992). Residents' use of humanistic skills and content of resident discussions in a support group. *American Journal of the Medical Sciences, 303,* 227–232.
Simner, M. L. (1971). Newborn response to the cry of another infant. *Developmental Psychology, 5,* 136–140.
Simpson, M., Buckman, R., Stewart, M., Maguire, P., Kipkin, M., Novack, D., & Till, J. (1991). Doctor-patient communication: The Toronto consensus statement. *British Medical Journal, 303,* 1385–1387.
Sims, A. (1988). *Symptoms in the mind: An introduction to descriptive psychotherapy.* London: Baillier, Tindall, W. B. Saunders.
Singer, T., Seymour, B., O'Doherty, J., Kaube, H., Dolan, R. J., & Frith, C. D. (2004). Empathy for pain involves the affective but not sensory components of pain. *Science, 303,* 1157–1162.
Singer, T., Seymour, B., O'Doherty, J., Stephan, K. E., Dolan, R. J., & Frith, C. (2006). Empathic neural responses are modulated by the perceived fairness of others. *Nature, 439* (7075), 466–469.
Singer, T., & Frith, C. (2005). The painful side of empathy. *Nature Neuroscience, 8,* 845–846.
Skeff, K. M., & Mutha, S. (1998). Role models: Guiding the future of medicine. *New England Journal of Medicine, 339,* 2015–2017.
Skelton, J. R., Macleod, J. A. A., & Thomas, C. P. (2000). Teaching literature and medicine to medical students, Part II: Why literature and medicine? *Lancet, 356,* 2001–2003.
Slipp, S. (2000). Subliminal stimulation research and its implications for psychoanalytic theory and treatment. *Journal of the American Academy of Psychoanalysis, 28,* 305–320.
Sloan, F. A., Mergenhagen, P. M., Burfield, W. B., Bovjerg, R. R., & Hassan, M. (1989). Medical malpractice experience of physicians: Predictable or haphazard? *Journal of the American Medical Association, 262,* 3291–3297.
Smith, B. H. (1981). Narrative versions, narrative theories. In W. J. T. Mitchell (Ed.), *On narrative* (pp. 209–232). Chicago: University of Chicago Press.
Smith, G. R. (1991). *Somatization disorder in the medical setting.* Washington, DC: American Psychiatric Press.
Smith, R. C. (1984). Teaching interviewing skills to medical students: The issue of countertransference. *Journal of Medical Education, 59,* 582–588.
Smolarz, B. G. (2005). *Determining the relationship between medical student empathy and undergraduate college major.* Unpublished manuscript, University of Virginia, Charlottsville.
Smotherman, W. P., & Robinson, S. R. (1994). Milk as the proximal mechanism for behavioral change in the newborn. *Acta Pædiatrica Scandinavica, 397,* 64–70.
Smyth, J., Stone, A., Hurewitz, A., & Kaell, A. (1999). Effects of writing about stressful experiences on symptom reduction in patients with asthma or rheumatoid arthritis: A randomized trial. *Journal of the American Medical Association, 281,* 1304–1309.
Sochting, I., Skoe, E. E., & Marcia, J. E. (1994). Care-oriented moral reasoning and prosocial behavior: A question of gender role orientation. *Sex Roles, 31,* 131–147.
Solomon, R. C. (1976). *The passion.* New York: Anchor/Doublely.
Sommer, R. (1969). *Personal space.* Englewood Cliffs, NJ: Prentice-Hall.
Sorce, J. F., Emde, R. N., Campos, J., & Klinnert, M. D. (1985). Maternal emotional signaling: Its effect on the visual cliff behavior of 1-year-olds. *Developmental Psychology, 21,* 195–200.

Sotile, W. M., & Sotile, M. O. (1996). *The medical marriage: A couple's survival manual.* New York: Carol Publication.
Southard, E. E. (1918). The empathic index in the diagnosis of mental diseases. *Journal of Abnormal Psychology, 13,* 199–214.
Sox, H. C. (2002). Medical professionalism in the new millennium: A physician charter. *Annals of Internal Medicine, 136,* 243–246.
Speedling, E. J., & Rose, D. N. (1985). Building an effective doctor-patient relationship: From patient satisfaction to patient participation. *Social Science & Medicine, 21,* 115–120.
Spelke, E. S. (2005). Sex differences in intrinsic aptitude for mathematics and science? A critical review. *American Psychologist, 60,* 950–958.
Spiegel, D. (1990). Can psychotherapy prolong cancer survival? *Psychosomatics, 31,* 361–366.
Spiegel, D. (1993). *Living beyond limits: New hope and help for facing life-threatening illness.* New York: Times Books.
Spiegel, D. (1994). Health caring: Psychological support for patients with cancer. *Cancer, 74,* 1453–1457.
Spiegel, D. (2004). Mind matters—Group therapy and survival in breast cancer. *The New England Journal of Medicine, 345,* 1–3.
Spiegel, D., & Bloom, J. R. (1983). Group therapy and hypnosis reduce metastatic breast carcinoma pain. *Psychosomatic Medicine, 45,* 333–339.
Spiegel, D., Bloom, J. R., Kraemer, H. C., & Gottheil, E. (1989). Effect of psychosocial treatment on survival of patients with metastatic breast cancer. *Lancet, 2,* 888–891.
Spiegel, D., Bloom, J. R., & Yalom, I. D. (1981). Group support for patients with metastatic breast cancer. *Archives of General Psychiatry, 38,* 527–533.
Spinella, M. (2002). A relationship between smell identification and empathy. *International Journal of Neuroscience, 112,* 605–612.
Spiro, H. (1998). *The power of hope: A doctor's perspective.* New Haven: Yale University Press.
Spiro, H. (1992). What is empathy and can it be taught? *Annals of Internal Medicine, 116,* 843–846.
Spiro, H. M. (1986). *Doctors, patients and placebos.* New Haven: Yale University Press.
Spiro, H. M., McCrea Curnen, M. G. M., Peschel, E., & St. James, D. (1993). *Empathy and the practice of medicine: Beyond pills and the scalpel.* New Haven: Yale University Press.
Squier, R. W. (1990). A model of empathic understanding and adherence to treatment regimens in practitioner-patient relationships. *Social Science & Medicine, 30,* 325–339.
Stamps, P. L., & Boley Cruz, N. T. (1994). *Issues in physician satisfaction: New perspectives.* Ann Arbor, MI: Health Administration Press.
Starcevic, V., & Piontek, C. M. (1997). Empathic understanding revisited: Conceptualization, controversies, and limitations. *American Journal of Psychotherapy, 51,* 317–328.
Starfield, B., Wray, C., Hess, K., Gross, R., Birk, P., & D'Lugoff, B. (1981). The influence of patient-practitioner agreement on outcome of care. *American Journal of Public Health, 71,* 127–131.
Starr, P. (1982). *Social transformation of American medicine.* New York: Basic Books.
Staub, E. (1978). *Positive social behavior and morality: Social and personal influences.* (Vol. 1), New York: Academic Press.
Staudenmayer, H., & Lefkowitz, M. S. (1981). Physician-patient psychological characteristics influencing medical decision-making. *Social Science & Medicine, 15,* 77–81.
Stebbins, C. A. (2005). Enhancing empathy in medical students using Flex Care™ communication training. Doctoral dissertation completed at Iowa State University. Dissertation Abstracts International, 66(4-B), p. 1962.
Stein, M. D., Fleisman, J., Mor, V., & Dresser, M. (1993). Factors associated with patient satisfaction among HIV-infected persons. *Medical Care, 31,* 182–188.
Steinbrook, R. (2002). Nursing in the crossfire. *New England Journal of Medicine, 346,* 1757–1766.
Steiner, J. F. (2005). The use of stories in clinical research and health policy. *Journal of the American Medical Association, 294,* 2901–2904.
Stepien, K. A. & Baernstien, A. (2006). Educating for empathy: A review. *Journal of General Internal Medicine, 21,* 524–530.
Stephan, W. G., & Finlay, K. (1999). The role of empathy in improving inter-group relations. *Journal of Social Issues, 55,* 729–743.

Stern, D. (1985). *The interpersonal world of the infant: A view from psychoanalysis and developmental psychology*. New York: Basic Books.

Stern, D. T., Frohna, A. Z., & Gruppen, L. A. (2005). The prediction of professional behaviour. *Medical Education, 39*, 75–82.

Sternberg, R. J. (2004). Culture and intelligence. *American Psychologist, 59*, 325–338.

Stewart, M. A. (1996). Effective physician-patient communication and health outcomes: A review. *Canadian Medical Association Journal, 152*, 1423–1433.

Stiles, W., Putman, S., Wolfe, M., & James, S. (1979). Interaction exchange structure and patient satisfaction with medical interview. *Medical Care, 17*, 667–679.

Stokes, J. (1980). Grief and the performing arts: A brief experiment in humanistic medical education. *Journal of Medical Education, 55*, 215.

Stotland, E. (1969). Exploratory investigation of empathy. In Berkowitz. L. (Ed.), *Advances in experimental social psychology* (pp. 271–314). New York: Academic Press.

Stotland, E. (1978). Fantasy-empathy research: An integration. In E. Stotland, K. E. Matthews, Jr., S. E. Sherman, R. O. Hansson, & B. Z. Richardson (Eds.), *Empathy, fantasy, and helping* (pp. 103–122). Beverly Hills, CA: Sage.

Stotland, E., Mathews, K. E. Jr., Sherman, S. E., Hansson, R. O., & Richardson, B. Z. (1978). *Empathy, fantasy and helping* (Vol. 65), Beverly Hills: Sage.

Strauss, M. B. (1968). *Familiar medical quotations*. Boston: Little, Brown.

Streit-Forest, U. (1982). Differences in empathy: A preliminary analysis. *Journal of Medical Education, 57*, 65–67.

Streit, U. (1980). Attitudes toward psycho-social factors in medicine: An appraisal of the ATSIM scale. *Medical Education, 14*, 259–266.

Stuss, D. T. (2001). The right frontal lobes are necessary for theory of mind. *Brain, 124*, 279–286.

Suchman, A. L., Markakis, K., Beckman, H. B., & Frankel, R. (1997). A model of empathic communication in the medical interview. *Journal of the American Medical Association, 277*, 678–682.

Sullivan, P. (1990). Pay more attention to your own health, physicians warned. *Canadian Medical Association Journal, 142*, 1309–1310.

Surrey, J. L., & Bergman, S. J. (1994). Gender differences in rational development: Implications for empathy in the doctor-patient relationship. In L. S. More & M. A. Milligan (Eds.), *The empathic practitioner: Empathy, gender, and medicine* (pp. 113–131). New Brunswick, NJ: Rutgers University Press.

Sutherland, J. A. (1993). The nature and evolution of phenomenological empathy in nursing: An historical treatment. *Archives of Psychiatric Nursing, 7*, 369–376.

Szalita, A. B. (1976). Some thoughts on empathy. The eighteenth annual Frieda Fromm-Reichmann memorial lecture. *Psychiatry, 39*, 142–152.

Taragin, M. I., Sonnenberg, F. A., Karns, M. E., Trout, R., Shapiro, S., & Carson, J. L. (1994). Does physician performance explain interspecialty differences in malpractice claim rates? *Medical Care, 32*, 661–667.

Tausch, R. (1988). The relationship between emotions and cognitions: Implications for therapist empathy. *Person-Centered Review, 3*, 277–291.

Taylor, S. E., Klein, L. C., Gruenewald, T. L., Gurung, R. A. R., & Fernandes-Taylor, S. (2003). Affiliation, social support and biobehavioral response to stress. In J. Suls & K. A. Wallston (Eds.), *Social psychological foundations of health and illness* (pp. 314–331). Malden,MA: Blackwell.

Taylor, S. E., Klein, L. C., Lewis, B. P., Gruenewald, T. L., Gurung, R. A., Regan, A. R., & Updegraff, J. (2000). Biobehavioral responses to stress in females: Tend-and-befriend, not fight-or-flight. *Psychological Review, 107*, 411–429.

Therrien, M. E. (1979). Evaluating empathy skills training for parents. *Social Work, 24*, 417–419.

Thom, D. H., Hall, M. A., & Pawlson, L. G. (2004). Measuring patients' trust in physicians when assessing quality of care. *Health Affairs, 23*, 124–132.

Thomas, L. (1985). *The youngest science*. Oxford University Press.

Thompson, B. M., Hearn, G. N., & Collins, M. J. (1992). Patient perceptions of health professional interpersonal skills. *Australian Psychologist, 27*, 91–95.

Titchener, E. B. (1909). *Lectures on the experimental psychology of the thought-processes*. New York: Macmillan.

Titchener, E. B. (1915). *A beginner's psychology.* New York: Macmillan.
Tomkins, S. S. (1962). *Affect, imagery, consciousness, Vol. I: The positive effects.* New York: Springer.
Tomkins, S. S. (1963). *Affect, imagery, consciousness, Vol. II: The negative effects.* New York: Springer.
Tomkins, S. S. (1987). Script theory. In J. Aronoff, A. J. Rubin, & R. A. Zucker (Eds.), *The emergence of personality.* (pp. 147–216). New York: Springer.
Trautmann Banks, J. (2002). The story inside. In R. Charon & M. Montello (Eds.), *Stories matter: The role of narrative in medical ethics* (pp. 219–226). New York: Routledge.
Triandis, H. C. (1995). *Individualism & collectivism.* Boulder, CO: Westview Press.
Trivers, R. L. (1972). Parental investment and sexual selection. In B. Campbell (Ed.), *Sexual selection and the descent of man* (pp. 136–179). Chicago, IL: Aldine.
Trommsdorff, G. (1991). Child-rearing and children's empathy. *Perceptual & Motor Skills, 72,* 387–390.
Trommsdorff, G. (1995). Person-context relations as developmental conditions for empathy and prosocial action: A cross-cultural analysis. In T. A. Kindermann & J. Valsiner (Eds.), *Development of person-context relations* (pp. 189–208). Hillsdale, NJ: Erlbaum.
Tronick, E., Als, H., Adamson, L., Wise, S., & Brazelton, T. B. (1978). The infant's response to entrapment between contradictory messages in face-to-face interaction. *Journal of the American Academy of Child Psychiatry, 17,* 1–13.
Trout, D. L., & Rosenfeld, H. M. (1980). The effect of postural lean and body congruence on the judgment of psychotherapeutic rapport. *Journal of Nonverbal Behavior, 4,* 176–190.
Truax, C. B., Altmann, H., & Millis, W. A. (1974). Therapeutic relationships provided by various professionals. *Journal of Community Psychology, 2,* 33–36.
Truax, C. B., & Carkhuff, R. (1967). *Towards effective counseling and psychotherapy: Training and practice.* Chicago: Aldine.
Turner, J. A., Deyo, R. A., Loeser, J. D., von Korff, M., & Fordyce, W. E. (1994). The importance of placebo effect on pain treatment and research. *Journal of the American Medical Association, 271,* 1609–1614.
Umilta, M. A., Kohler, E., Gallese, V., Fogassi, L., Fadiga, L., Keysers, C., & Rizzolatti, G. (2001). I know what you are doing: A neurophysiological study. *Neuron, 31,* 155–165.
Underwood, B., & Moore, B. (1982). Perspective-taking and altruism. *Psychological Bulletin, 91,* 143–173.
Uvnas-Moberg, K. (1997). Physiological and endocrine effects of social contact. *Annals of the New York Academy of Sciences, 807,* 146–163.
Valliant, G. E. (1977). *Adaptation to life.* Boston: Little, Brown.
Van Orum, W., Foley, J. M., Burns, P. R., DeWolfe, A. S., & Kennedy, E. C. (1981). Empathy, altruism, and self-interest in college students. *Adolescence, 16,* 799–808.
Vaughan, K. B., & Lanzetta, J. T. (1981). The effect of modification of expressive displays on vicarious emotional arousal. *Journal of Experimental Social Psychology, 17,* 16–30.
Velicer, W. F., & Fava, J. L. (1998). Effects of variables and subject sampling on factor pattern recovery. *Psychological Methods, 3,* 231–251.
Veloski, J. J., & Hojat, M. (2006). Measuring specific elements of professionalism: Empathy, teamwork and lifelong learning. In D. T. Stern (Ed.), *Measurement of Professionalism in Medicine* (pp. 117–145). Oxford: Oxford University Press.
Verbrugge, L. M. (1979). Marital status and health. *Journal of Marriage and the Family, 41,* 267–285.
Viviani, P. (2002). Motor competence in the perception of dynamic events: A tutorial. In W. Prinz & B. Hommel (Eds.), *Common mechanisms in perception and action* (pp. 406–442). New York: Oxford University Press.
Wagner, H. L., Buck, R., & Winterbotham, M. (1993). Communication of specific emotions: Gender differences in sending accuracy and communication measures. *Journal of Nonverbal Behavior, 17,* 29–53.
Waisman, M. (1966). Listening with the third ear in eczematous eruptions. *Medical Times, 94,* 1108–1113.
Wallace, D. S., Paulson, R. M., Lord, C. G., & Bond, C. F., Jr. (2005). Which behaviors do attitudes predict? Meta-analyzing the effects of social pressure and perceived difficulty. *Review of General Psychology, 9,* 214–227.

Wasserman, R. C., Inui, T. S., Barriatua, R. D., Carter, W. B., & Lippincott, P. (1984). Pediatric clinicians' support for patients makes a difference: An outcome-based analysis of clinician-parent interaction. *Pediatrics, 74,* 1047–1053.

Watson, J. B. (1924). *Behaviorism.* New York: W. W. Norton.

Watson, J. C. (2002). Re-visioning empathy. In D. Cain & J. Seeman (Eds.), *Humanistic psychotherapies: Handbook of research and practice* (pp. 445–471). Washington, DC: American Psychological Association.

Watson, P. J., Grisham, S. O., Trotter, M. V., & Biderman, M. D. (1984). Narcissism and empathy: Validity evidence for the Narcissistic Personality Inventory. *Journal of Personality Assessment, 48,* 301–305.

Waxler-Morrison, N., Anderson, J. M., & Richardson, E. (1990). *Cross-cultural caring: A handbook for health professionals in Western Canada.* Vancouver: University of British Columbia Press.

Wear, D., & Aultman, J. M. (2005). The limits of narrative: Medical student resistance to confronting inequality and oppression in literature and beyond. *Medical Education, 39,* 1056–1065.

Weaver, M. J., Ow, C. L., Walker, D. J., & Degenhardt, E. F. (1993). A questionnaire for patients' evaluations of their physicians' humanistic behaviors. *Journal of General Internal Medicine, 8,* 135–139.

Webb, C. (1996). Caring, curing, coping: Toward an integrated model. *Journal of Advanced Nursing, 23,* 960.

Weinberg, M. K., Tronick, E. Z., & Cohn, J. F. (1999). Gender differences in emotional expressivity and self-regulation during early infancy. *Developmental Psychology, 35,* 175–188.

Weinberg, M. K., & Tronik, E. Z. (1996). Infant affective reaction to the resumption of maternal interaction after the still-face. *Child Development, 67,* 905–914.

Weisman, C. S., & Teitlebaum, M. A. (1985). Physician gender and the physician-patient relationship: Recent evidence and relevant questions. *Social Science & Medicine, 20,* 1119–1127.

Weisman, J. S., Betancourt, J., Campbell, E. G., Park, E. R., Kim, M., Clarridge, B., et al. (2005). Resident physicians' preparedness to provide cross-cultural care. *Journal of the American Medical Association, 294,* 1058–1067.

Weiss, R. F., Boyer, J. L., Lombardo, J. P., & Stich, M. H. (1973). Altruistic drive and altruistic reinforcement. *Journal of Personality and Social Psychology, 25,* 390–400.

Weissman, S. H., Haynes, R. A., Killan, C. D., & Robinowitz, C. (1994). A model to determine the influence of medical school on students' career choices. *Academic Medicine, 69,* 58–59.

Wellman, B. (1998). Social network. In H. S. Friedman (Ed.), *Encyclopedia of mental health* (pp. 525–544). San Diego, CA: Academic Press.

Wellman, H. (1991). *The child's theory of mind.* Cambridge, MA: Bradford Books/MIT Press.

Werner, A., & Schneider, J. M. (1974). Teaching medical students interactional skills: A research-based course in doctor-patient relationship. *New England Journal of Medicine, 290,* 1232–1237.

Wester, W. C., & Smith, A. H. J. (1984). *Clinical hypnosis: A multidisciplinary approach.* Philadelphia: Lippincott.

Westerman, M. A. (2005). What is interpersonal behavior? Post-cartesian approach to problematic interpersonal pattern and psychotherapy process. *Review of General Psychology, 9,* 16–34.

White, K. L. (1991). *Healing the schism: Epidemiology, medicine, and the public's health.* New York: Springer-Verlag.

Whittemore, P. B., Burstein, A. G., Loucks, S., & Schoenfeld, L. S. (1985). A longitudinal study of personality changes in medical students. *Journal of Medical Education, 60,* 404–405.

Whorf, B. L. (1956). *Language, thought, and reality: Selected writings of Benjamin Lee Whorf.* New York: John Wiley & Sons.

Wicker, B., Keysers, C., Plailly, J., Royet, J. P., Gallese, V., & Rizzolatti, G. (2003). Both of us disgusted in my insula: The common neural basis of seeing and feeling disgust. *Neuron, 40,* 655–664.

Wickramasekera, I. E., & Szylk, J. P. (2003). Could empathy be a predictor of hypnotic ability? *International Journal of Clinical & Experimental Hypnosis, 51,* 390–399.

Wiehe, V. R. (2003). Empathy and narcissism in a sample of child abuse perpetrators and a comparison sample of foster parents. *Child Abuse & Neglect, 27,* 541–555.

Wiesenfeld, A. R., Whitman, P. B., & Malatesta, C. Z. (1984). Individual differences among adult women in sensitivity to infants: Evidence in support of an empathy concept. *Journal of Personality and Social Psychology, 46,* 118–124.

Wiklund, I., Oden, A., & Sanne, H. (1988). Prognostic importance of somatic and psychosocial variables after a first myocardiac infarction. *American Journal of Epidemiology, 128,* 786–795.

Wilkes, M., Milgrom, E., & Hoffman, J. R. (2002). Toward more empathic medical students: A medical student hospitalization experience. *Medical Education, 36,* 528–533.

Williams, C. A. (1989). Empathy and burnout in male and female helping professionals. *Research in Nursing & Health, 12,* 169–178.

Williams, R. B., Barefoot, J. C., Califf, R. M., Haney, T. L., Saunders, W. B., & Pryor, D. B. (1992). Prognostic importance of social and economic resources among medically treated patients with angiographically documented coronary artery disease. *Journal of the American Medical Association, 267,* 524.

Willingham, W. W., & Cole, N. S. (1997). *Gender and fair assessment.* Hillsdale, NJ: Erlbaum.

Wilmer, H. A. (1968). The doctor-patient relationship and issues of pity, sympathy and empathy. *British Journal of Medical Psychology, 41,* 243–248.

Windholz, M. J., Marmar, C. R., & Horowitz, M. J. (1985). A review of research in conjugal bereavement: Impact on health and efficacy of intervention. *Comprehensive Psychiatry, 26,* 433–447.

Winefield, H. R., & Chur-Hansen, A. (2000). Evaluating the outcome of communication skill teaching for entry-level medical students: Does knowledge of empathy increase? *Medical Education, 34,* 90–94.

Winnicott, D. W. (1987). *Babies and their mothers.* Reading, MA: Addison-Wesley.

Wispe, L. (1978). *Altruism, sympathy, and helping: Psychological and sociological principles.* New York: Academic Press.

Wispe, L. (1986). The distinction between sympathy and empathy: To call forth a concept, a word is needed. *Journal of Personality and Social Psychology, 50,* 314–321.

Wittstein, I. S., Thiemann, D. R., Lima, J. A. C., Baughman, K. L., Schulman, S. P., Gerstenblith, G., Wu, K. C., Rade, J. J., Bivalacqua, T. J., & Chapman, H. C. (2005). Neurohormunal features of myocardial stunning due to sudden emotional stress. *New England Journal of Medicine, 352,* 539–548.

Wolf, E. S. (1980). The dutiful physician: The central role of empathy in psychoanalysis, psychotherapy, and medical practice. *Hillside Journal of Clinical Psychiatry, 2,* 41–56.

Wolf, S. (1992). Prediction of myocardiac infarction over a span of 30 years in Rosato, Pennsylvania. *Integrative physiological & Behavioral Science, 27,* 246–257.

Wolf, T. M., Balson, P. M., Faucett, J. M., & Randall, H. M. (1989). A retrospective study of attitude change during medical education. *Medical Education, 23,* 19–23.

Wolfgang, A. (1979). *Nonverbal behavior: Applications and cultural implications.* New York: Academic Press.

World Health Organization. (1948). *World Health Organization Constitution: Basic documents.* Geneva: Author.

Wright, S. (1996). Examining what residents look for in their role models. *Academic Medicine, 71,* 290–292.

Yarnold, P. R, Bryant, F. B., Nightingale, S. D., & Martin, G. J. (1996). Assessing physician empathy using the Interpersonal Reactivity Index: A measurement model and cross-sectional analysis. *Psychology, Health & Medicine, 1,* 207–221.

Yarnold, P. R, Greenberg, M. S., & Nightingale, S. D. (1991). Comparing resource use of sympathetic and empathetic physicians. *Academic Medicine, 66,* 709–710.

Yarnold, P. R., Martin, G. J., & Soltysik, R. C. (1993). Androgyny predicts empathy for trainees in medicine. *Perceptual & Motor Skills, 77,* 576–578.

Yates, S. (2001). Finding your funny bone: Incorporating humour into medical practice. *Australian Family Physician, 30,* 22–24.

Yedidia, M. J., Gillespie, C. C., Kachur, E., Schwartz, M. D., Ockene, J., Chepaitis, A. E., Snyder, C. W., Lazare, A., & Lipkin, M. (2003). Effect of communications training on medical student performance. *Journal of the American Medical Association, 290,* 1157–1165.

Younger, J. B. (1990). Literary works as a mode of knowing. *Journal of Nursing Scholarship, 22,* 39–43.

Zachariae, R., Pedersen, C. G., Jensen, A. B., Ehrnrooth, E., Rossen, P. B., & von der Maase, H. (2003). Association of percieved physician communication style with patient satisfaction, distress, cancer-related self-efficacy, and perceived control over the disease. *British Journal of Cancer, 88*, 658–665.

Zahn-Waxler, C., Radke-Yarrow, M., & King, R. A. (1979). Child rearing and children's prosocial initiations toward victims of distress. *Child Development, 50*, 319–330.

Zahn-Waxler, C., Robinson, J. L., & Emde, R. N. (1992). The development of empathy in twins. *Developmental Psychology, 28*, 1038–1047.

Zeldow, P. B., & Daugherty, S. R. (1987). The stability and attitudinal correlates of warmth and caring in medical students. *Medical Education, 21*, 353–357.

Zeleznik, C., Hojat, M., Goepp, C. E., Amadio, P., Kowlessar, O. D., & Borenstein, B. D. (1988). Measurement of certainty in medical school examination: A pilot study on non-cognitive dimensions of test-taking behavior. *Journal of Medical Education, 63*, 881–891.

Zeleznik, C., Hojat, M., & Veloski, J. J. (1983). Levels of recommendation for students and academic performance in medical school. *Psychological Reports, 52*, 851–858.

Zhou, Q., Eisenberg, N., Losoya, S. H., Fabes, R. A., Reiser, M., Guthrie, I. K., Murphy, B. C., Cumberland, A. J., & Shepard, S. A. (2002). The relations of parental warmth and positive expressiveness to children's empathy-related responding and social functioning: A longitudinal study. *Child Development, 73*, 893–915.

Zhou, Q., Valiente, C., & Eisenberg, N. (2003). Empathy and its measurement. In S. J. Lopez & C. R. Snyder (Eds.), *Positive psychological assessment: A handbook of models and measures* (pp. 269–284). Washington, DC: American Psychological Association.

Zinn, W. (1990). Transference phenomenon in medical practice: Being whom the patient needs. *Annals of Internal Medicine, 113*, 298.

Zuckerman, M. (2002). Zuckerman-Kuhlman Personality Questionnaire (ZKPQ): An alternative five-factor model. In B. DeRaad & M. Perugini (Eds.), *Big five assessment* (pp. 377–396). Seattle, WA: Hogrefe & Huber.

Zuckerman, M., DePauls, B. M., & Rosenthal, R. (1981). Verbal and nonverbal communication of deception. In L. Berkowitz (Ed.), *Advances in experimental social psychology* (Vol. 14). New York: Academic Press.

Zuger, A. (2004). Dissatisfaction with medical practice. *New England Journal of Medicine, 350*, 69–75.

Author Index

Subject Index

About the Author

Mohammadreza Hojat, Ph.D., is Research Professor of Psychiatry and Human Behavior and Director of the Jefferson Longitudinal Study of Medical Education at Jefferson Medical College of Thomas Jefferson University in Philadelphia, Pennsylvania. He was born in Mashhad, Iran, received his bachelor's degree from Pahlavi University (currently University of Shiraz), his master's degree from the University of Tehran in Iran, and his doctoral degree from the University of Pennsylvania. Dr. Hojat is a licensed psychologist in the Commonwealth of Pennsylvania and has published more than 170 articles in peer-reviewed journals on educational, psychological, and social issues. Dr. Hojat is a manuscript referee for several American and European professional journals and has served as a co-editor of two books: *Loneliness: Theory, Research, and Applications* (Sage, 1987), and *Assessment Measures in Medical School, Residency, and Practice: The Connections* (Springer, 1993).

Printed in the United States
119053LV00003B/291/A

9 780387 336077